Teen Health Series

Fitness and Exercise

SOURCEBOOK

Fourth Edition

Health Reference Series

Fourth Edition

Fitness and Exercise
SOURCEBOOK

*Basic Consumer Health Information about the
Benefits of Physical Fitness, Including Strength, Endur-
ance, Longevity, Weight Loss, Bone Health, and Stress
Management, with Exercise Guidelines for People of All
Ages and Tips for Maintaining Motivation, Measuring
Exercise Intensity, Preventing Injuries, and
Exercising with a Health Condition*

*Along with Information on Different Types of
Exercises and Exercise Equipment, a Glossary of
Related Terms, and a Directory of Resources for
Additional Help and Information*

Edited by
Laura Larsen

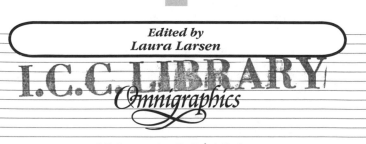

Omnigraphics

P.O. Box 31-1640, Detroit, MI 48231

GV
436
.F53
2011
C.2

Bibliographic Note

Because this page cannot legibly accommodate all the copyright notices, the Bibliographic Note portion of the Preface constitutes an extension of the copyright notice.

Edited by Laura Larsen

Health Reference Series

Karen Bellenir, *Managing Editor*
David A. Cooke, MD, FACP, *Medical Consultant*
Elizabeth Collins, *Research and Permissions Coordinator*
Cherry Edwards, *Permissions Assistant*
EdIndex, Services for Publishers, *Indexers*

* * *

Omnigraphics, Inc.

Matthew P. Barbour, *Senior Vice President*
Kevin M. Hayes, *Operations Manager*

* * *

Peter E. Ruffner, *Publisher*

Copyright © 2011 Omnigraphics, Inc.

ISBN 978-0-7808-1142-3

Library of Congress Cataloging-in-Publication Data

Fitness and exercise sourcebook : basic consumer health information about the benefits of physical fitness, including strength, endurance, longevity, weight loss, bone health, and stress management, with exercise guidelines for people of all ages and tips for maintaining motivation, measuring exercise intensity, preventing injuries, and exercising with a health condition ... / edited by Laura Larsen. -- 4th ed.
    p. cm.
Includes bibliographical references and index.
ISBN 978-0-7808-1142-3 (hardcover : alk. paper) 1. Physical fitness--Handbooks, manuals, etc. 2. Exercise--Handbooks, manuals, etc. I. Larsen, Laura.
GV436.F53 2010
613.7--dc22

2010037345

Table of Contents

Visit www.healthreferenceseries.com to view *A Contents Guide to the Health Reference Series*, a listing of more than 15,000 topics and the volumes in which they are covered.

v

Part II: Guidelines for Lifelong Physical Fitness

Part IV: Exercise Basics

Part VI: Physical Fitness for People with Health Conditions

Part VII—Additional Help and Information

Preface

About This Book

Regular physical activity provides numerous health benefits, including a reduced risk of diabetes, osteoporosis, obesity, some cancers, and heart disease, as well as increased mental well-being, longevity, and life satisfaction. Beginning a physical fitness program is important at any age, and it can provide a lifelong love of fitness in children, increased strength and endurance in adults, and improved balance and flexibility in the elderly. Yet, according to the Centers for Disease Control and Prevention, almost 39% of Americans engage in no leisure-time physical activity.

Fitness and Exercise Sourcebook, Fourth Edition provides updated information about the health benefits of physical activity. It discusses the guidelines for physical activity in people of all ages and diverse fitness levels—including those with disabilities, chronic diseases, or other challenges. It describes ways to make exercise fun and offers suggestions for incorporating fitness into everyday activities. Ways to maintain motivation and set fitness goals are described, and different types of physical activity—including aerobic, strength, balance, and mind-body—are detailed. Information on safety concerns, nutrition and hydration, and equipment needs is included, and an end section offers a glossary of related terms and a directory of organizations that provide information about physical fitness and exercise.

How to Use This Book

This book is divided into parts and chapters. Parts focus on broad areas of interest. Chapters are devoted to single topics within a part.

Part I: The Health Benefits of Physical Activity details the consequences of inactivity and the health and mental benefits of physical activity, including life satisfaction, disease prevention, increased mental health, and a healthy weight. It also explores a possible genetic contribution to physical inactivity.

Part II: Guidelines for Lifelong Physical Fitness offers readers specific fitness suggestions, age-appropriate guidelines, and tips for promoting physical activity among children, teenagers, adults, mid-life persons, and the elderly. It concludes with a discussion of ways in which a community's environment can promote physical fitness.

Part III: Start Moving explores practical suggestions for adding activity to everyday life and for beginning an exercise program. It explains how to create a fitness plan, overcome barriers to exercise, find a fitness club or workout partners, and measure and track exercise intensity and calorie expenditure. It also evaluates the reality behind advertising claims exercise equipment manufacturers sometimes make.

Part IV: Exercise Basics includes facts about specific forms of exercise, from basics—such as aerobics and strength training—to individual activities—such as walking, biking, running, kickboxing, racquet sports, dancing, aquatic exercise, boot camp, and even the Wii. Mind-body exercises, such as yoga and Pilates, are also discussed, and cross training, interval training, and power training are explained.

Part V: Fitness Safety offers suggestions about how to be safe during physical activity through warming up, avoiding common mistakes, choosing safe and comfortable equipment, eating and hydrating properly, and preventing sports injuries. It also discusses the risks of overtraining and compulsive exercise and offers tips for exercising safely out of doors.

Part VI: Physical Fitness for People with Health Conditions describes specific steps to physical fitness for people with disabilities, people who are overweight, and people with other health challenges, such as heart disease, bone disorders, breathing difficulties, diabetes, or cancer.

Part VII: Additional Help and Information includes a glossary of important terms and a directory of organizations able to provide information on physical fitness and exercise topics.

Bibliographic Note

This volume contains documents and excerpts from publications issued by the following U.S. government agencies: Centers for Disease Control and Prevention (CDC); Consumer Product Safety Commission (CPSC); National Cancer Institute (NCI); National Center for Complementary and Alternative Medicine; National Heart, Lung, and Blood Institute (NHLBI); National Institute of Arthritis and Musculoskeletal and Skin Diseases (NIAMS); National Institute of Diabetes and Digestive and Kidney Diseases (NIDDK); National Institute on Aging (NIA); National Institutes of Health (NIH); President's Council on Physical Fitness and Sports; U.S. Department of Health and Human Services (HHS); and U.S. Department of Homeland Security.

In addition, this volume contains copyrighted documents from the following organizations: Allergy and Asthma Network Mothers of Asthmatics; American College of Sports Medicine; American Council on Exercise; American Heart Association; American Orthopaedic Foot and Ankle Society; American Podiatric Medical Association; American Psychological Association; Aquatic Exercise Association; Asthma and Allergy Foundation of America; Boys Town Pediatrics; Cleveland Clinic; ExRx.net; Government of Ontario Ministry of the Environment; Harvard Health Publications; Helpguide (Center for Healthy Aging); IDEA Health & Fitness Association; Indiana University Office of University Communications; National Association for Sport and Physical Education; National Strength and Conditioning Association; Nemours Foundation; OrthoIndy; Oxford University Press; Rails-to-Trails Conservancy; United States Professional Tennis Association; University of Michigan Health System; University of Oxford; Wisconsin Department of Health and Family Services; Wolters Kluwer Health; Women's Sports Foundation; and World Health Organization (WHO).

Full citation information is provided on the first page of each chapter or section. Every effort has been made to secure all necessary rights to reprint the copyrighted material. If any omissions have been made, please contact Omnigraphics to make corrections for future editions.

Acknowledgements

Thanks go to the many organizations, agencies, and individuals who have contributed materials for this *Sourcebook* and to medical consultant Dr. David Cooke and document engineer Bruce Bellenir. Special thanks go to managing editor Karen Bellenir and research and permissions coordinator Liz Collins for their help and support.

About the Health Reference Series

The *Health Reference Series* is designed to provide basic medical information for patients, families, caregivers, and the general public. Each volume takes a particular topic and provides comprehensive coverage. This is especially important for people who may be dealing with a newly diagnosed disease or a chronic disorder in themselves or in a family member. People looking for preventive guidance, information about disease warning signs, medical statistics, and risk factors for health problems will also find answers to their questions in the *Health Reference Series*. The *Series*, however, is not intended to serve as a tool for diagnosing illness, in prescribing treatments, or as a substitute for the physician/patient relationship. All people concerned about medical symptoms or the possibility of disease are encouraged to seek professional care from an appropriate health care provider.

A Note about Spelling and Style

Health Reference Series editors use *Stedman's Medical Dictionary* as an authority for questions related to the spelling of medical terms and the *Chicago Manual of Style* for questions related to grammatical structures, punctuation, and other editorial concerns. Consistent adherence is not always possible, however, because the individual volumes within the *Series* include many documents from a wide variety of different producers and copyright holders, and the editor's primary goal is to present material from each source as accurately as is possible following the terms specified by each document's producer. This sometimes means that information in different chapters or sections may follow other guidelines and alternate spelling authorities. For example, occasionally a copyright holder may require that eponymous terms be shown in possessive forms (Crohn's disease *vs.* Crohn disease) or that British spelling norms be retained (leukaemia *vs.* leukemia).

Locating Information within the Health Reference Series

The *Health Reference Series* contains a wealth of information about a wide variety of medical topics. Ensuring easy access to all the fact sheets, research reports, in-depth discussions, and other material contained within the individual books of the *Series* remains one of our highest priorities. As the *Series* continues to grow in size and scope, however, locating the precise information needed by a reader may become more challenging.

A Contents Guide to the Health Reference Series was developed to direct readers to the specific volumes that address their concerns. It presents an extensive list of diseases, treatments, and other topics of general interest compiled from the Tables of Contents and major index headings. To access *A Contents Guide to the Health Reference Series*, visit www.healthreferenceseries.com.

Medical Consultant

Medical consultation services are provided to the *Health Reference Series* editors by David A. Cooke, MD, FACP. Dr. Cooke is a graduate of Brandeis University, and he received his M.D. degree from the University of Michigan. He completed residency training at the University of Wisconsin Hospital and Clinics. He is board-certified in Internal Medicine. Dr. Cooke currently works as part of the University of Michigan Health System and practices in Ann Arbor, MI. In his free time, he enjoys writing, science fiction, and spending time with his family.

Our Advisory Board

We would like to thank the following board members for providing guidance to the development of this *Series*:

- Dr. Lynda Baker, Associate Professor of Library and Information Science, Wayne State University, Detroit, MI

- Nancy Bulgarelli, William Beaumont Hospital Library, Royal Oak, MI

- Karen Imarisio, Bloomfield Township Public Library, Bloomfield Township, MI

- Karen Morgan, Mardigian Library, University of Michigan-Dearborn, Dearborn, MI

- Rosemary Orlando, St. Clair Shores Public Library, St. Clair Shores, MI

Health Reference Series Update Policy

The inaugural book in the *Health Reference Series* was the first edition of *Cancer Sourcebook* published in 1989. Since then, the *Series* has been enthusiastically received by librarians and in the medical community. In order to maintain the standard of providing high-quality health information for the layperson the editorial staff at Omnigraphics felt it was necessary to implement a policy of updating volumes when warranted.

Medical researchers have been making tremendous strides, and it is the purpose of the *Health Reference Series* to stay current with the most recent advances. Each decision to update a volume is made on an individual basis. Some of the considerations include how much new information is available and the feedback we receive from people who use the books. If there is a topic you would like to see added to the update list, or an area of medical concern you feel has not been adequately addressed, please write to:

Editor
Health Reference Series
Omnigraphics, Inc.
P.O. Box 31-1640
Detroit, MI 48231
E-mail: editorial@omnigraphics.com

Part One

The Health Benefits of Physical Activity

Chapter 1

Physical Activity Has Many Health Benefits

All Americans should be regularly physically active to improve overall health and fitness and to prevent many adverse health outcomes. The benefits of physical activity occur in generally healthy people, in people at risk of developing chronic diseases, and in people with current chronic conditions or disabilities. This chapter gives an overview of research findings on physical activity and health.

Physical activity affects many health conditions, and the specific amounts and types of activity that benefit each condition vary. In developing public health guidelines, the challenge is to integrate scientific information across all health benefits and identify a critical range of physical activity that appears to have an effect across the health benefits. One consistent finding from research studies is that once the health benefits from physical activity begin to accrue, additional amounts of activity provide additional benefits.

Although some health benefits seem to begin with as little as 60 minutes (1 hour) a week, research shows that a total amount of 150 minutes (2 hours and 30 minutes) a week of moderate-intensity aerobic activity, such as brisk walking, consistently reduces the risk of many chronic diseases and other adverse health outcomes.

Excerpted from "Chapter 2. Physical Activity Has Many Health Benefits," *Physical Activity Guidelines for Americans,* U.S. Department of Health and Human Services (www.hhs.gov), October 16, 2008.

Examining the Relationship between Physical Activity and Health

In many studies covering a wide range of issues, researchers have focused on exercise, as well as on the more broadly defined concept of physical activity. Exercise is a form of physical activity that is planned, structured, repetitive, and performed with the goal of improving health or fitness. So, although all exercise is physical activity, not all physical activity is exercise.

Studies have examined the role of physical activity in many groups—men and women, children, teens, adults, older adults, people with disabilities, and women during pregnancy and the postpartum period. These studies have focused on the role that physical activity plays in many health outcomes, including the following:

- Premature (early) death

- Diseases such as coronary heart disease, stroke, some cancers, type 2 diabetes, osteoporosis, and depression

- Risk factors for disease, such as high blood pressure and high blood cholesterol

- Physical fitness, such as aerobic capacity and muscle strength and endurance

- Functional capacity (the ability to engage in activities needed for daily living)

- Mental health, such as depression and cognitive function

- Injuries or sudden heart attacks

These studies have also prompted questions as to what type and how much physical activity is needed for various health benefits. To answer this question, investigators have studied three main kinds of physical activity: aerobic, muscle strengthening, and bone strengthening. Investigators have also studied balance and flexibility activities.

Aerobic Activity

In this kind of physical activity (also called an endurance activity or cardio activity), the body's large muscles move in a rhythmic manner for a sustained period of time. Brisk walking, running, bicycling, jumping rope, and swimming are all examples. Aerobic activity causes a person's heart to beat faster than usual.

Aerobic physical activity has three components:

- Intensity, or how hard a person works to do the activity—the intensities most often examined are moderate intensity (equivalent in effort to brisk walking) and vigorous intensity (equivalent in effort to running or jogging)

- Frequency, or how often a person does aerobic activity

- Duration, or how long a person does an activity in any one session

Although these components make up a physical activity profile, research has shown that the total amount of physical activity (minutes of moderate-intensity physical activity, for example) is more important for achieving health benefits than is any one component (frequency, intensity, or duration).

Muscle-Strengthening Activity

This kind of activity, which includes resistance training and lifting weights, causes the body's muscles to work or hold against an applied force or weight. These activities often involve relatively heavy objects, such as weights, which are lifted multiple times to train various muscle groups. Muscle-strengthening activity can also be done by using elastic bands or body weight for resistance (climbing a tree or doing push-ups, for example).

Muscle-strengthening activity also has three components:

- Intensity, or how much weight or force is used relative to how much a person is able to lift

- Frequency, or how often a person does muscle-strengthening activity

- Repetitions, or how many times a person lifts a weight (analogous to duration for aerobic activity)

The effects of muscle-strengthening activity are limited to the muscles doing the work. It's important to work all the major muscle groups of the body: the legs, hips, back, abdomen, chest, shoulders, and arms.

Bone-Strengthening Activity

This kind of activity (sometimes called weight-bearing or weight-loading activity) produces a force on the bones that promotes bone growth and strength. This force is commonly produced by impact with the ground. Examples of bone-strengthening activity include jumping jacks, running, brisk walking, and weight-lifting exercises. As these examples illustrate, bone-strengthening activities can also be aerobic and muscle strengthening.

The Health Benefits of Physical Activity

Studies clearly demonstrate that participating in regular physical activity provides many health benefits. These benefits are summarized here. Many conditions affected by physical activity occur with increasing age, such as heart disease and cancer. Reducing the risk of these conditions may require years of participation in regular physical activity. However, other benefits, such as increased cardiorespiratory fitness, increased muscular strength, and decreased depressive symptoms and blood pressure, require only a few weeks or months of participation in physical activity.

Health Benefits Associated with Regular Physical Activity

Children and Adolescents

There is strong evidence for the following:

- Improved cardiorespiratory and muscular fitness
- Improved bone health
- Improved cardiovascular and metabolic health biomarkers
- Favorable body composition

There is moderate evidence for reduced symptoms of depression.

Adults and Older Adults

There is strong evidence for the following:

- Lower risk of early death
- Lower risk of coronary heart disease
- Lower risk of stroke
- Lower risk of high blood pressure
- Lower risk of adverse blood lipid profile
- Lower risk of type 2 diabetes

- Lower risk of metabolic syndrome
- Lower risk of colon cancer
- Lower risk of breast cancer
- Prevention of weight gain
- Weight loss, particularly when combined with reduced calorie intake
- Improved cardiorespiratory and muscular fitness
- Prevention of falls
- Reduced depression
- Better cognitive function (for older adults)

There is moderate to strong evidence for the following:

- Better functional health (for older adults)
- Reduced abdominal obesity

There is moderate evidence for the following:

- Lower risk of hip fracture
- Lower risk of lung cancer
- Lower risk of endometrial cancer
- Weight maintenance after weight loss
- Increased bone density
- Improved sleep quality

Note: The Advisory Committee rated the evidence of health benefits of physical activity as strong, moderate, or weak. To do so, the committee considered the type, number, and quality of studies available, as well as consistency of findings across studies that addressed each outcome. The committee also considered evidence for causality and dose response in assigning the strength-of-evidence rating.

The Beneficial Effects of Increasing Physical Activity: It's About Overload, Progression, and Specificity

Overload is the physical stress placed on the body when physical activity is greater in amount or intensity than usual. The body's structures and functions respond and adapt to these stresses. For example, aerobic physical activity places a stress on the cardiorespiratory system and muscles, requiring the lungs to move more air and the heart to pump more blood and deliver it to the working muscles. This increase in demand increases the efficiency and capacity of the lungs, heart, circulatory system, and exercising muscles. In the same way, muscle-strengthening and bone-strengthening activities overload muscles and bones, making them stronger.

Progression is closely tied to overload. Once a person reaches a certain fitness level, he or she progresses to higher levels of physical activity by continued overload and adaptation. Small, progressive changes in overload help the body adapt to the additional stresses while minimizing the risk of injury.

Specificity means that the benefits of physical activity are specific to the body systems that are doing the work. For example, aerobic physical activity largely benefits the body's cardiovascular system.

The health benefits of physical activity are seen in children and adolescents, young and middle-aged adults, older adults, women and men, people of different races and ethnicities, and people with disabilities and chronic conditions. The health benefits of physical activity are generally independent of body weight. Adults of all sizes and shapes gain health and fitness benefits by being habitually physically active. The benefits of physical activity also outweigh the risk of injury and sudden heart attacks, two concerns that prevent many people from becoming physically active.

The following sections provide more detail on what is known from research studies about the specific health benefits of physical activity and how much physical activity is needed to get the health benefits.

Premature Death

Strong scientific evidence shows that physical activity reduces the risk of premature death (dying earlier than the average age of death for a specific population group) from the leading causes of death, such as heart disease and some cancers, as well as from other causes of death. This effect is remarkable in two ways:

- First, only a few lifestyle choices have as large an effect on mortality as physical activity. It has been estimated that people who are physically active for approximately 7 hours a week have a 40% lower risk of dying early than those who are active for less than 30 minutes a week.

- Second, it is not necessary to do high amounts of activity or vigorous-intensity activity to reduce the risk of premature death. Studies show substantially lower risk when people do 150 minutes of at least moderate-intensity aerobic physical activity a week.

Research clearly demonstrates the importance of avoiding inactivity. Even low amounts of physical activity reduce the risk of dying prematurely. The most dramatic difference in risk is seen between those who are inactive (30 minutes a week) and those with low levels of activity (90 minutes or 1 hour and 30 minutes a week). The relative risk of dying prematurely continues to be lower with higher levels of reported moderate- or vigorous-intensity leisure-time physical activity.

All adults can gain this health benefit of physical activity. Age, race, and ethnicity do not matter. Men and women younger than 65 years as well as older adults have lower rates of early death when they are physically active than when they are inactive. Physically active people of all body weights (normal weight, overweight, obese) also have lower rates of early death than do inactive people.

Cardiorespiratory Health

The benefits of physical activity on cardiorespiratory health are some of the most extensively documented of all the health benefits. Cardiorespiratory health involves the health of the heart, lungs, and blood vessels.

Heart diseases and stroke are two of the leading causes of death in the United States. Risk factors that increase the likelihood of cardiovascular diseases include smoking, high blood pressure (called hypertension), type 2 diabetes, and high levels of certain blood lipids (such as low-density lipoprotein, or LDL, cholesterol). Low cardiorespiratory fitness also is a risk factor for heart disease.

People who do moderate- or vigorous-intensity aerobic physical activity have a significantly lower risk of cardiovascular disease than do inactive people. Regularly active adults have lower rates of heart disease and stroke and have lower blood pressure, better blood lipid profiles, and greater levels of fitness. Significant reductions in risk of cardiovascular disease occur at activity levels equivalent to 150 minutes a week of moderate-intensity physical activity. Even greater benefits are seen with 200 minutes (3 hours and 20 minutes) a week. The evidence is strong that greater amounts of physical activity result in even further reductions in the risk of cardiovascular disease.

Everyone can gain the cardiovascular health benefits of physical activity. The amount of physical activity that provides favorable cardiorespiratory health and fitness outcomes is similar for adults of various ages, including older people, as well as for adults of various races and ethnicities. Aerobic exercise also improves cardiorespiratory fitness in individuals with some disabilities, including people who have lost the use of one or both legs and those with multiple sclerosis, stroke, spinal cord injury, and cognitive disabilities.

Moderate-intensity physical activity is safe for generally healthy women during pregnancy. It increases cardiorespiratory fitness without increasing the risk of early pregnancy loss, preterm delivery, or low birth weight. Physical activity during the postpartum period also improves cardiorespiratory fitness.

Metabolic Health

Regular physical activity strongly reduces the risk of developing type 2 diabetes as well as the metabolic syndrome. The metabolic syndrome is defined as a condition in which people have some combination of high blood pressure, a large waistline (abdominal obesity), an adverse blood lipid profile (low levels of high-density lipoprotein [HDL] cholesterol, raised triglycerides), and impaired glucose tolerance.

People who regularly engage in at least moderate-intensity aerobic activity have a significantly lower risk of developing type 2 diabetes than do inactive people. Although some experts debate the usefulness of defining the metabolic syndrome, good evidence exists that physical activity reduces the risk of having this condition, as defined in various ways. Lower rates of these conditions are seen with 120 to 150 minutes (2 hours to 2 hours and 30 minutes) a week of at least moderate-intensity aerobic activity. As with cardiovascular health, additional levels of physical activity seem to lower risk even further. In addition, physical activity helps control blood glucose levels in persons who already have type 2 diabetes.

Physical activity also improves metabolic health in youth. Studies find this effect when young people participate in at least three days of vigorous aerobic activity a week. More physical activity is associated with improved metabolic health, but research has yet to determine the exact amount of improvement.

Obesity and Energy Balance

Overweight and obesity occur when fewer calories are expended, including calories burned through physical activity, than are taken in through food and beverages. Physical activity and caloric intake both must be considered when trying to control body weight. Because of this role in

10

energy balance, physical activity is a critical factor in determining whether a person can maintain a healthy body weight, lose excess body weight, or maintain successful weight loss. People vary a great deal in how much physical activity they need to achieve and maintain a healthy weight. Some need more physical activity than others to maintain a healthy body weight, to lose weight, or to keep weight off once it has been lost.

Strong scientific evidence shows that physical activity helps people maintain a stable weight over time. However, the optimal amount of physical activity needed to maintain weight is unclear. People vary greatly in how much physical activity results in weight stability. Many people need more than the equivalent of 150 minutes of moderate-intensity activity a week to maintain their weight.

Over short periods of time, such as a year, research shows that it is possible to achieve weight stability by doing the equivalent of 150 to 300 minutes (5 hours) a week of moderate-intensity walking at about a four-mile-an-hour pace. Muscle-strengthening activities may help promote weight maintenance, although not to the same degree as aerobic activity.

People who want to lose a substantial (more than 5% of body weight) amount of weight and people who are trying to keep a significant amount of weight off once it has been lost need a high amount of physical activity unless they also reduce their caloric intake. Many people need to do more than 300 minutes of moderate-intensity activity a week to meet weight-control goals.

Regular physical activity also helps control the percentage of body fat in children and adolescents. Exercise training studies with overweight and obese youth have shown that they can reduce their body fatness by participating in physical activity that is at least moderate intensity on three to five days a week, for 30 to 60 minutes each time.

Musculoskeletal Health

Bones, muscles, and joints support the body and help it move. Healthy bones, joints, and muscles are critical to the ability to do daily activities without physical limitations.

Preserving bone, joint, and muscle health is essential with increasing age. Studies show that the frequent decline in bone density that happens during aging can be slowed with regular physical activity. These effects are seen in people who participate in aerobic, muscle-strengthening, and bone-strengthening physical activity programs of moderate or vigorous intensity. The range of total physical activity for these benefits varies widely. Important changes seem to begin at 90 minutes a week and continue up to 300 minutes a week.

11

Hip fracture is a serious health condition that can have life-changing negative effects for many older people. Physically active people, especially women, appear to have a lower risk of hip fracture than do inactive people. Research studies on physical activity to prevent hip fracture show that participating in 120 to 300 minutes a week of physical activity that is of at least moderate intensity is associated with a reduced risk. It is unclear, however, whether activity also lowers risk of fractures of the spine or other important areas of the skeleton.

Building strong, healthy bones is also important for children and adolescents. Along with having a healthy diet that includes adequate calcium and vitamin D, physical activity is critical for bone development in children and adolescents. Bone-strengthening physical activity done three or more days a week increases bone-mineral content and bone density in youth.

Regular physical activity also helps people with arthritis or other rheumatic conditions affecting the joints. Participation in 130 to 150 minutes (2 hours and 10 minutes to 2 hours and 30 minutes) a week of moderate-intensity, low-impact physical activity improves pain management, function, and quality of life. Researchers don't yet know whether participation in physical activity, particularly at low to moderate intensity, reduces the risk of osteoarthritis. Very high levels of physical activity, however, may have extra risks. People who participate in very high levels of physical activity, such as elite or professional athletes, have a higher risk of hip and knee osteoarthritis, mostly due to the risk of injury involved in competing in some sports.

Progressive muscle-strengthening activities increase or preserve muscle mass, strength, and power. Higher amounts (through greater frequency or higher weights) improve muscle function to a greater degree. Improvements occur in younger and older adults. Resistance exercises also improve muscular strength in persons with such conditions as stroke, multiple sclerosis, cerebral palsy, spinal cord injury, and cognitive disability. Though it doesn't increase muscle mass in the same way that muscle-strengthening activities do, aerobic activity may also help slow the loss of muscle with aging.

Functional Ability and Fall Prevention

Functional ability is the capacity of a person to perform tasks or behaviors that enable him or her to carry out everyday activities, such as climbing stairs or walking on a sidewalk. Functional ability is key to a person's ability to fulfill basic life roles, such as personal care, grocery shopping, or playing with his or her grandchildren. Loss of functional ability is referred to as functional limitation.

Middle-aged and older adults who are physically active have lower risk of functional limitations than do inactive adults. It appears that greater physical activity levels can further reduce risk of functional limitations.

Older adults who already have functional limitations also benefit from regular physical activity. Typically, studies of physical activity in adults with functional limitations tested a combination of aerobic and muscle strengthening activities, making it difficult to assess the relative importance of each type of activity. However, both types of activity appear to provide benefit.

In older adults at risk of falls, strong evidence shows that regular physical activity is safe and reduces this risk. Reduction in falls is seen for participants in programs that include balance and moderate-intensity muscle-strengthening activities for 90 minutes a week plus moderate-intensity walking for about an hour a week. It's not known whether different combinations of type, amount, or frequency of activity can reduce falls to a greater degree. Tai chi exercises also may help prevent falls.

Cancer

Physically active people have a significantly lower risk of colon cancer than do inactive people, and physically active women have a significantly lower risk of breast cancer. Research shows that a wide range of moderate-intensity physical activity—between 210 and 420 minutes a week (3 hours and 30 minutes to 7 hours)—is needed to significantly reduce the risk of colon and breast cancer; currently, 150 minutes a week does not appear to provide a major benefit. It also appears that greater amounts of physical activity lower risks of these cancers even further, although exactly how much lower is not clear.

Although not definitive, some research suggests that the risk of endometrial cancer in women and lung cancers in men and women also may be lower among those who are regularly active compared to those who are inactive.

Finally, cancer survivors have a better quality of life and improved physical fitness if they are physically active, compared to survivors who are inactive.

Mental Health

Physically active adults have lower risk of depression and cognitive decline (declines with aging in thinking, learning, and judgment skills). Physical activity also may improve the quality of sleep. Whether physical activity reduces distress or anxiety is currently unclear.

Mental health benefits have been found in people who do aerobic or a combination of aerobic and muscle-strengthening activities three to five days a week for 30 to 60 minutes at a time. Some research has shown that even lower levels of physical activity also may provide some benefits.

Regular physical activity appears to reduce symptoms of anxiety and depression for children and adolescents. Whether physical activity improves self-esteem is not clear.

Adverse Events

Some people hesitate to become active or increase their level of physical activity because they fear getting injured or having a heart attack. Studies of generally healthy people clearly show that moderate-intensity physical activity, such as brisk walking, has a low risk of such adverse events.

The risk of musculoskeletal injury increases with the total amount of physical activity. For example, a person who regularly runs 40 miles a week has a higher risk of injury than a person who runs 10 miles each week. However, people who are physically active may have fewer injuries from other causes, such as motor vehicle collisions or work-related injuries. Depending on the type and amount of activity that physically active people do, their overall injury rate may be lower than the overall injury rate for inactive people.

Participation in contact or collision sports, such as soccer or football, has a higher risk of injury than participation in noncontact physical activity, such as swimming or walking. However, when performing the same activity, people who are less fit are more likely to be injured than people who are fitter.

Cardiac events, such as a heart attack or sudden death during physical activity, are rare. However, the risk of such cardiac events does increase when a person suddenly becomes much more active than usual. The greatest risk occurs when an adult who is usually inactive engages in vigorous-intensity activity (such as shoveling snow). People who are regularly physically active have the lowest risk of cardiac events both while being active and overall.

The bottom line is that the health benefits of physical activity far outweigh the risks of adverse events for almost everyone.

Chapter 2

The Health Burden of Physical Inactivity

Facts

- Appropriate regular physical activity is a major component in preventing the growing global burden of chronic disease.

- At least 60% of the global population fails to achieve the minimum recommendation of 30 minutes moderate intensity physical activity daily.

- The risk of getting a cardiovascular disease increases by 1.5 times in people who do not follow minimum physical activity recommendations.

- Inactivity greatly contributes to medical costs—by an estimated $75 billion in the United States in 2000 alone.

- Increasing physical activity is a societal, not just an individual, problem and demands a population-based, multi-sectoral, multi-disciplinary, and culturally relevant approach.

Appropriate regular daily physical activity is a major component in preventing chronic disease, along with a healthy diet and not smoking. For individuals, it is a powerful means of preventing chronic diseases; for nations, it can provide a cost-effective way of improving public

"Physical Activity," http://www.who.int/dietphysicalactivity/media/en/gsfs_pa.pdf. © 2003 World Health Organization. Reprinted with permission. Reviewed by David A. Cooke, MD, FACP, March 2010.

health across the population. Available experience and scientific evidence show that regular physical activity provides people, both male and female, of all ages and conditions—including disabilities—with a wide range of physical, social, and mental health benefits. Physical activity interacts positively with strategies to improve diet, discourage the use of tobacco, alcohol, and drugs, helps reduce violence, enhances functional capacity, and promotes social interaction and integration.

Extent of the Problem

Physical inactivity was estimated to cause 1.9 million deaths worldwide annually, according to *World Health Report [WHR] 2002*. Globally, it is estimated to cause about 10–16% of cases each of breast cancer, colon cancers, and diabetes, and about 22% of ischemic heart disease. Estimated attributable fractions are similar in men and women. Opportunities for people to be physically active exist in the four major domains of their day. These are:

- at work (whether or not the work involves manual labor);
- for transport (walking or cycling to work, to shop, etc.);
- during domestic duties (housework, gathering fuel, etc.);
- in leisure time (sports and recreational activities).

The global estimate for the prevalence of physical inactivity among adults is 17%. Estimates for prevalence of some, but insufficient, activity (<2.5 hours per week of moderate activity) ranged from 31% to 51%, with a global average of 41% across the sub-regions. *WHR 2002* used a number of direct and indirect data sources and a range of survey instruments and methodologies to estimate activity levels in these four domains. The most data was available for leisure time activity, with less direct data available on occupational activity, and little direct data available for activity related to transport and domestic tasks. In addition, the *WHR 2002* data only estimates the prevalence of physical inactivity among people aged 15 years and over, which suggests the total figures could be higher. Physical activity declines with age, falling off from adolescence, and physical activity and physical education is declining in schools worldwide. Inactivity is generally higher amongst girls and women.

Why Is Regular Physical Activity Necessary?

Physical inactivity, along with other key risk factors, is a significant contributor to the global burden of chronic disease. Regular physical activity reduces the risk of heart disease, stoke, and breast and colon cancers. These benefits are mediated through a number of mechanisms. In general, physical activity improves glucose metabolism, reduces body fat, and lowers blood pressure; these are the main ways in which it is thought to reduce the risk of CVD [cardiovascular disease] and diabetes. It can also help manage and mitigate the effects of these diseases. Physical activity may also reduce the risk of colon cancer by its effects on prostaglandins, reduced intestinal transit time, and higher antioxidant levels.

Physical activity is associated with a lower risk of breast cancer, which may be the result of effects on hormonal metabolism. Participation in physical activity can also improve musculoskeletal health, control body weight, and reduce symptoms of depression. The possible beneficial effects on musculoskeletal conditions such as lower back pain, osteoporosis, and falls, as well as on obesity, depression, anxiety, and stress, have been well reported in a number of studies. Beyond the direct medical benefits, increasing physical activity through an integrated program, which takes into account transportation and urban planning policy, makes other broader contributions, increasing social interaction throughout the life course, providing recreational enjoyment, and reducing violence, urban traffic congestion, and pollution.

Physical activity also has economic benefits, especially in terms of reduced health care costs, increased productivity, and healthier physical and social environments. Data from developed countries indicate that the direct costs of inactivity are enormous. The costs associated with inactivity and obesity accounted for some 9.4% of the national U.S. health expenditure in 1995. Physically active individuals in the United States save an estimated $500 per year in health care costs according to 1998 data. Inactivity alone may have contributed as much as $75 billion to U.S. medical costs in the year 2000. In Canada, physical inactivity accounts for about 6% of total health care costs.

What Can We Do about It?

While different amounts are needed for various outcomes, the optimal combination of type, frequency, and intensity for different populations is not known. There is, however, clear consensus in recommending at least 30 minutes daily of moderate intensity activity. Increased benefits come from doing more, especially more vigorous activities, and these are highly recommended for youth to support healthy bones and muscles. Physical activity does not necessarily mean running a strenuous marathon or playing competitive sports. Rather, for many people, it is about walking the children to school, or taking a brisk stroll in the park. It means taking the stairs, instead of the elevator, or getting off the bus two stops early.

Currently 60% of the world's population is estimated to not get enough physical activity to achieve even this modest recommendation, with adults in developed countries most likely to be inactive. Patterns of physical activity acquired during childhood and adolescence are more likely to be maintained throughout the life span, providing the basis for active and healthy life. Unhealthy lifestyles—including sedentary behavior, poor diet, and substance abuse, adopted at a young age, are likely to persist. Physical activity is not merely about individual behavior. Multi-sectoral policies and initiatives are needed to create environments that help people to be physically active. These should be:

- Population-based collective actions, involving various stakeholders, including public and private sector groups and NGOs [nongovernmental organizations].

- These should involve multiple sectors—especially health, sport, education, transport, and culture and recreation ministries, as well as urban planners and local governments/municipalities.

- They should be culturally relevant and partnership based.

- They should promote physical activity in all life settings.

- They should make use of major sport, health, and cultural events.

Action Is Underway

- The WHO [World Health Organization]'s development of a Global Strategy on Diet, Physical Activity, and Health reflects Member States' increasing recognition that physical activity must be considered alongside diet in combating the growing chronic disease burden.

- WHO dedicated World No Tobacco Day 2002 to "Tobacco Free Sports: Play it Clean."

- WHO and other agencies are actively collaborating with sports bodies in programs such as Sports for All, aimed at increasing access to sport across population groups.

- A special focus is being placed upon partnership-based action to promote physical activity and sport among both boys and girls, in and out of schools.

Chapter 3

Physical Activity and Life Satisfaction

Moderate training of an endurance nature, but also other exercise activities, not only has a preventive effect on various illnesses and pre-illness states such as the metabolic syndrome and cancer, but is also effective in treating patients in the rehabilitation phase after illness, e.g. cardiovascular or cancer. Our investigation demonstrates that even low level physical activity has a very good preventive effect too, which is enhanced when it is accompanied by mental activity and psychological well-being. In total, we investigated 13,000 people on the basis of socioeconomic panel polls with respect to life contentment, health status, and leisure-time activities. Life contentment is positively linked to contentment with labor, which seems to be an essential aspect with regard to the increasing number of unemployed people in Europe. The second important factor is health-promoting activities during leisure time. Exercise, especially, has a significant influence on life satisfaction as a feeling of physical fitness is regarded as synonymous with good health. The results underline the psycho-neuroimmunological network, which stabilizes our health and shows that different activities in older adults have a significant effect on the aging process and age-related illnesses. Besides the various activities that are important in this arena, namely muscle and mental mobility ("brawn and brain"), a

Jennen, Christiane and Gerhard Uhlenbruck. Exercise and Life-Satisfactory-Fitness: Complementary Strategies in the Prevention and Rehabilitation of Illnesses. *Evidence-based Complementary and Alternative Medicine,* 2004, 157–165, Volume 1, Issue 2. Reprinted by permission of Oxford University Press, © 2004. Reviewed by David A. Cooke, MD, FACP, March 2010.

third component must be taken into consideration: life contentment in the form of a successful retrospective view and a positive outlook, embedded in a psychosocial family environment ("brood") and integrated in a stress-free biotope, where life does make sense. Alternative and complementary strategies should be considered in light of these three aspects when we think about additional anti-inflammatory strategies in preventing diseases or treating them and their relapses.

Sport has made a few healthy people ill, but sport has also made a good few of ill people healthy! (Gerhard Uhlenbruck, Aphorisms)

Summary and Discussion

In order to determine the influence of bodily and mental exercise on fitness and wellness in the older adult population, polls were taken in 1990 and 1991 with about 9,400 and 13,600 people, respectively. These "socioeconomic" panel polls were analyzed with respect to contentment with life, health, and leisure time.

Men and women were equally satisfied with life; percentage figures increased for both at age 60 and higher. In a time of unemployment in Europe, it is important to note that contentment with life is positively linked to contentment with labor. Being employed or having a good job seems to be a stabilizing health factor.

Satisfaction with leisure-time activities is closely connected to general life satisfaction. Contentment with life improves the more people engage in artistic and cultural activities, which is also true for those engaged in handicrafts or house repair.

There is a significant positive link between contentment with life and health. Women, however, are, in general, less satisfied with their health than men. As our special interest is focused on exercise activity, it was interesting to note the percentage of 47.7% non-active persons. It was also astonishing that at the time of the investigation (1990/1991) only 4.1% performed daily exercise, this percentage being even smaller in the over-50 population (2.2–2.7%). The percentage of non-active persons also rises linearly in the over-50 population, which is probably due to orthopedic or other health problems. However, a general limitation on exercise with respect to aging does not exist. On the contrary, in recent years we have found an increase in preventative exercise for older persons in order to prevent heart disease, metabolic syndrome, diabetes, high blood pressure, osteoporosis, and cancer. Accordingly, the share of exercise-performing persons over 59 years was raised in our study up to 21.0%.

Nearly half of the people interviewed never engaged in exercise or sport activities. The percentage of those exercising daily was nearly the same in every age category, whereas the percentage of those exercising only occasionally (once a week, once a month, or seldom) declines with increasing age. Men engage in exercise more often than women. The more often people exercise, the more satisfied they are with their life, regardless of age. Regular exercise obviously leads to increased fitness, which apparently has a positive influence on the immune system and, therefore, is greatly related to enjoyment of other life activities.

It was to be expected that the percentages of men with respect to exercise training would be higher than the figures for women, and consequently the number of daily active men was 64.8%, compared with 57.0% of women who perform no exercise at all. It can be assumed that professional and family stress contributes to this large latter figure. Otherwise, in certain sport groups, especially those for women (osteoporosis prevention and post breast cancer care groups), women are well accepted whereas in the coronary and heart exercise groups the men play a dominant role.

Life satisfaction was very dependent on the frequency of active exercise training. It was lowered from 65.8% down to 48.1% the less exercise was performed. This is in agreement with a study by E. Emrich who found that high exercise activity can be seen in a positive correlation with life contentment. In this connection we can confirm that the share of those who are content with their health rises from 36.9% up to 66.8%, the more frequently exercise is performed. Therefore, exercise has a positive influence on health satisfaction, if it is fully integrated into one's lifestyle. The number of men content with their health is significantly higher in the exercise groups than in those who never exercise, and is also higher with women in the exercise groups. Generally, the fitness feeling is much better in men doing exercise than in woman who are active. It is remarkable that a medical prescription or advice of a medical doctor (GP) is extremely important for the motivation of various people to join an exercise group, because otherwise there are certain mental inhibitions towards exercising within such groups.

Those content with their health are significantly more satisfied with labor and leisure time than those who are not content with their health.

The more often a leisure activity is undertaken the higher the percentage of those satisfied with health. Among those engaging in handicrafts or house repair, health satisfaction is also the highest when done at least once a month. The data demonstrate the important influence of mental activity on health satisfaction. Thus, mental health can positively influence physical health and vice versa, as is already known from the field of psycho-neuroimmunology.

Furthermore, there is a significant relationship between contentment with health and frequency of exercising. The more often people exercised the more content they were with their health; this influence was higher among males than among females.

Contentment with leisure time is equal for males and females and it increases with aging. Satisfaction with leisure time is positively linked to satisfaction with labor, since leisure seems to be regarded as a "reward" for hard work. The more often exercise activity was undertaken, the more content people were with their leisure time; this is also true for those engaging in handicrafts.

There is a significant relationship between contentment with leisure time and satisfaction with health. Satisfaction with leisure time increases with the frequency of exercise engagement. The share of those who are content with their health of those content with their leisure time is only 10.7% higher than those who are not content with their leisure time. The health aspect of leisure time seems to be not as significant as expected on the basis of exercise activity. The percentage of men content with their leisure time is about 9.6% higher than for women (53.3% versus 45.7%). The share of those content with the scale of their leisure time decreases by 15.6% with decreasing exercise activity: from 51.9% of the daily active persons down to 36.3% of those who seldom exercise. In the never-exercise group, the percentage of those content with the scale of their leisure time rises from this low point by 10.3% up to 46.6% in cases where people enjoy other hobbies and leisure-time activities besides sport. With regard to contentment with leisure time, there is a 27.3% difference between the figures for those who exercise daily (71.2% content) and those exercising seldom (43.9% content). Accordingly, exercise has a high value with respect to a satisfying leisure time. In spite of this fact, those who never exercised were also content with the use of their leisure time. From our data it could be deduced that women are more motivated with respect to exercise than men. This can be especially observed when looking at the activity of female walking groups nowadays. On the other hand, women are not satisfied when they are inhibited by other work from performing exercise.

An important aspect for aging nowadays is that people need to keep fit in order to avoid premature nursing. The ability to take care of oneself becomes a critical aspect for one's social, medical, and financial well-being. Thus, strategies for good health and general fitness need to be developed and realized. An interesting byproduct of this study was the contentment with life in relation to the existence of grandchildren and the closeness to them.

People not satisfied with their health more frequently had more children. Life satisfaction is higher only for grandparents at age 60 and up, whether the connection to the grandchildren is close or not. Health-contentment of those with grandchildren is higher only in persons aged 80 years and above. The feeling of biological survival apparently influences life satisfaction.

The percentage of those satisfied with leisure time is higher for those with children than for childless individuals. This percentage decreases with an increase in hours spent daily in child care. Grandparents are more content with leisure time than people without grandchildren. The closer the relationship to grandchildren (parents who are employed or grandparents living in the near neighborhood or in the same house), the more content are the grandparents with their leisure time. Older people are quite eager to fulfill the new roles associated with grandchildren, which includes more physical and mental activities. Obviously, having meaningful tasks to undertake makes people of 60 and older more content then those having meaningless perspectives.

So far, our findings imply that a meaningful task, an optimistic outlook on life, a promising perspective, a perceived successful life, as well as the wish to remain healthy and fit, positively influence life satisfaction.

Summarizing the results of the study, the following suggestions can be postulated in order to ensure physical and psychological well-being, not only in older adults but also as complementary strategies for ill people and those in rehabilitation programs, as well as in psychological coping techniques with patients:

i.   Regular, daily if possible, exercise routines should be performed in order to ensure general well-being and the ability to look after oneself.

ii. On the basis of several investigations it is suggested that exercise sufficient to burn 2,000–2,500 kcal per week (1 min jogging = ~10 kcal) should be performed three to four times a week. In addition, life-style change should also include reduction of the BMI and a change in nutritional behavior.

iii. Daily mental training (not by passive TV watching), e.g. participation in cultural events or personal hobbies such as arts and crafts, should be engaged in, because the immune system has its origin in the brain and accordingly can be influenced by the central nervous system.

iv. A good relationship with children and grandchildren should be established ("grand family feeling") in order to ensure the feeling of having necessary tasks, the safety of a nest, and the enjoying of the "sunset feeling" of a successful life. In addition, the vision of a biological immortality may strengthen health.

It is assumed that these suggestions stabilize the psycho-neuroimmunological network, slow down the physical and mental aging processes, prevent premature disabilities, and may be very useful in treating patients during, and especially after, severe illnesses, the results of which are reported by Beuth. As the costs of clinical and geriatric care are becoming more expensive, regular exercise, mental fitness, and psychosocial interests are of increasing importance for coping not only with the "stress" of belonging to the "old, but useless people," but also with respect to a promising and successful rehabilitation strategy as is already known from heart sport groups and those sport groups dealing with cancer survivors: the number of the latter in Germany amounts to ~350.

Chapter 4

Physical Activity and Disease Prevention

Chapter Contents

Section 4.1

Physical Fitness and a Healthy Immune System

Sir William Osler, the famous Canadian medical doctor, once quipped, "There's only one way to treat the common cold—with contempt." And for good reason. The average adult has two to three respiratory infections each year. That number jumps to six or seven for young children.

Whether or not you get sick with a cold after being exposed to a virus depends on the many factors that affect your immune system. Old age, cigarette smoking, mental stress, poor nutrition, and lack of sleep have all been associated with impaired immune function and increased risk of infection.

Keeping the Immune System in Good Shape

Research has established a link between moderate, regular exercise and a strong immune system. Early studies reported that recreational exercisers reported fewer colds once they began running. Moderate exercise has been linked to a positive immune system response and a temporary boost in the production of macrophages, the cells that attack bacteria. It is believed that regular, consistent exercise can lead to substantial benefits in immune system health over the long term.

More recent studies have shown that there are physiological changes in the immune system as a response to exercise. During moderate exercise, immune cells circulate through the body more quickly and are better able to kill bacteria and viruses. After exercise ends, the immune system generally returns to normal within a few hours, but consistent, regular exercise seems to make these changes a bit more long-lasting.

According to professor David Nieman, Dr. PH., of Appalachian State University, when moderate exercise is repeated on a near-daily basis there is a cumulative effect that leads to a long-term immune response.

His research showed that those who perform a moderate-intensity walk for 40 minutes per day had half as many sick days due to colds or sore throats as those who don't exercise.

On the other hand, there is also evidence that too much intense exercise can reduce immunity. Research shows that more than 90 minutes of high-intensity endurance exercise can make athletes susceptible to illness for up to 72 hours after the exercise session. This is important information for those who compete in longer events such as marathons or triathlons. Intense exercise seems to cause a temporary decrease in immune system function. During intense physical exertion, the body produces certain hormones that temporarily lower immunity. Cortisol and adrenaline, known as the stress hormones, raise blood pressure and cholesterol levels and suppress the immune system.

Should You Exercise When Sick?

Fitness enthusiasts and endurance athletes alike are often uncertain of whether they should exercise or rest when sick. Most sports-medicine experts in this area recommend that if you have symptoms of a common cold with no fever (that is, symptoms are above the neck), moderate exercise such as walking is probably safe.

Intensive exercise should be postponed until a few days after the symptoms have gone away. However, if there are symptoms or signs of the flu (fever, extreme tiredness, muscle aches, swollen lymph glands), then at least two weeks should probably be allowed before you resume intensive training.

Staying in Shape to Exercise

For athletes who are training intensely for competition, the following guidelines can help reduce their odds of getting sick.

Eat a well-balanced diet—The immune system depends on many vitamins and minerals for optimal function. However, at this time, there is no good data to support supplementation beyond 100% of the Recommended Dietary Allowances.

Avoid rapid weight loss—Low-calorie diets, long-term fasting, and rapid weight loss have been shown to impair immune function. Losing weight while training heavily is not good for the immune system.

Obtain adequate sleep—Major sleep disruptions (getting three hours less than normal) have been linked to immune suppression.

Avoid overtraining and chronic fatigue—Space vigorous workouts and race events as far apart as possible. Keep "within yourself" and don't push beyond your ability to recover.

Section 4.2

The Link Between Fitness and Longevity in Older Adults

"Fitness Predicts Longevity in Older Adults," National
Institutes of Health (www.nih.gov), December 17, 2007.

Being physically fit after age 60 helps you live longer, regardless of
your body's fat content, according to a new study.

Although earlier research had suggested that obesity and low physical fitness each can increase the risk of dying during middle age, it was
unclear whether this was also true in later years. In a new report from
an ongoing study, Dr. Xuemei Sui of the University of South Carolina
and her colleagues examined the links between fitness, fatness, and
mortality in older adults.

The scientists looked at more than 2,600 men and women, age 60
or older, who were participating in the Aerobics Center Longitudinal
Study, funded by the National Institute of Health (NIH)'s National
Institute on Aging (NIA) and National Heart, Lung, and Blood Institute
(NHLBI). Participants walked on a treadmill to determine their fitness
levels. Their fat levels, or adiposity, were assessed by measuring their
waist circumference, percent body fat, and body mass index (a ratio of
weight to height). The results were reported in the December 5, 2007,
issue of the *Journal of the American Medical Association*.

During an average follow-up period of 12 years, 450 of the participants
died. They were generally older, had lower fitness levels, and had more
cardiovascular risk factors, such as high blood pressure, high cholesterol,
and diabetes, than survivors. The percent of body fat did not appear to
be related to the risk of dying. However, greater fitness, lower body mass
index, and lower waist circumference each reduced the risk of death.

The researchers grouped the participants into five categories based
on their fitness levels. The least-fit group had a death rate four times
higher than the fittest. Even those in the low-fitness group fared much
better than the least-fit; the least-fit participants were twice as likely
to die as those in the low-fitness group. In most cases, the death rates
for those with higher fitness levels were less than half of the rates for
those who were least fit but weighed similar amounts.

The researchers say their findings suggest that you don't need to be thin to benefit from regular physical activity. Regular activity—like brisk walking for at least 30 minutes most days of the week—will keep most older adults out of the lowest fitness category and possibly help prolong their lives. A key to healthy aging is being physically active, regardless of your weight.

Section 4.3

The Link Between Mortality and Physical Inactivity

"Mortality Linked to Physical Activity Levels in Unfit Individuals,"
News release, © 2009. Reprinted with permission of the American
College of Sports Medicine (www.acsm.org).

The least-fit segment of the population has twice the mortality risk of even those who are just a bit more in shape, according to a study published in the official journal of the American College of Sports Medicine.

A research team from Stanford University led by Victor F. Froelicher, MD, and Jonathan Myers, PhD, FACSM, performed exercise tests and followed more than 4,300 subjects from 1986 to 2006, none of whom had a history of heart disease. Fitness and physical activity levels were measured using treadmill tests and questionnaires, and mortality rates were tracked during the 20-year study period.

Sandra Mandic, PhD, and the research team from Stanford analyzed the results, and found that the mortality rate for the least-fit individuals was twice that of the second least-fit group, and more than four times the rate of the most-fit group. Fitness was the strongest predictor of mortality in this group of healthy individuals.

The study suggests that reduced recent physical activity, rather than differences in health status, contributes to the striking difference in mortality rates between the least-fit individuals and those who are just a bit more fit. Nearly two-thirds of the least-fit individuals were not meeting the minimum recommended amount of physical activity

29

(at least 150 minutes per week, or 30 minutes per day, five days per week). Yet, this group achieves the greatest health benefits from increasing fitness.

"Given the considerable survival benefit associated with improving fitness in the least-fit group, increasing fitness through regular physical activity should be a priority in unfit individuals," Mandic said. "Health professionals should consider a sedentary lifestyle and poor fitness as treatable and major risk factors."

The study's findings are consistent with Exercise is Medicine™, a multi-organizational effort to make physical activity a standard part of the health care paradigm. The program encourages health care providers to talk to their patients about physical activity and, conversely, for patients to talk to their physician about how to get active.

The American College of Sports Medicine is the largest sports medicine and exercise science organization in the world. More than 35,000 international, national, and regional members and certified professionals are dedicated to advancing and integrating scientific research to provide educational and practical applications of exercise science and sports medicine.

Section 4.4

Physical Activity Promotes Bone Health

"Exercise and Bone Health," National Institute of Arthritis and
Musculoskeletal and Skin Diseases (www.niams.nih.gov), January 2009.

Vital at every age for healthy bones, exercise is important for treating and preventing osteoporosis. Not only does exercise improve your bone health, it also increases muscle strength, coordination, and balance, and it leads to better overall health.

Why Exercise?

Like muscle, bone is living tissue that responds to exercise by becoming stronger. Young women and men who exercise regularly generally achieve greater peak bone mass (maximum bone density and strength) than those who do not. For most people, bone mass peaks during the third decade of life. After that time, we can begin to lose bone. Women and men older than age 20 can help prevent bone loss with regular exercise. Exercising allows us to maintain muscle strength, coordination, and balance, which in turn helps to prevent falls and related fractures. This is especially important for older adults and people who have been diagnosed with osteoporosis.

The Best Bone-Building Exercise

The best exercise for your bones is the weight-bearing kind, which forces you to work against gravity. Some examples of weight-bearing exercises include weight training, walking, hiking, jogging, climbing stairs, tennis, and dancing. Examples of exercises that are not weight-bearing include swimming and bicycling. Although these activities help build and maintain strong muscles and have excellent cardiovascular benefits, they are not the best way to exercise your bones.

Exercise Tips

If you have health problems—such as heart trouble, high blood pressure, diabetes, or obesity—or if you are age 40 or older, check with your doctor before you begin a regular exercise program.

31

According to the Surgeon General, the optimal goal is at least 30 minutes of physical activity on most days, preferably daily.

Listen to your body. When starting an exercise routine, you may have some muscle soreness and discomfort at the beginning, but this should not be painful or last more than 48 hours. If it does, you may be working too hard and need to ease up. Stop exercising if you have any chest pain or discomfort, and see your doctor before your next exercise session.

If you have osteoporosis, ask your doctor which activities are safe for you. If you have low bone mass, experts recommend that you protect your spine by avoiding exercises or activities that flex, bend, or twist it. Furthermore, you should avoid high-impact exercise to lower the risk of breaking a bone. You also might want to consult with an exercise specialist to learn the proper progression of activity, how to stretch and strengthen muscles safely, and how to correct poor posture habits. An exercise specialist should have a degree in exercise physiology, physical education, physical therapy, or a similar specialty. Be sure to ask if he or she is familiar with the special needs of people with osteoporosis.

A Complete Osteoporosis Program

Remember, exercise is only one part of an osteoporosis prevention or treatment program. Like a diet rich in calcium and vitamin D, exercise helps strengthen bones at any age. But proper exercise and diet may not be enough to stop bone loss caused by medical conditions, menopause, or lifestyle choices such as tobacco use and excessive alcohol consumption. It is important to speak with your doctor about your bone health. Discuss whether you might be a candidate for a bone mineral density test. If you are diagnosed with low bone mass, ask what medications might help keep your bones strong.

Section 4.5

The Effect of Physical Activity on the Risk for Coronary Heart Disease

"Physical Activity and Weight Affect Coronary Heart Disease Risk,"
National Institutes of Health (www.nih.gov), May 12, 2008.

Researchers have long known that both physical activity and excess weight affect the risk of coronary heart disease. However, it's been hard to tease apart how much each contributes. A new study found that being physically active can considerably, but not completely, lower the risk of cardiovascular disease associated with being overweight or obese.

The research stems from the Women's Health Study, begun in 1992 by NIH's National Cancer Institute (NCI) and NHLBI. Its original goals were to evaluate the effects of vitamin E and low-dose aspirin on cardiovascular disease and cancer in healthy women. Recognizing the value of the data they were collecting, the researchers extended the study to do more follow-up and evaluate other cardiovascular risk factors.

Dr. Amy Weinstein at the Beth Israel Deaconess Medical Center in Boston and colleagues at Brigham and Women's Hospital analyzed data collected in the Women's Health Study on almost 39,000 women who were 45 and older. They compared the participants' body mass index (BMI—a ratio of weight to height) and physical activity levels at the start of the study with cardiovascular outcomes (such as heart attacks) over an average of 11 years of follow-up.

In the April 28, 2008, issue of *Archives of Internal Medicine*, the researchers reported that the group had 948 cases of coronary heart disease during the follow-up period. The risk of coronary heart disease, they found, increased as BMI increased. Obese women were over twice as likely to have a coronary event as women in the normal weight category.

Overall, the women who were physically active were 31% less likely to have coronary heart disease than those who weren't active. After the researchers adjusted the data to account for other known influences—such as alcohol use, smoking, and diet—the physically active women still had an 18% lower risk of coronary heart disease. In particular, the researchers found that physical activity significantly reduced the risk of coronary heart disease in the overweight and obese women.

The researchers also looked at the time the women spent walking and found that the more the women walked, the lower their risk for coronary heart disease. The greatest drop, for each weight category, was between those who didn't walk for exercise or recreation and those who walked 1–1.5 hours per week.

This study adds to a growing body of evidence showing that physical activity can help you live longer, regardless of whether you have excess weight. A half hour of moderate physical activity every day significantly reduces your risk of chronic disease, and more than 30 minutes further reduces the risk.

Although walking and physical activity significantly reduced the risk of coronary heart disease among the overweight and obese women in this study, their risk didn't drop as low as normal-weight women. Both weight control and physical activity are important for preventing coronary heart disease.

Section 4.6

Physical Fitness Improves Asthma Management in Children

"Physical Fitness Improves Asthma Management in Children,"
News release, © 2007. Reprinted with permission of the American
College of Sports Medicine (www.acsm.org).

Children with asthma who improve their physical fitness are likely to experience beneficial effects on disease control and quality of life, according to a study published recently in *Medicine & Science in Sports & Exercise®*, the official journal of the American College of Sports Medicine (ACSM). The results show aerobic training to be effective in improving cardiopulmonary fitness and decreasing daily use of inhaled steroids in asthmatic children, outcomes that should have positive implications for disease management in a group that tends to have lower cardiorespiratory fitness than their healthy counterparts.

"Children who experience breathing restrictions caused by asthma sometimes fear inducing breathlessness by exercise, which can cause physical deconditioning over time," said Celso Carvalho, PhD, an author on the study. "This is where we often see patients with asthma having lower fitness levels. Physical training, properly supervised, is not only a possibility for this group, but also a management strategy for their symptoms."

The study enrolled 38 children with moderate-to-severe persistent asthma, randomly assigned to either a training group or a control group. Exercise performance and exercise-induced bronchoconstriction was evaluated 16 weeks apart, while daily doses of inhaled steroids and Pediatric Asthma Quality of Life Questionnaire (PAQLQ) scores also were recorded.

Asthmatic children, even with moderate to severe disease, showed significant improvements in their aerobic capacity after the training program and a reduction in exercise-induced bronchoconstriction, which induces breathlessness and is a characteristic response to exercise present in most patients. Daily doses of inhaled steroids were reduced in trained patients by 52% but remained unchanged or increased in the control (untrained) group. When compared to controls, these children also reported a significant improvement in health-related quality of life.

The authors emphasize that training should be supervised and performed in children properly medicated, and the actual impact of physical training on clinical indicators of disease control is unknown. While these data suggest an adjunct role of physical conditioning on clinical management of patients with more advanced disease, additional research is warranted to discover the contribution of exercise on asthma symptoms and its manifestations.

The American College of Sports Medicine is the largest sports medicine and exercise science organization in the world. More than 20,000 international, national, and regional members are dedicated to advancing and integrating scientific research to provide educational and practical applications of exercise science and sports medicine.

Chapter 5

Physical Activity and Mental Health

Chapter Contents

Section 5.1

Physical Activity Helps Control Stress

People who exercise regularly will tell you they feel better. Some will say it's because chemicals called neurotransmitters, which are produced in the brain, are stimulated during exercise. Since it's believed that neurotransmitters mediate people's moods and emotions, they can make you feel better and less stressed.

While there's no scientific evidence to conclusively support the neurotransmitter theory, there is plenty to show that exercise provides stress-relieving benefits.

There are four ways in which exercise controls stress:

- **Exercise can help you feel less anxious:** Exercise is being prescribed in clinical settings to help treat nervous tension. Following a session of exercise, clinicians have measured a decrease in electrical activity of tensed muscles. People are often less jittery and hyperactive after an exercise session.

- **Exercise can relax you:** One exercise session generates 90 to 120 minutes of relaxation response. Some people call this post-exercise euphoria or endorphin response. Many neurotransmitters, not just endorphins, are involved. The important thing, though, is not what they're called, but what they do: They improve your mood and leave you relaxed.

- **Exercise can make you feel better about yourself:** Think about those times when you've been physically active. Haven't you felt better about yourself? That feeling of self-worth contributes to stress relief.

- **Exercise can make you eat better:** People who exercise regularly tend to eat more nutritious food. And it's no secret that good nutrition helps your body manage stress better.

It's Time to Get Started

Now that you know exercise can make a big difference in controlling stress, make some time for regular physical activity. We'll help you get started by listing three activities you can choose from:

- **Aerobic activity:** All it takes is 20 minutes, six to seven days a week. Twenty minutes won't carve a big chunk out of your day, but it will significantly improve your ability to control stress.

- **Yoga:** In yoga or yoga-type activities, your mind relaxes progressively as your body increases its amount of muscular work. Studies have shown that when large muscle groups repeatedly contract and relax, the brain receives a signal to release specific neurotransmitters, which in turn make you feel relaxed and more alert.

- **Recreational sports:** Play tennis, racquetball, volleyball, or squash. These games require the kind of vigorous activity that rids your body of stress-causing adrenaline and other hormones.

Not Just Any Exercise WIll Do

Don't try exercising in your office. Outdoors or away from the office is the best place to find a stress-free environment. Even a corporate fitness center can trigger too many work-related thoughts for some people.

Stay away from overcrowded classes. If you work surrounded by people, a big exercise class may be counterproductive. Solo exercise may be more relaxing for you. If, however, you work alone, you may enjoy the social benefit of exercising in a group. A lot depends on your personality and what causes stress for you.

Don't skip a chance to exercise. Take a break every 90 minutes and you'll be doing yourself a favor. Ninety-minute intervals are a natural work-break period. And four 10-minute exercise breaks will burn about as many calories as a solid 40-minute session. Work-break exercises can be as simple as walking or climbing stairs, stretching, or doing calisthenics.

Controlling stress comes down to making the time to exercise. You're worth it!

Section 5.2

Exercise Fights Dementia

Based on a review of studies on exercise and its effect on brain functioning in human and animal populations, researchers find that physical exercise may slow aging's effects and help people maintain cognitive abilities well into older age. Animals seem to benefit from exercise too and perform spatial tasks better when they are active. Furthermore, fitness training—an increased level of exercise—may improve some mental processes even more than moderate activity, say the authors of the review.

Findings from the review will be presented at the 114th Annual Convention of the American Psychological Association (APA).

Varying opinions still exist on the benefits of exercise and activity, said authors Arthur F. Kramer, PhD, Kirk I. Erickson, PhD, and Stanley J. Colcombe of the University of Illinois at Urbana–Champaign, "but our review of the last 40 years of research does offer evidence that physical exercise can have a positive influence on cognitive and brain functions in older animal and human subjects." Different methodologies were examined to comprehensively study what effects exercise can have.

The researchers first examined the epidemiological literature of diseases to determine whether exercise and physical activity can at certain points in a person's lifetime improve cognitive ability and decrease the likelihood of age-related neurological diseases, like Alzheimer's. The authors then reviewed longitudinal randomized trial studies to see if specific fitness training had an effect on cognition and brain function in older adults. Finally, animal studies were examined to understand the molecular and cellular mechanisms responsible for exercise effects on the brain as well as on learning and memory.

Based on a review of the epidemiological literature, the authors found a significant relationship between physical activity and later cognitive function and decreased occurrence of dementia. And the benefits may last several decades. In a few of the studies that examined men and women over 65 years old, the findings showed that those who exercised for at least 15–30 minutes at a time three times a week were less likely to develop Alzheimer's disease, even if they were genetically predisposed to the disease.

By examining the human intervention studies, a relationship was also found between fitness training and improved cognition, more efficient brain function, and retained brain volume in older people, said Kramer. He cautions that different fitness training regimens and aspects of mental functions need further study to solidify a causal relationship. But, he added, there are some preliminary positive findings. In a four-year study looking at the relationship between physical activity on cognition and brain function in 62- to 70-year-olds, "those who continued to work and retirees who exercised showed sustained levels of cerebral blood flow and superior performance on general measures of cognition as compared to the group of inactive retirees," said Kramer.

Other studies confirmed the evidence that fitness does have positive effects on brain function in older adults. A study of older adults who were randomly assigned to either a walking group or a stretching and toning control group for six months found that those in the walking group were better able to ignore distracting information in a distractibility task than those in the control group. "Aerobically trained older adults showed increased neural activities in certain parts of the brain that involved attention and reduced activity in other parts of the brain that are sensitive to behavioral conflict," said Kramer.

Animal studies also provide support for the aging benefits of physical activity. Analyzing the effects of exercise in animal populations provides a unique window into learning about exercise-induced neurological and cognitive plasticity—the ability of parts of the brain to function in place of other parts of the brain, said Dr. Kramer. Some of the animal studies reviewed used voluntary wheel-running experiments to show the existence of performance benefits of wheel running on hippocampus-related spatial learning tasks. Moreover, a few studies found that aged rodents that exercised in a water maze learned and retained information about a hidden platform better than age-matched controls.

Exercise also protected both young and aged animals from developing some age-related diseases as indicated by increases in certain neurochemical levels that can offset or prevent certain pathological diseases.

"From this review we have found that physical and aerobic exercise training can lower the risk for developing some undesirable age-related changes in cognitive and brain functions," said Dr. Kramer, "and also help the brain maintain its plasticity—ability to cover one function if another starts failing later in life."

More research is needed to know exactly how much and what types of exercise produce the most rapid and significant effects on thinking and the brain, how long exercise effects last following the end of training, or how much exercise is needed to get continued benefits, said Kramer.

Presentation: "Fitness Training and the Brain: From Molecules to Minds," Arthur F. Kramer, PhD, Stanley J. Colcombe, PhD, Kirk Erickson, PhD, and Paige Scalf, PhD, University of Illinois at Urbana–Champaign.

Session 2028: Invited Symposium: Optimal Aging and Cognition—Moderators of Cognitive Change and Decline, 8:00–9:50 a.m., Friday, August 11, [2006], Morial Convention Center, Second Level, Meeting Room 278.

Section 5.3

Physical Activity, Mood, and Serious Mental Illness

"Physical Activity, Mood, and Serious Mental Illness," reprinted with permission from the Indiana University Office of University Communications. © 2009 Trustees of Indiana University.

A new study from Indiana University [IU] suggests that even meager levels of physical activity can improve the mood of people with serious mental illnesses (SMI) such as bipolar disorder, major depression, and schizophrenia. The study, published in the November [2008] issue of the *International Journal of Social Psychiatry*, both reinforces earlier findings that people with SMI demonstrate low levels of physical activity and supports the consideration of physical activity as a regular part of psychiatric rehabilitation. "We found a positive association between physical activity level and positive mood when low to moderate levels of physical activity are considered," said study author Bryan McCormick, associate professor in IU's Department of Recreation, Park, and Tourism Studies. "Physical activity interventions that require lower levels of exertion might be more conducive to improving transitory mood, or the ups and downs people with SMI experience throughout the day." McCormick said physical activity often is advocated in addition to psychiatric treatment for people with SMI because of the significant health concerns common to this population. The low levels of physical activity also common to this population poses a major hurdle, however. For this study, physical activity is considered most forms of sustained movement, such as house cleaning, gardening, walking for transportation, or formal exercise. "The challenge is how to use naturally motivating activities that people have in their everyday lives to get them out and engaged," McCormick said.

About the Study

- For seven consecutive days, researchers randomly paged study participants, who then filled out questionnaires about their mood and recent activities. The responses were matched with data collected during the previous 10 minutes using small light-weight accelerometers worn by the study participants. The equipment measured activity levels and duration. McCormick said this is the first time these research methods were combined, allowing researchers to look at study participants' daily ups and downs as they occur rather than trying to average the experiences.

- The study involved 11 people from the United States and 12 people from Serbia. Central Europe is experiencing a shift from institutional care to community care for its citizens with SMI, similar to the shift seen in the United States in the 1970s. Mc-Cormick's research has been examining this, too, in comparison to U.S. populations. The findings were surprising in this particular study. "I was expecting a higher level of physical activity within the population of Eastern Europeans," he said. "We didn't see any differences."

- The average physical activity level for both groups was comparable to that of sedentary adults, less than that of adults with a developmental disability, and considerably less than that of active adults, according to earlier research by study co-author Georgia Frey, associate professor in IU's Department of Kinesiology.

- The least active experiences captured in this study correlated with less positive moods.

The study notes that walking is one of the most frequently advocated forms of physical activity in psychiatric rehabilitation programs. Such programs, according to the study, would appear to afford both physiological and psychological benefits.

Co-authors include Frey; Chien-Tsung Lee, IU Department of Kinesiology, School of Health, Physical Education, and Recreation; Sanghee Chun, IU School of HPER's Department of Recreation, Park, and Tourism Studies; Jim Sibthorp, University of Utah, Salt Lake City; Tomislav Gajic, MD, Branka Stamatovic-Gajic, MD, and Milena Maksimovich, Department of Psychiatry, Health Centre Valjevo, Valjevo, Serbia.

Journal citation: "Predicting Transitory Mood from Physical Activity Level among People with Severe Mental Illness in Two Cultures," *International Journal of Social Psychiatry*. 2008, 54: 527–538.

Chapter 6

Physical Activity and a Healthy Weight

Chapter Contents

Section 6.1

Physical Activity for Weight Loss

"Physical Activity for a Healthy Weight," Centers for Disease Control and Prevention (www.cdc.gov), January 27, 2009.

Why is physical activity important?

Regular physical activity is important for good health, and it's especially important if you're trying to lose weight or to maintain a healthy weight.

- When losing weight, more physical activity increases the number of calories your body uses for energy or "burns off." The burning of calories through physical activity, combined with reducing the number of calories you eat, creates a "calorie deficit" that results in weight loss.

- Most weight loss occurs because of decreased caloric intake. However, evidence shows the only way to maintain weight loss is to be engaged in regular physical activity.

- Most importantly, physical activity reduces risks of cardiovascular disease and diabetes beyond that produced by weight reduction alone.

Physical activity also helps accomplish the following:

- Maintain weight
- Reduce high blood pressure
- Reduce risk for type 2 diabetes, heart attack, stroke, and several forms of cancer
- Reduce arthritis pain and associated disability
- Reduce risk for osteoporosis and falls
- Reduce symptoms of depression and anxiety

How much physical activity do I need?

When it comes to weight management, people vary greatly in how much physical activity they need. Here are some guidelines to follow:

To maintain your weight: Work your way up to 150 minutes of moderate-intensity aerobic activity, 75 minutes of vigorous-intensity aerobic activity, or an equivalent mix of the two each week. Strong scientific evidence shows that physical activity can help you maintain your weight over time. However, the exact amount of physical activity needed to do this is not clear since it varies greatly from person to person. It's possible that you may need to do more than the equivalent of 150 minutes of moderate-intensity activity a week to maintain your weight.

To lose weight and keep it off: You will need a high amount of physical activity unless you also adjust your diet and reduce the amount of calories you're eating and drinking. Getting to and staying at a healthy weight requires both regular physical activity and a healthy eating plan.

What do moderate and vigorous intensity mean?

Moderate: While performing the physical activity, if your breathing and heart rate are noticeably faster but you can still carry on a conversation, it's probably moderately intense. Examples include the following:

- Walking briskly (a 15-minute mile)
- Light yard work (raking/bagging leaves or using a lawn mower)
- Light snow shoveling
- Actively playing with children
- Biking at a casual pace

Vigorous: If your heart rate is increased substantially and you are breathing too hard and fast to have a conversation, it's probably vigorously intense. Examples include the following:

- Jogging/running
- Swimming laps
- Rollerblading/inline skating at a brisk pace
- Cross-country skiing
- Most competitive sports (football, basketball, or soccer)
- Jumping rope

How many calories are used in typical activities?

The table 6.1 shows calories used in common physical activities at both moderate and vigorous levels.

Table 6.1. Calories Used per Hour in Common Physical Activities

Moderate Physical Activity	Approximate Calories/30 Minutes for a 154-lb Person[1]	Approximate Calories/Hr for a 154-lb Person[1]
Hiking	185	370
Light gardening/yard work	165	330
Dancing	165	330
Golf (walking and carrying clubs)	165	330
Bicycling (<10 mph)	145	290
Walking (3.5 mph)	140	280
Weight lifting (general light workout)	110	220
Stretching	90	180

Vigorous Physical Activity	Approximate Calories/30 Minutes for a 154-lb Person[1]	Approximate Calories/Hr for a 154-lb Person[1]
Running/jogging (5 mph)	295	590
Bicycling (>10 mph)	295	590
Swimming (slow freestyle laps)	255	510
Aerobics	240	480
Walking (4.5 mph)	230	460
Heavy yard work (chopping wood)	220	440
Weight lifting (vigorous effort)	220	440
Basketball (vigorous)	220	440

1. Calories burned per hour will be higher for persons who weigh more than 154 lbs (70 kg) and lower for persons who weigh less.

Source: Adapted from *Dietary Guidelines for Americans,* U.S. Department of Health and Human Services, 2005, page 16, Table 4, at http://www.health.gov/dietaryguidelines/dga2005/document/html/chapter3.htm#table4.

Section 6.2

Exercise Does Not Over-Stimulate Appetite

"Experts Debunk Myth about Exercise, Weight Loss," News release, © 2009. Reprinted with permission of the American College of Sports Medicine (www.acsm.org).

Leading experts in exercise and weight management have taken strong exception to assertions that exercise can inhibit weight loss by over-stimulating the appetite.

According to John Jakicic, PhD, FACSM, "There is strong evidence from the majority of the scientific literature that physical activity is an important component for initial weight loss."

Responding to a statement recently published online and in print, Jakicic added that "The statement 'in general, for weight loss, exercise is pretty useless' is not supported by the scientific evidence when there is adherence to a sufficient dose of physical activity in overweight and obese adults." Jakicic chairs a committee on obesity prevention and treatment for the American College of Sports Medicine (ACSM) and helped write an ACSM Position Stand on strategies for weight loss and prevention of weight regain for adults.

According to Jakicic and other experts, overwhelming evidence belies the assertion that exercise doesn't necessarily help people lose weight and may even make the task harder.

"Again, it is clear in this regard that physical activity is one of the most important behavioral factors in enhancing weight loss maintenance and improving long-term weight loss outcomes," Jakicic said. In fact, his own research, published in 2008, showed a high dose of physical activity (275 minutes above baseline levels) contributed to the greatest observed weight loss after a 24-month intervention. He noted that the scientific literature includes additional evidence to support physical activity, adding that a growing body of literature suggests the importance of physical activity to improve long-term weight loss following bariatric surgery.

Another noted expert and ACSM member, Timothy Church, MD, PhD, described how his professional opinions were misrepresented in a recent news article. According to Church, the article should have touched on the following key concepts:

- Weight maintenance is different from weight loss, and should have been discussed. Virtually all people who lose weight and keep it off are exercising to maintain weight.

- Comments about children and physical activity were misleading. Studies have shown that kids are not necessarily more active after school (and therefore need a good in-school physical education program), and that the focus with children should be on physical activity and prevention of excess weight gain. (Adults, however, more often must deal with losing excess weight.)

- Exercise and diet go together. Weight management is most successful when careful attention is given to both physical activity and proper nutrition.

Janet Rankin, PhD, FACSM, an expert in nutrition and exercise, supplemented the bountiful scientific evidence with a simple observation: "A practical response to the claim that exercise makes you eat more and gain weight is to look around. If this were the case, wouldn't those who regularly exercise be the fattest? Obviously that isn't the case."

ACSM experts stressed that, particularly when so many struggle with the health consequences of overweight and obesity, it is important that Americans have accurate information based on science and evidence.

The American College of Sports Medicine is the largest sports medicine and exercise science organization in the world. More than 35,000 international, national, and regional members and certified professionals are dedicated to advancing and integrating scientific research to provide educational and practical applications of exercise science and sports medicine.

Section 6.3

The Effect of Exercise on Metabolism

"Does Exercise Affect Resting Metabolism?" by Chris Melby, DrPH, reprinted with permission of the American College of Sports Medicine, ACSM Fit Society® Page, Summer 2004, pp 4–5, and "Maximizing Metabolism for Weight Loss," by Greg S. Miller and Lisa K. Lloyd, PhD. Reprinted with permission of the American College of Sports Medicine, ACSM Fit Society® Page, Summer 2004, pp 5–6. Reviewed by David A. Cooke, MD, FACP, March 2010.

Does Exercise Affect Resting Metabolism?

It is rare these days to pick up a health or fitness magazine from a grocery store shelf without our attention being drawn to an article proclaiming to have the latest information on the best way to exercise in order to boost metabolism. With the high risk for obesity in America, it would seem foolish to pass up reading an expose on newly discovered secrets about how to change our metabolism from a "warm glow" to a "raging fire." Unfortunately, we are often exposed to considerable misinformation that can leave us frustrated when our implementation of these latest "secrets" falls short of all the metabolic benefits promised.

Components of Energy Expenditure

Metabolism is a word that, for our purposes, describes the burning of calories necessary to supply the body with the energy it needs to function. There are three major ways we burn calories during the day: resting metabolic rate (RMR), the thermic effect of food (TEF), and physical activity energy expenditure (PAEE). RMR is the number of calories we burn to maintain our vital body processes in a resting state. It is usually determined by measuring your body's oxygen utilization (which is closely tied to calorie burning) while you lay or sit quietly in the early morning before breakfast after a restful night's sleep. RMR typically accounts for about 65–75% of your total daily calorie expenditure. The TEF results from eating food and is the increase in energy expended above your RMR that results from digestion, absorption, and storage of the food you eat. It typically accounts for about 5–10% of the total calories you burn in a day. The last component, PAEE, accounts for the remainder of your daily energy expenditure and, as the name suggests, is the increase in our calorie burning above RMR resulting from any physical activity. Included in PAEE is the energy expended in exercise, the activities of daily living, and even fidgeting. PAEE can vary considerably depending on how much you move throughout the day. For example, your PAEE would be high on a day that you participate in several hours of vigorous sports competition or exercise, while the calories you burn in physical activity would be quite low the next day if you choose to rest and recover.

Your total daily energy expenditure is the sum of these three components—if it is less than your energy intake, you will store most of the surplus energy, especially as body fat. If it is more than your energy intake, you will burn some body stores of energy to provide the needed energy not available from your food.

Is My Metabolic Rate Elevated following Exercise?

Your calorie expenditure obviously increases above your resting rate when you exercise, with the magnitude of this increase dependent on how long and hard you exercise. One frequently asked question is "Do we continue to burn 'extra' calories after we finish exercising?" In other words, does our energy expenditure remain elevated above RMR for a period of time after we stop the exercise, and if so, does it contribute significantly to our total energy expenditure on the day we exercise? Research has clearly shown that energy expenditure does not return to pre-exercise resting baseline levels immediately following exercise. The amount of this post-exercise elevation of energy expenditure depends primarily on how hard you exercise (i.e., intensity) and to a lesser degree on how long you exercise (i.e., duration).

Endurance Exercise: Exercise of the intensity and duration commonly performed by recreational exercisers (e.g., walking for 30–60 minutes or jogging at a pace of 8–10 minutes per mile for 20–30 minutes) typically results in a return to baseline of energy expenditure well within the first hour of recovery. The post-exercise calorie bonus for this type of exercise probably accounts for only about 10–30 additional calories burned beyond the exercise bout itself. In athletes performing high intensity, long duration exercise, the post-exercise energy expenditure may remain elevated for a longer period and could contribute significantly to total daily calorie burning. Ironically, such athletes are typically less concerned about this "extra" calorie burning and its implications for body weight regulation than are the recreational exercisers. The average person who does considerably less strenuous exercise will likely experience little meaningful contribution of this post-exercise bonus to their total daily calorie expenditure.

Weight-Lifting Exercise: A number of recent studies suggest that vigorous weight-lifting exercise may elevate calorie burning above usual resting values for several hours after exercise. However, the average person at the gym who rests for several minutes between sets of exercise will likely not experience a prolonged elevation of post-exercise energy expenditure.

Does Exercise Training Increase My RMR?

Endurance Exercise: A number of studies have found endurance-trained athletes to exhibit higher RMR than non-athletes. It appears likely that the combination of high exercise energy expenditure and high energy intake in these athletes can temporarily, but not permanently, elevate their RMR when measured the next morning after exercise. However, there is little evidence that the amount of physical activity performed by recreational exercisers for the purpose of weight control and health promotion will produce any increases in RMR, with the possible exception of such exercise in older individuals. It is clear that for both athletes and non-athletes, young and old, the major impact of exercise on total daily energy expenditure occurs during the activity itself, and not from increases in RMR.

Weight-Lifting Exercise: Some fitness enthusiasts have promoted the idea that because regular weight lifting can increase skeletal muscle mass, such exercise will dramatically increase RMR. However, it is estimated that each pound of muscle burns about 5–10 calories per day while at rest, so you would have to bulk up quite a bit to increase your RMR. Most people who lift weights for health rather than for bodybuilding will not increase their muscle mass enough to have a major effect on RMR.

Summary

Regular exercise has many benefits and plays an important role in increasing our daily energy expenditure. However, despite what we may read in many popular magazines, the increase in energy expenditure from exercise occurs primarily while we are exercising, rather than due to any sizeable exercise-induced elevations in our resting energy expenditure.

Maximizing Metabolism for Weight Loss

Recent reports from the Centers for Disease Control and Prevention indicate that 64.5% of American adults are overweight or obese. Body mass index (BMI), a measure of body fat based on height and weight, is commonly used to determine whether a person is overweight or obese. (To find out your BMI, visit www.cdc.gov/healthyweight/assessing/bmi/adult_bmi/english_bmi_calculator/bmi_calculator.html.) If you fall into the overweight or obese category, you are not alone. There are several reasons that may explain your weight status. One thing is for sure … weight gain does not happen overnight. An inactive lifestyle coupled with excessive eating and/or drinking can lead to gradual weight gain over time. Most people, despite their best efforts, struggle to control their body weight. Many get discouraged and give up, while others look for that "miracle" pill or diet plan to control their body weight. Why is this? We live in a fast-paced world and desire quick results with little to no effort. As a result, pharmaceutical corporations and book publishers promote their products as cures for obesity. Sadly, people buy into this marketing hype and the obesity problem continues to worsen.

Metabolism and Weight Loss

A more viable and realistic solution is to help people understand metabolism's role in weight loss. Metabolism, by definition, is the total of all cellular reactions that occur in the body. Basically, metabolism involves two processes: anabolism and catabolism. Simply stated, anabolic reactions result in the building of cellular structures and the storing of energy. For example, if you lift weights regularly, a portion of the protein that you ingest is used to build muscle tissue via anabolic reactions. On the other hand, catabolic reactions refer to the breaking down of molecules for energy. For example, if you exercise regularly and eat less than your body needs, your body will break down fat stores for energy via catabolic reactions.

The key to weight loss is to speed up metabolism by increasing both anabolic and catabolic reactions. Simply stated, through exercise and dietary modification, both anabolic and catabolic reactions can be increased, thereby increasing your likelihood of achieving a healthy body weight and optimal body composition.

To fully grasp how to increase metabolism, we must further explore catabolism. Energy is stored in food. For instance, one gram of carbohydrate and one gram of protein each contain four calories of energy, whereas one gram of fat contains nine calories of energy. When any of these are consumed, an anabolic or catabolic reaction occurs. If you exercise regularly and do not eat excessively, then the fats and carbohydrates that you eat undergo catabolic reactions (keep in mind that under these conditions, proteins undergo anabolic reactions and are used to maintain or build muscle tissue). These fats and carbohydrates are broken down and their energy is used to: 1) carry out life's necessary functions, such as breathing; 2) perform daily tasks, such as combing hair; 3) digest food; and 4) exercise. It's been estimated that active females and males require 2,200 and 2,900 calories per day, respectively, to satisfy the catabolic demands placed on the body. Based on these estimates, for example, an active female who consumes about 2,200 calories per day will more than likely maintain her weight. On the other hand, if she is not physically active and eats too many fats, proteins, and/or carbohydrates, then her body will store any unused energy as fat. If this is getting a little too overwhelming, just remember this:

If you consistently take in:

- more calories than you need, then your body will store the extra calories as fat;

- the same amount of calories as your body needs, then you will not gain or lose weight;

- less calories than your body needs, then you will lose weight.

To achieve a healthy body weight and optimal body composition, the key is to maximize your metabolism and reduce your caloric intake. To increase your metabolism, you should: 1) increase your muscle mass by performing resistance exercise two to three days per week (e.g., working out with elastic bands, weights, stability balls, body bars, etc.); 2) work up to at least 200 minutes of aerobic exercise per week (e.g., walking, jogging, bicycling, step aerobics, etc.); and 3) eat a low- (but not too low) calorie diet. Eating less than 1,200 calories per day has been shown to decrease your metabolism. Although everyone is different, to lose about one to two pounds per week, active men should eat about 1,800 calories per day and active women should eat about 1,500 calories per day. Remember, there is no miracle pill or other "quick-fix" solution for jump-starting a person's metabolism. One who is willing to make simple lifestyle changes and be consistent in their application will reap the future benefits of a healthy body weight and composition.

Chapter 7

Is Physical Inactivity Genetic?

Introduction

To understand whether genes can influence physical activity, let's begin by making a distinction between *physical inactivity* and *level of physical activity*. Physical inactivity is a construct of great importance for a proper understanding of the relationships between behavior and risks for a number of diseases and even premature death. Indeed, a sedentary lifestyle, which is dominated by physical inactivity, has been recognized as a major risk factor for hypertension, coronary heart disease, stroke, type 2 diabetes, obesity, and other conditions. The other important concept, level of physical activity, reflects the variation in activity from a small amount of light exercise performed occasionally to a large amount executed every day. Research has clearly shown that an active lifestyle, with even a moderate amount of physical activity almost every day, is quite beneficial in terms of prevention of cardiovascular events, type 2 diabetes, and premature death.

Human variation in degree of physical inactivity or amount of physical activity in a typical day is quite large. For instance, physical inactivity is the way of life in quadriplegic individuals, is almost complete in people who are bedridden for some reasons or who have lost some of their mobility because of disease or senescence, and is

This chapter excerpted from "Are People Physically Inactive Because of Their Genes?" President's Council on Physical Fitness and Sports (www.fitness.gov), June 2006. The full publication, including references, is available at www.fitness.gov/digests/digest-june2006-lo.pdf.

pervasive in people who have a sedentary occupation. For instance, the amount of energy expended at rest in the reclining or sitting position is about 1,500 kcal per day in a 165-pound young adult male, but energy expenditure for physical activity of any kind may range from as low as about 100 kcal (for a bedridden patient) to almost 300 kcal or so for a couch potato, a very sedentary individual. In contrast, the range of energy expenditure associated with physical activity is much larger for people who engage in voluntary regular exercise. Thus, a young male may typically expend a total of 400 to 500 kcal when he exercises for about 30 minutes at moderate intensity, while a professional cyclist with the same body mass competing in very demanding races (such as the Tour de France) may expend as many as 6,000 kcal per day.

Even though this enormous range of physical activity level (and related energy expenditure) is best represented by a more or less normal distribution, it is useful for a number of purposes to categorize people in two activity phenotype groups: the physically inactive (or sedentary) group and the physically active group. It is also relevant for research and perhaps clinical purposes to use a third category, based on the distinction between those who are physically active and those who are engaging in very demanding exercise programs. However, for the purpose of this review and considering the dearth of data on the topic in general, we will focus only on the former: the physical inactivity and moderate level of physical activity phenotypes (as measured behavioral traits). The fundamental question that we will address is whether human genetic variation contributes to the observation that there are individuals who are reliably physically inactive and others who readily adopt and maintain a physically active lifestyle.

Challenging the Common Dogma

Research on the determinants of a sedentary lifestyle or level of physical activity is typically rooted in paradigms that incorporate social factors, economic circumstances, time constraint, equipment and facilities, education level, etc. Despite the fact that it is never stated as such, the behaviorists engaged in this field of research assume by and large that biology has little to do with human variation in physical activity level or the adoption of a physically inactive lifestyle. To oversimplify, the underlying assumption is that individuals are born with a blank slate, with an almost infinite ability to learn and adopt desirable behavior. For quite some time, we have expressed the view that these research paradigms needed to be broadened and enriched to include biological determinants, including genetic factors and epigenetic events as well. Unfortunately, the interest in the biological basis of physical activity does not have a long history.

Several lines of evidence can be invoked to support the hypothesis that biology plays a role among the determinants of physical inactivity and physical activity levels.

- First, current models that do not incorporate biological influences account for only a moderate fraction of the variance in physical activity levels and do not discriminate fully between sedentary and physically active people.

- Second, most people who begin to exercise with the goal of becoming more physically active revert to a sedentary lifestyle. Low adherence rates diminish the public health value of regular physical activity and the preventive and therapeutic potential of regular exercise.

- Third, there are family lines with high rates of sedentary behavior as opposed to others in which all members are quite active as shown by a whole series of twin and family studies.

- Fourth, the heritability coefficients (quantitative indicators of the contribution of genetic inheritance to human variation in a trait) for physical activity level and sedentarism are statistically significant and meaningful from a behavioral perspective.

- Fifth, the genome-wide screening studies in animal models and in one human study have identified several regions on chromosomes that appear to harbor genes and DNA sequence variants that contribute to variation in activity levels among individuals.

- Sixth, a few genes exhibiting DNA sequence differences among people have already been associated with human variation in activity level or physical inactivity.

- Seventh, there is highly suggestive evidence from animal studies that maternal nutritional status and other in utero or perinatal factors cause alterations (epigenetic events) in the levels of gene expression without altering DNA sequence, thus setting the stage for stable changes in physiology.

Reviewing the evidence for these seven lines of evidence is beyond the scope of this chapter. However, we will highlight what we believe are the important findings and key relevant studies in the following paragraphs with an emphasis on the genetic and epigenetic aspects of the central question.

Evidence from Twin Studies

Much can be learned from observations made in pairs of identical (monozygotic) and fraternal (dizygotic) twins. Quite informative are the studies in which such observations were made on twin brothers or sisters who were separated for a variety of reasons early in life and who have lived apart ever since. Unfortunately no such studies have been reported for physical inactivity or level of physical activity. On the other hand, more than a dozen studies have been conducted with pairs of twin raised together and the findings from these studies have been reviewed elsewhere. To illustrate the major findings from these twin observational studies, we will rely on the one performed with the largest sample size.

In a large cohort of monozygotic and dizygotic male twin pairs over 18 years of age from the Finnish Twin Registry, information on intensity and duration of activity, years of participation in a given activity, and physical activity on the job was obtained from a questionnaire. A physical activity score was generated from these variables, which was then used to compute correlations within pairs of brothers of each twin type. The correlation for the physical activity score reached 0.57 in 1,537 pairs of monozygotic twins and 0.26 in 3,507 pairs of dizygotic twins. The results indicated that heritability accounted for 62% of the physical activity score. Other twin studies have generated higher heritability estimates for indicators of physical activity levels but many more have yielded heritability values in the 40% to 50% range.

Evidence from Family Studies

Physical activity levels and patterns in children and their parents tend to be similar. A good number of studies have been reported on the relationships between the level of physical activity and a few on the level of sedentarism in parents and their offspring. Only a few examples will be mentioned here.

Detailed analyses of the questionnaire on physical activity habits available on 18,073 individuals living in households from the 1981 Canada Fitness Survey and from a three-day diary obtained in 1,610 subjects from 375 families in Phase 1 of the Québec Family Study generated familial correlations that ranged from 0.2 to 0.3 for various indicators of physical activity. More recently, it was reported that maximal heritabilities reached 25% for an indicator of physical inactivity and 19% for a total physical activity score.

In an interesting study, 100 children, aged four to seven years, and 99 mothers and 92 fathers from the Framingham Children's Study were monitored with an accelerometer for about 10 hours per day for more than one week in children and parents over the course of one year. Active fathers were 3.5 times more likely to have active offspring and active mothers were 2.0 times more likely to have active offspring than inactive fathers or mothers, respectively. When both parents were active, the children were 5.8 times more likely to be active as children of two inactive parents. These results are thus compatible with the notion that genetic or other factors transmitted across generations predispose a child to be active or inactive.

Evidence from Animal Models

Experimental studies in informative animal models provide several examples of how naturally occurring DNA mutations and laboratory-induced changes in key genes may affect physical activity levels and patterns. For example, mice lacking the dopamine transporter gene exhibit marked hyperactivity, whereas dopamine receptor D2-deficient mice are characterized by reduced physical activity levels. Likewise, disruption of genes within the melanin-concentrating hormone pathway leads to hyperactivity.

An intriguing example of the strong effect of a mutation in a single gene on physical activity regulation comes from the fruit fly. In two populations of flies, each exhibiting a distinct activity pattern in terms of food-search behavior, those defined as rovers move about twice the distance while feeding compared to those qualified as sitters. This activity pattern is genetically determined and is regulated by a single gene, dg2, which encodes a cGMP-dependent protein kinase. The activity of this gene product is significantly higher in wild-type rovers than in wild-type and mutant sitters, and activation of this gene reverts foraging behavior from the sitter to rover phenotype. Furthermore, overexpression of the gene in sitters changed their behavior and made them behave more like rovers.

Evidence from Genome-Wide Explorations

The only genome-wide linkage scan for physical activity traits available to date was carried out in the Québec Family Study cohort. The scan was based on 432 DNA markers across the human genome (except the sex chromosomes) that were genotyped in 767 subjects from 207 families. Physical activity measures were derived from a three-day activity diary that yielded three traits of interest—total daily activity, inactivity, and moderate to strenuous activity—and from a questionnaire used to assess weekly physical activity during the past year. The strongest evidence for the presence of a gene influencing physical inactivity scores was detected on chromosome 2. Suggestive linkages with physical inactivity were also reported with markers on chromosomes 7 and 20. Several regions of the genome were linked with indicators of physical activity, including regions on chromosomes 4, 9, 11, 13, and 15.

Are There Epigenetic Effects?

In recent years, a growing body of evidence has emphasized that DNA sequence variation is extremely important in accounting for individual differences in behavior, physiology, and response to drugs or lifestyle interventions. More recently, another and very significant line of evidence indicates that chemical modification of DNA and histone proteins could translate in nongenetic phenotypic differences that often remarkably mimic those associated with DNA sequence variants. These DNA and nucleoprotein alterations have been collectively referred to as "epigenetic events." They begin to occur early after fertilization, are thought to take place in utero and even throughout the lifespan, are typically stable, and influence gene expression. Is there any evidence for a contribution of epigenetics to human variation in physical activity levels or physical inactivity?

No direct evidence exists for a contribution of any epigenetic alterations to physical activity level for the simple reason that the issue has not been considered yet. However, there are experimental data that are highly compatible with the hypothesis that epigenetics can influence the spontaneous level of physical activity. For instance, in one such experiment, performed in a leading New Zealand laboratory, maternal undernutrition throughout pregnancy resulted in differences in postnatal locomotor behavior. Female Wistar rats received only 30% of the ad libitum intake of the control females during pregnancy. The offspring of restricted mothers were significantly smaller at birth. At ages 35 days, 145 days, and 420 days, the voluntary locomotor activity of the offspring of the two groups were assessed. At all ages, the offspring of the undernourished mothers were significantly less active. These results suggested that the effects of undernutrition during pregnancy persisted during postnatal life. This effect persisted even when offspring were overnourished during postnatal life. One possible mechanism for such an effect of maternal undernutrition is via alterations in either the level of production or the sensitivity to endogenous hormones or other secreted factors during pregnancy. It is not unreasonable to hypothesize that chemical modifications superimposed on the DNA, without altering its sequence, could have played a role in the lower spontaneous physical activity level and its persistence throughout the life of the animal exposed to severe undernutrition during fetal life.

Other lines of research suggest that high-fat diets, protein restriction, and other maternal dietary manipulations before and during pregnancy also have considerable consequences on the physiology and behavior of the offspring. The implications of fetal life exposures and epigenetic events on the propensity to be sedentary or physically active remain to be understood.

Summary

Research indicates that the inclination to be physically active or sedentary has a biological foundation. Twin and family studies confirm that physical activity–related traits are characterized by familial aggregation and influenced by genetic factors. Results from animal model studies indicate that single genes can markedly influence physical activity–related behavior.

The first molecular genetic studies on physical activity traits in humans have been published during the last few years. They support the notion that it is possible to detect relatively small, yet biologically important genetic effects impacting the tendency to be sedentary or physically active at the molecular level. We are beginning to appreciate that the in utero environment and epigenetic events may play a role in postnatal physiology and behavior, but their impact on physical inactivity or physical activity level remains to be determined.

Part Two

Guidelines for Lifelong Physical Fitness

Chapter 8

Prevalence of Self-Reported Physically Active Adults

The report *2008 Physical Activity Guidelines for Americans* (2008 Guidelines), released in October by the U.S. Department of Health and Human Services, provides new guidelines for aerobic physical activity (i.e., activity that increases breathing and heart rate) and muscle strengthening physical activity.[1] Under the 2008 Guidelines, the minimum recommended aerobic physical activity required to produce substantial health benefits in adults is 150 minutes of moderate-intensity activity per week, or 75 minutes of vigorous-intensity activity per week, or an equivalent combination of moderate- and vigorous-intensity physical activity. Recommendations for aerobic physical activity in the 2008 Guidelines differ from those used in *Healthy People 2010* (HP2010) objectives, which call for adults to engage in at least 30 minutes of moderate-intensity activity, five days per week, or 20 minutes of vigorous-intensity activity, three days per week.[2] To establish baseline data for the 2008 Guidelines and compare the percentage of respondents who reported meeting these guidelines with the percentage who reported meeting HP2010 objectives, CDC [Centers for Disease Control and Prevention] analyzed data from the 2007 Behavioral Risk Factor Surveillance System (BRFSS) survey. This chapter summarizes the results of that analysis, which indicated that, overall, 64.5% of respondents in 2007 reported meeting the 2008 Guidelines, and 48.8% of the same respondents reported meeting HP2010 objectives. Public health

"Prevalence of Self-Reported Physically Active Adults—United States, 2007," *Morbidity and Mortality Weekly Report*, Centers for Disease Control and Prevention (www.cdc.gov), December 5, 2008.

officials should be aware that, when applied to BRFSS data, the two sets of recommendations yield different results. Additional efforts are needed to further increase physical activity.

BRFSS is a state-based, random-digit-dialed telephone survey of the noninstitutionalized U.S. civilian population aged >18 years. Data for the 2007 BRFSS survey were collected from 430,912 respondents (median response rate: 50.6%; median cooperation rate: 72.1%*) and reported by the 50 states, District of Columbia, Puerto Rico, and U.S. Virgin Islands. Response rates were calculated using guidelines from the Council of American Survey and Research Organizations (CASRO). A total of 31,805 respondents with missing physical activity data were excluded, resulting in a final sample of 399,107.

Since 2001, in alternate years, BRFSS surveys have included the same questions regarding participation in moderate-intensity and vigorous-intensity physical activities. In 2007, to assess participation in moderate activities, respondents were asked, "When you are not working, in a usual week, do you do moderate activities for at least 10 minutes at a time, such as brisk walking, bicycling, vacuuming, gardening, or anything else that causes some increase in breathing or heart rate?" Respondents who answered yes were then asked, "How many days per week do you do these moderate activities for at least 10 minutes at a time?" Finally, they were asked, "On days when you do moderate activities for at least 10 minutes at a time, how much total time per day do you spend doing these activities?" To assess participation in vigorous-intensity activities, respondents were asked, "When you are not working, in a usual week, do you do vigorous activities for at least 10 minutes at a time, such as running, aerobics, heavy yard work, or anything else that causes large increases in breathing or heart rate?" Respondents who answered yes were then asked, "How many days per week do you do these vigorous activities for at least 10 minutes at a time?" Finally, they were asked, "On days when you do vigorous activities for at least 10 minutes at a time, how much total time per day do you spend doing these activities?"

Using the 2008 Guidelines, respondents were classified as physically active if they reported at least 150 minutes per week of moderate-intensity activity, or at least 75 minutes per week of vigorous-intensity activity, or a combination of moderate-intensity and vigorous-intensity activity (multiplied by two) totaling at least 150 minutes per week. Using the HP2010 objectives, respondents were classified as physically active if they reported at least 30 minutes of moderate activity, five or more days per week, or at least 20 minutes of vigorous activity, three or more days per week.[†] Data were analyzed by selected characteristics, age adjusted to the 2000 U.S. standard population, and weighted to provide overall estimates; 95% confidence intervals were calculated. Statistically significant differences in prevalence were determined by t-test (p<0.05).

Using the 2008 Guidelines, 64.5% of U.S. adults were classified as physically active in 2007, including 68.9% of men and 60.4% of women. By age group, the percentage classified as physically active ranged from 51.2% (>65 years) to 74.0% (18–24 years). Among racial/ethnic populations, prevalence was lower for non-Hispanic blacks (56.5%) than for non-Hispanic whites (67.5%, p<0.01). By education level, prevalence was lowest for persons with less than a high school diploma (52.2%) and highest among college graduates (70.3%). By U.S. census region,[§] prevalence was lowest among respondents in the South (62.3%) and highest among those in the West (67.8%). A smaller percentage of persons classified as obese (57.1%) were physically active than persons classified as overweight (67.3%, p<0.01) or of normal weight (68.8%, p<0.01).[¶]

Applying the HP2010 objectives to the same respondents, the percentage of U.S. adults overall in 2007 classified as physically active was 48.8%, including 50.7% of men and 47.0% of women. Greater prevalence estimates were noted across all variables when comparing the 2008 Guidelines with the HP2010 objectives; patterns by sex, age group, race/ethnicity, education level, census region, and weight classification were similar.

CDC Editorial Note

The findings in this report indicate that 64.5% of U.S. adults reported meeting the minimum level of aerobic physical activity in the 2008 Guidelines using BRFSS 2007 data. When HP2010 physical activity objectives were assessed using the same respondents, 48.8% reported meeting minimum levels of physical activity, a difference of 15.7 percentage points. Prevalence patterns by demographic variables were consistent with those reported previously for physical activity.[3,4] Similar to findings in this report, a 2000 study noted a greater prevalence of physically active persons by using >150 minutes per week as the criteria, compared with six other criteria for moderate activity.[5] The 2008 Guidelines reflect the most recent major scientific review of the health benefits of physical activity. Officials at state and local health departments and other agencies and organizations that promote physical activity can utilize these evidence-based guidelines in developing physical activity initiatives. Findings from this report can serve as a baseline comparison with future estimates of physical activity using survey data.

Analysis of the findings in this report identified two main reasons why a higher proportion of respondents were classified as physically active based on the 2008 Guidelines than based on the HP2010 objectives: 1) removal of the frequency and duration requirement (i.e., 30 minutes of moderate activity, five days per week, or 20 minutes of vigorous activity, three days per week) and 2) addition of the criteria enabling respondents to meet the guidelines with a combination of moderate and vigorous (multiplied by two) activity. The report from the Physical Activity Guidelines Advisory Committee** emphasized total volume of activity for health benefits, independent of frequency. As explained in the 2008 Guidelines, existing scientific evidence cannot determine whether the health benefits of 30 minutes of activity, five days per week, are any different from the benefits of 50 minutes, three days per week. As a result, the 2008 Guidelines allow a person to accumulate 150 minutes a week in various combinations.[1] Nonetheless, the 2008 Guidelines add that aerobic activity should be performed in periods of at least 10 minutes, and preferably, those periods should be spread throughout the week.

The findings in this study are subject to at least three limitations. First, BRFSS data are self-reported and subject to recall and social-desirability bias; compared with accelerometer-measured physical activity, higher levels of self-reported physical activity were reported.[6] Second, BRFSS is a landline telephone survey and excludes persons in households without telephone access or persons who use only cellular telephones. Finally, the mean CASRO response rate was 50.6%, and low response rates can result in response bias; however, BRFSS estimates generally are comparable with estimates from surveys based on face-to-face interviews. In addition, weighting adjustments that account for sex, age group, and race/ethnicity attempt to minimize nonresponse, noncoverage, and undercoverage.[7,8]

Approximately one third of U.S. adults did not report meeting minimum levels of aerobic physical activity as defined by the 2008 Guidelines. Minimum levels were analyzed for this report because they provided the most direct comparison with *Healthy People 2010* objectives. However, more extensive health benefits can be attained by engaging in physical activity beyond these levels.[1] Increasing physical activity among U.S. adults can be accomplished through informational, behavioral, and environmental evidence-based approaches, such as those recommended in the *Guide to Community Preventive Services*.[††] Strong evidence of increased physical activity has been documented for communitywide campaigns, targeted health-behavior change programs, school-based physical education, nonfamily social support, and increased access to locations for physical activity combined with information outreach activities. Evidence of increased physical activity also has been documented for use of point-of-decision prompts and for community-scale and street-scale urban design and land-use policies and practices.[9,10]

References

1. U.S. Department of Health and Human Services. *2008 physical activity guidelines for Americans.* Hyattsville, MD: US Department of Health and Human Services; 2008. Available at www.health.gov/paguidelines.

2. U.S. Department of Health and Human Services. Objectives 22-2 and 22-3. In *Healthy people 2010* (conference ed, in 2 vols). Washington, DC: U.S. Department of Health and Human Services; 2000. Available at www.healthypeople.gov.

3. CDC. Prevalence of physical activity, including lifestyle activities among adults—United States, 1994–2004, *MMWR* 2003;52:764–9.

4. CDC. Prevalence of regular physical activity among adults—United States, 2001 and 2005, *MMWR* 2007;56:1209–12.

5. Brownson RC, Jones DA, Pratt M, Blanton C, Smith GW. Measuring physical activity with the behavioral risk factor surveillance system. *Med Sci Sports Exerc* 2000;32:1913–8.

6. Troiano RP, Berrigan D, Dodd KW, Masse LC, Tilert T, McDowell M. Physical activity in the United States measured by accelerometer. *Med Sci Sports Exerc* 2008;40:181–8.

7. Fahimi M, Link M, Schwartz D, Levy P, Mokdad A. Tracking chronic disease and risk behavior prevalence as survey participation declines: Statistics from the Behavioral Risk Factor Surveillance System and other national surveys. *Prev Chronic Dis* 2008;5(3). Available at www.cdc.gov/pcd/issues/2008/jul/07_0097.htm.

8. CDC. *Comparability of data: BRFSS 2007.* Atlanta, GA: U.S. Department of Health and Human Services, CDC; 2007. Available at www.cdc.gov/brfss/technical_infodata/surveydata/2007/compare_07.rtf.

9. CDC. Increasing physical activity: A report on recommendations of the Task Force on Community Preventive Services. *MMWR* 2001;50(No. RR-18).

10. Heath GW, Brownson RC, Kruger J, Miles R, Powell KE, Ramsey LT, Task Force on Community Preventive Services. The effectiveness of urban design and land use and transport policies and practices to increase physical activity: A systematic review. *J Phys Act Health* 2006;3(Suppl 1):S55–76.

* The response rate is the percentage of persons who completed interviews among all eligible persons, including those who were not successfully contacted. The cooperation rate is the percentage of persons who completed interviews among all eligible persons who were contacted.

† For example, both of the following persons would be considered physically active under the 2008 Guidelines but would not be considered physically active under HP2010 objectives: a person who did moderate activity for 25 minutes, seven days per week, and a person who did vigorous activity for 40 minutes, two days per week.

§ West: Alaska, Arizona, California, Colorado, Hawaii, Idaho, Montana, Nevada, New Mexico, Oregon, Utah, Washington, and Wyoming; Midwest: Illinois, Indiana, Iowa, Kansas, Michigan, Minnesota, Missouri, Nebraska, North Dakota, Ohio, South Dakota, and Wisconsin; Northeast: Connecticut, Maine, Massachusetts, New Hampshire, New Jersey, New York, Pennsylvania, Rhode Island, and Vermont; and South: Alabama, Arkansas, Delaware, District of Columbia, Florida, Georgia, Kentucky, Louisiana, Maryland, Mississippi, North Carolina, Oklahoma, South Carolina, Virginia, West Virginia, Tennessee, and Texas.

¶ Normal, overweight, and obese classifications are on the basis of body mass index, which is weight (kg) / height (m)^2. Normal: 18.5–24.9, overweight: 25.0–29.9, and obese: >30.0.

** Available at www.health.gov/paguidelines/report.

†† Available at www.thecommunityguide.org/pa.

Chapter 9

Introduction to Fitness Guidelines

Being physically active is one of the most important steps that Americans of all ages can take to improve their health. This inaugural *Physical Activity Guidelines for Americans* provides science-based guidance to help Americans aged six and older improve their health through appropriate physical activity.

The U.S. Department of Health and Human Services (HHS) issues the *Physical Activity Guidelines for Americans*. The content of *the Physical Activity Guidelines* complements the *Dietary Guidelines for Americans*, a joint effort of HHS and the U.S. Department of Agriculture (USDA). Together, the two documents provide guidance on the importance of being physically active and eating a healthy diet to promote good health and reduce the risk of chronic diseases.

Why and How the Guidelines Were Developed

The Rationale for Physical Activity Guidelines

We clearly know enough now to recommend that all Americans should engage in regular physical activity to improve overall health and to reduce risk of many health problems. Physical activity is a leading example of how lifestyle choices have a profound effect on health. The choices we make about other lifestyle factors, such as diet, smoking,

---

"Chapter 1. Introducing the 2008 Physical Activity Guidelines for Americans," *Physical Activity Guidelines for Americans,* U.S. Department of Health and Human Services (www.hhs.gov), October 16, 2008.

and alcohol use, also have important and independent effects on our health.

The primary audiences for the *Physical Activity Guidelines for Americans* are policymakers and health professionals. The Guidelines are designed to provide information and guidance on the types and amounts of physical activity that provide substantial health benefits. This information may also be useful to interested members of the public. The main idea behind the Guidelines is that regular physical activity over months and years can produce long-term health benefits. Realizing these benefits requires physical activity each week.

These Guidelines are necessary because of the importance of physical activity to the health of Americans, whose current inactivity puts them at unnecessary risk. *Healthy People 2010* set objectives for increasing the level of physical activity in Americans over the decade from 2000 to 2010. Unfortunately, the latest information shows that inactivity among American adults and youth remains relatively high and that little progress has been made in meeting these objectives.

The Development of the Physical Activity Guidelines for Americans

Since 1995, the *Dietary Guidelines for Americans* has included advice on physical activity. However, with the development of a firm science base on the health benefits of physical activity, HHS began to consider whether separate physical activity guidelines were appropriate. With the help of the Institute of Medicine, HHS convened a workshop in October 2006 to address this question. The workshop's report affirmed that advances in the science of physical activity and health justified the creation of separate physical activity guidelines.

The steps used to develop the *Physical Activity Guidelines for Americans* were similar to those used for the *Dietary Guidelines for Americans*. In 2007, HHS Secretary Mike Leavitt appointed an external scientific advisory committee called the Physical Activity Guidelines Advisory Committee. The Advisory Committee conducted an extensive analysis of the scientific information on physical activity and health. The *Physical Activity Guidelines Advisory Committee Report, 2008* and meeting summaries are available at www.health.gov/PAGuidelines/.

HHS primarily used the Advisory Committee's report but also considered comments from the public and government agencies when writing the Guidelines.

The Framework for the Physical Activity Guidelines for Americans

The Advisory Committee report provided the content and conceptual underpinning for the Guidelines. The main elements of this framework are described in the following sections.

Baseline Activity versus Health-Enhancing Physical Activity

Physical activity has been defined as any bodily movement produced by the contraction of skeletal muscle that increases energy expenditure above a basal level. However, in this chapter, the term "physical activity" will generally refer to bodily movement that enhances health. Bodily movement can be divided into two categories:

- **Baseline activity** refers to the light-intensity activities of daily life, such as standing, walking slowly, and lifting lightweight objects. People vary in how much baseline activity they do. People who do only baseline activity are considered to be inactive. They may do very short episodes of moderate- or vigorous-intensity activity, such as climbing a few flights of stairs, but these episodes aren't long enough to count toward meeting the Guidelines.

- **Health-enhancing physical activity** is activity that, when added to baseline activity, produces health benefits. In this chapter, the term "physical activity" generally refers to health-enhancing physical activity. Brisk walking, jumping rope, dancing, lifting weights, climbing on playground equipment at recess, and doing yoga are all examples of physical activity. Some people (such as postal carriers or carpenters on construction sites) may get enough physical activity on the job to meet the Guidelines.

We don't understand enough about whether doing more baseline activity results in health benefits. Even so, efforts to promote baseline activities are justifiable. Encouraging Americans to increase their baseline activity is sensible for several reasons:

- Increasing baseline activity burns calories, which can help in maintaining a healthy body weight.

- Some baseline activities are weight-bearing and may improve bone health.

- There are reasons other than health to encourage more baseline activity. For example, walking short distances instead of driving can help reduce traffic congestion and the resulting air pollution.

75

- Encouraging baseline activities helps build a culture where physical activity in general is the social norm.

- Short episodes of activity are appropriate for people who were inactive and have started to gradually increase their level of activity and for older adults whose activity may be limited by chronic conditions.

The availability of infrastructure to support short episodes of activity is therefore important. For example, people should have the option of using sidewalks and paths to walk between buildings at a worksite, rather than having to drive. People should also have the option of taking the stairs instead of using an elevator.

Health Benefits versus Other Reasons to Be Physically Active

Although the Guidelines focus on the health benefits of physical activity, these benefits are not the only reason why people are active. Physical activity gives people a chance to have fun, be with friends and family, enjoy the outdoors, improve their personal appearance, and improve their fitness so that they can participate in more intensive physical activity or sporting events. Some people are active because they feel it gives them certain health benefits (such as feeling more energetic) that aren't yet conclusively proven for the general population.

The Guidelines encourage people to be physically active for any and all reasons that are meaningful for them. Nothing in the Guidelines is intended to mean that health benefits are the only reason to do physical activity.

Focus on Disease Prevention

The Guidelines focus on preventive effects of physical activity, which include lowering the risk of developing chronic diseases such as heart disease and type 2 diabetes. Physical activity also has beneficial therapeutic effects and is commonly recommended as part of the treatment for medical conditions.

Health-Related versus Performance-Related Fitness

The Guidelines focus on reducing the risk of chronic disease and promoting health-related fitness, particularly cardiovascular and muscular fitness. People can gain this kind of fitness by doing the amount and types of activities recommended in the Guidelines.

The Guidelines do not address the types and amounts of activity necessary to improve performance-related fitness. Athletes need this kind of fitness when they compete. People who are interested in training programs to increase performance-related fitness should seek advice from other sources. Generally, these people do much more activity than required to meet the Guidelines.

Lifespan Approach

The best way to be physically active is to be active for life. Therefore, the Guidelines take a lifespan approach and provide recommendations for three age groups: children and adolescents, adults, and older adults.

The Physical Activity Guidelines are for Americans aged six and older. The Advisory Committee report did not review evidence for children younger than age six. Physical activity in infants and young children is, of course, necessary for healthy growth and development. Children younger than six should be physically active in ways appropriate for their age and stage of development.

Individualized Health Goals

The Guidelines generally explain the amounts and types of physical activity needed for health benefits. Within these overall parameters, individuals have many choices about appropriate types and amounts of activity.

To make these choices, American adults need to set personal goals for physical activity. Setting these goals involves questions like, "How physically fit do I want to be?" "How important is it to me to reduce my risk of heart disease and diabetes?" "How important is it to me to reduce my risk of falls and hip fracture?" "How much weight do I want to lose and keep off?"

People can meet the Guidelines and their own personal goals through different amounts and types of activity. Written materials, health care providers, and fitness professionals can provide useful information and help people set and carry out specific goals.

Four Levels of Physical Activity

The Advisory Committee report provides the basis for dividing the amount of aerobic physical activity an adult gets every week into four categories: inactive, low, medium, and high (see following table). This classification is useful because these categories provide a rule of thumb of how total amount of physical activity is related to health benefits. Low amounts of activity provide some benefits; medium amounts provide substantial benefits; and high amounts provide even greater benefits.

Table 9.1. Classification of Total Weekly Amounts of Aerobic Physical Activity into Four Categories

Levels of Physical Activity	Range of Moderate-Intensity Minutes a Week	Summary of Over-all Health Benefits	Comment
Inactive	No activity beyond baseline	None	Being inactive is unhealthy.
Low	Activity beyond baseline but fewer than 150 minutes a week	Some	Low levels of activity are clearly preferable to an inactive lifestyle.
Medium	150 minutes to 300 minutes a week	Substantial	Activity at the high end of this range has additional and more extensive health benefits than activity at the low end.
High	More than 300 minutes a week	Additional	Current science does not allow researchers to identify an upper limit of activity above which there are no additional health benefits.

Putting the Guidelines into Practice

Although the Advisory Committee did not review strategies to promote physical activity, action is needed at the individual, community, and societal levels to help Americans become physically active. Publications such as the *Guide to Community Preventive Services* (www .thecommunityguide.org/pa/) and the recommendations of the U.S. Preventive Services Task Force (www.ahrq.gov/clinic/cps3dix.htm) summarize evidence-based strategies for promoting physical activity on the community level and through primary health care.

Assessing Whether Physical Activity Programs Are Consistent with the Guidelines

Programs that provide opportunities for physical activity, such as classes or community activities, can help people meet the Guidelines. These programs do not have to provide all, or even most, of the recommended weekly activity. For example, a mall walking program for older adults may meet only once a week yet provide useful amounts of activity, as long as people get the rest of their weekly recommended activity on other days.

Programs that are consistent with the Guidelines meet the following criteria:

- Provide advice and education consistent with the Guidelines

- Add episodes of activity that count toward meeting the Guidelines

- May also include activities, such as stretching or warming up and cooling down, whose health benefits are not yet proven but that are often used in effective physical activity programs

Chapter 10

Physical Fitness and Children

Chapter Contents

Section 10.1

Statistics on Physical Activity in Children

Reprinted from the *Shape of the Nation Report,* © 2006, with permission from the National Association for Sport and Physical Education (NASPE), 1900 Association Drive, Reston, VA 20191-1599.

Overweight among Youth

- The percentage of young people who are overweight has more than tripled since 1980. Among children and teens aged 6 to 19 years, 16% (over 9 million young people) are overweight.[1]

- About 10% of children aged 2 to 5 years are overweight.[2]

- Four in 10 Mexican-American and African-American youth age 6 to 19 are overweight or at risk of being overweight.[2]

- Approximately 60% of obese children ages 5 to 10 years have at least one cardiovascular disease risk factor, such as elevated total cholesterol, triglycerides, insulin, or blood pressure, and 25% have two or more risk factors.[3]

- Children and adolescents who are overweight by the age of 8 are 80% more likely to become overweight or obese adults.

Participation in Physical Activity by Young People

- More than a third of young people in grades 9 to 12 do not regularly engage in vigorous physical activity.[4]

- One-third of young people in grades 9 to 12 get an insufficient amount of moderate to vigorous physical activity.[4]

- Over 11% of high school students get no moderate to vigorous physical activity.[4]

- Participation in physical activity declines as children get older. Sixty-nine percent of 9th graders participate in vigorous physical activity on a regular basis, while only 55% of 12th graders participate in the same level of activity.[4]

- Overall, among high school students, males are more physically active than females and white students are more active than black and Hispanic students.[4]

Participation in School Physical Education

- Nationwide, the percentage of high school students enrolled in physical education was 56% in 2003 (71% of 9th graders, 61% of 10th graders, 46% of 11th graders, and 40% of 12th graders).[4]

- The percentage of students who attended a daily physical education class has dropped from 42% in 1991 to 28% in 2003.[5]

- The percentage of schools that require physical education in each grade declines from about 50% in grades 1 through 5 to 25% in grade 8, to only 5% in grade 12.[6]

- Eight percent of elementary schools, 6.4% of middle school/junior high schools, and 5.8% of senior high schools provide daily physical education or its equivalent (i.e., 150 minutes per week for elementary schools; 225 minutes per week for middle schools/junior high schools and senior high schools) for the entire school year for students in all grades in the school.[6]

Public Support for Physical Education

- Ninety-five percent of parents nationwide said that physical education should be included in the school curriculum for all students in kindergarten through grade 12.[7]

- Eighty-five percent of parents and 81% of teachers believe that students should be required to take physical education every day at every grade level and 92% of teens said that they should receive daily physical education.[7]

- More than 75% of parents and teachers believe that school boards should not eliminate physical education for budgetary reasons or because of the need to meet stricter academic standards.[8]

National Recommendations

School-age youth should participate daily in 60 minutes or more of moderate to vigorous physical activity that is developmentally appropriate, enjoyable, and involves a variety of activities.[9,10,11]

All elementary school students should participate in at least 150 minutes per week of physical education, and all middle and high school students should participate in at least 225 minutes of physical education, for the entire school year.[12,13,14,15,16]

Critical Elements of a Quality Physical Education Program

1. Physical education is delivered by certified/licensed physical education teachers.

2. Adequate time (i.e., 150 minutes per week for elementary school students; 225 minutes per week for middle and high school students) is provided for physical education at every grade, K to 12.

3. All states develop standards for student learning in physical education that reflect the National Standards for Physical Education.

4. All states set minimum standards for student achievement in physical education.

5. Successfully meeting minimum standards in physical education is a requirement for high school graduation.

Positive Physical Education Pledge (NASPE, 2004)

As a highly-qualified physical education teacher, I pledge to:

- establish a positive, safe learning environment for all students;
- teach a variety of physical activities that make physical education class fun and enjoyable;
- create maximum opportunities for students of all abilities to be successful;
- promote student honesty, integrity, and good sportsmanship;
- guide students into becoming skillful and confident movers;
- facilitate the development and maintenance of physical fitness;
- assist students in setting and achieving personal goals;
- provide specific, constructive feedback to help students master motor skills;

- afford opportunities for students to succeed in cooperative and competitive situations; and

- prepare and encourage students to practice skills and be active for a lifetime.

References

1. Hedley, A. A., Ogden, C. L., Johnson, C. L., Carroll, M. D., Curtin, L. R., & Flegal, K. M. (2004). Overweight and obesity among U.S. children, adolescents, and adults, 1999-2002. *Journal of the American Medical Association, 291*(23), 2847–2850.

2. Ogden, C. L., Flegal, K. M., Carroll, M. D., & Johnson, C. L. (2002). Prevalence and trends in overweight among U.S. children and adolescents, 1999-2000. *Journal of the American Medical Association, 288*(14), 1728–1732.

3. Freedman, D. S., Khan, L. K., Dietz, W. H., Srinivason, S. R., & Berenson, G. S. (2001). Relationship of childhood obesity to coronary heart disease risk factors in adulthood: The Bogalusa heart study. *Pediatrics, 108*(3), 712–718.

4. Grunbaum, J. A., Kann, L., Kinchen, S., Ross, J., Hawkins, J., Lowry, R., Harris, W. A., McManus, T., Chyen, D., & Collins, J. (2004). Youth risk behavior surveillance—United States, 2003. *Morbidity and Mortality Weekly Report, 53*(SS-2), 1–95.

5. Centers for Disease Control and Prevention. (2004). Participation in high school physical education—United States, 1991–2003. *Morbidity and Mortality Weekly Report, 53*(36), 844–847.

6. Burgeson, C. R., Wechsler, H., Brener, N. D., Young, J. C., & Spain, C. G. (2001). Physical education and activity: Results from the School Health Policies and Programs Study, 2000. *Journal of School Health, 71*(7), 279–293.

7. National Association for Sport and Physical Education. (2003). *Parents' views of children's health & fitness: A summary of results [Executive summary]*. Reston, VA: Author.

8. Robert Wood Johnson Foundation. (2003). *National poll shows parents and teachers agree on solutions to childhood obesity [News release]*. Princeton, NJ: Author.

9. Strong, W. B., Malina, R. M., Bumkie, C. J. R., Daniels, S. R., Dishman, R. K., Gutin, B., Hergenroeder, A. C., Must, A., Nixon,

P. A., Pivarnik, J. M., Rowland, T., Trost, S., & Trudeau, F. (2005). Evidence based physical activity for school-age youth. *Journal of Pediatrics, 146,* 732–737.

10. U.S. Department of Agriculture & U.S. Department of Health and Human Services. (2000). *Nutrition and your health: Dietary guidelines for Americans* (5th ed.). Washington, DC: Author.

11. National Association for Sport and Physical Education. (2004). *Physical activity for children: A statement of guidelines for children ages 5–12* (2nd ed.). Reston, VA: Author.

12. National Association for Sport and Physical Education. (2000). *Opportunity to learn standards for elementary school physical education.* Reston, VA: Author.

13. National Association for Sport and Physical Education. (2004). *Opportunity to learn standards for middle school physical education.* Reston, VA: Author.

14. National Association for Sport and Physical Education. (2004). *Opportunity to learn standards for high school physical education.* Reston, VA: Author.

15. National Association of State Boards of Education. (2000). *Fit, healthy, and ready to learn: A school health policy guide. Part 1: Physical activity, healthy eating, and tobacco-use prevention.* Alexandria, VA: Author.

16. Centers for Disease Control and Prevention. (1997). Guidelines for school and community programs to promote lifelong physical activity among young people. *Morbidity and Mortality Weekly Report, 46*(No. RR-6), 1–36.

Section 10.2

Physical Activity from Birth to Age Five

Reprinted from *Active Start: A Statement of Physical Activity Guidelines for Children from Birth to Age 5,* 2nd Edition, © 2009, with permission from the National Association for Sport and Physical Education (NASPE), 1900 Association Drive, Reston, VA 20191-1599.

NASPE position statement: All children from birth to age five should engage daily in physical activity that promotes movement skillfulness and foundations of health-related fitness.

Purpose of the Guidelines

NASPE developed specific guidelines for the physical activity of children from birth to age five to support its position statement and to address the developing child's unique characteristics and needs. The guidelines reflect the best thinking of specialists in motor development, movement, and exercise about the physical activity needs of young children during the first years of life.

Guidelines

Guidelines for Infants

Guideline 1: Infants should interact with caregivers in daily physical activities that are dedicated to exploring movement and the environment.

Guideline 2: Caregivers should place infants in settings that encourage and stimulate movement experiences and active play for short periods of time several times a day.

Guideline 3: Infants' physical activity should promote skill development in movement.

Guideline 4: Infants should be placed in an environment that meets or exceeds recommended safety standards for performing large-muscle activities.

Guideline 5: Those in charge of infants' well-being are responsible for understanding the importance of physical activity and should promote movement skills by providing opportunities for structured and unstructured physical activity.

Guidelines for Toddlers

Guideline 1: Toddlers should engage in a total of at least 30 minutes of structured physical activity each day.

Guideline 2: Toddlers should engage in at least 60 minutes—and up to several hours—per day of unstructured physical activity and should not be sedentary for more than 60 minutes at a time, except when sleeping.

Guideline 3: Toddlers should be given ample opportunities to develop movement skills that will serve as the building blocks for future motor skillfulness and physical activity.

Guideline 4: Toddlers should have access to indoor and outdoor areas that meet or exceed recommended safety standards for performing large-muscle activities.

Guideline 5: Those in charge of toddlers' well-being are responsible for understanding the importance of physical activity and promoting movement skills by providing opportunities for structured and unstructured physical activity and movement experiences.

Guidelines for Preschoolers

Guideline 1: Preschoolers should accumulate at least 60 minutes of structured physical activity each day.

Guideline 2: Preschoolers should engage in at least 60 minutes—and up to several hours—of unstructured physical activity each day, and should not be sedentary for more than 60 minutes at a time, except when sleeping.

Guideline 3: Preschoolers should be encouraged to develop competence in fundamental motor skills that will serve as the building blocks for future motor skillfulness and physical activity.

Guideline 4: Preschoolers should have access to indoor and outdoor areas that meet or exceed recommended safety standards for performing large-muscle activities.

Guideline 5: Caregivers and parents in charge of preschoolers' health and well-being are responsible for understanding the importance of physical activity and for promoting movement skills by providing opportunities for structured and unstructured physical activity.

Section 10.3

Raising a Fit Preschooler

Preschoolers have a lot of energy, and they use it in a more organized way than when they were toddlers. Instead of just running around in the backyard, a preschooler has the physical skills and coordination to ride a tricycle or chase a butterfly.

Preschoolers are also discovering what it means to play with a friend instead of just alongside another child, as toddlers do. By being around other kids, a preschooler gains important social skills, such as sharing and taking turns. Despite occasional disputes, preschoolers learn to cooperate and interact during play.

Good Games for Your Growing Preschooler

- Play follow the leader.
- Kick a ball back and forth.
- Practice balance by pretending to be statues.
- Play freeze dance.

Helping Kids Learn New Skills

Preschoolers develop important motor skills as they grow. New skills your preschooler may be showing off include hopping, jumping forward, catching a ball, doing a somersault, skipping, and balancing on one foot. Help your child practice these skills by playing and exercising together.

When you go for a walk, your preschooler may complain about being tired, but most likely is just bored. A brisk walk can be dull for young kids, so try these ways to liven up your family stroll:

- Make your walk a scavenger hunt by giving your child something to find, like a red door, a cat, a flag, and something square.

- Sing songs or recite nursery rhymes while you walk.

- Mix walking with jumping, racing, hopping, and walking backwards.

- Make your walk together a mathematical experience as you emphasize numbers and counting: How many windows are on the garage door? What numbers are on the houses?

These kinds of activities are fun but also help to prepare kids for school.

How Much Activity Is Enough?

According to the 2005 dietary guidelines, all kids two years and older should get at least 60 minutes of moderate to vigorous exercise on most, preferably all, days of the week.

NASPE offers more specific recommendations for preschoolers, saying they should:

- accumulate at least 60 minutes of physical activity that's structured (meaning it's organized by you or another adult);

- engage in at least one hour—and up to several hours—of free play;

- not be inactive for more that one hour at a time, unless they are sleeping.

It's important to limit TV (including videos and DVDs) and computer time to no more than one to two hours per day.

Structured Play

Preschoolers are likely to get structured play at child care or in preschool programs through games like "Duck, Duck, Goose" and "London Bridge." Consider enrolling your child in a preschool tumbling or dance class.

Your preschooler can get structured outdoor play at home, too. Play together in the backyard or practice motor skills, such as throwing and catching a ball. Preschoolers also love trips to the playground.

Though many kids tend to gravitate toward the outdoors, lots of fun things can be organized indoors: a child-friendly obstacle course, a treasure hunt, or forts made out sheets and boxes or chairs. Designate a play area and clear the space of any breakables.

Here are some more ideas for structured play:

- Play bounce catch.

- Use paper airplanes to practice throwing.

- Balance a beanbag while walking—make this more challenging by setting up a simple slalom course.

- Play freeze dance.

- Play wheelbarrow by holding your child's legs while he or she walks forward on hands.

Many parents are eager to enroll their preschool child in organized sports. Although some leagues may be open to kids as young as four years old, organized and team sports are not recommended until a child is a little older. Preschoolers can't understand complex rules and often lack the attention span, skills, and coordination needed to play sports.

If you decide to enroll your preschooler in an organized team sport, such as T-ball or soccer, make sure the emphasis is on helping your child gain basic physical skills, like running, and fundamental social skills, like following rules and taking turns.

If your preschooler is not ready for the team or not interested in sports, consider focusing instead on helping him or her continue to work on fundamental skills—hopping on one foot, catching a ball, doing a somersault, and maybe riding a bicycle or tricycle.

To teach preschoolers to play baseball, start by teaching them basic skills, such as throwing, catching, and hitting off a T-ball stand. Then, if you play a game of whiffleball, don't worry if your child doesn't tag first base—it's enough to get kids running in the right direction.

Unstructured Play

Unstructured or free play is when kids are left more to their own devices—within a safe environment. During these times, they should be able to choose from a variety of activities, such as exploring, playing with toys, painting and drawing, doing a puzzle, or playing dress-up.

During pretend play, preschoolers often like to take on a gender-specific role because they are beginning to identify with members of the same gender. A girl might pretend to be her mother by "working" in the garden, while a boy might mimic his dad by pretending to cut the lawn.

It's clear your preschooler is keeping an eye on how you spend your time, so set a good example by exercising regularly. Kids who pick up on this as something parents do will naturally want to do it, too.

Safety Concerns

No matter what type of physical activity your child gets, it's important to keep safety concerns in mind. Remember that preschoolers are still developing coordination, balance, and judgment.

So as preschoolers play, a parent's challenge is to find a balance between letting them try new things and doing what is necessary to keep them safe and prevent injuries.

- A child on a tricycle or bike should always wear a helmet.

- If you haven't done so already, it's time to talk about street safety, because even the most cautious preschooler may dart into the street after a ball.

- A preschooler in a swimming pool needs constant adult supervision, even if he or she has learned to swim.

It's a tricky age because kids want more independence, and should have some, but cannot be left unsupervised. Preschoolers still need their parents to set limits.

Giving kids safe opportunities to play in both organized and unstructured ways builds a foundation for a fit lifestyle that can carry them through life.

Section 10.4

Fitness Guidelines for School-Aged Youth

This section excerpted from "Chapter 3. Active Children and Adolescents," *Physical Activity Guidelines for Americans*, U.S. Department of Health and Human Services (www.hhs.gov), October 16, 2008.

Regular physical activity in children and adolescents promotes health and fitness. Compared to those who are inactive, physically active youth have higher levels of cardiorespiratory fitness and stronger muscles. They also typically have lower body fatness. Their bones are stronger, and they may have reduced symptoms of anxiety and depression.

Youth who are regularly active also have a better chance of a healthy adulthood. Children and adolescents don't usually develop chronic diseases, such as heart disease, hypertension, type 2 diabetes, or osteoporosis. However, risk factors for these diseases can begin to develop early in life. Regular physical activity makes it less likely that these risk factors will develop and more likely that children will remain healthy as adults.

Youth can achieve substantial health benefits by doing moderate- and vigorous-intensity physical activity for periods of time that add up to 60 minutes (one hour) or more each day. This activity should include aerobic activity as well as age-appropriate muscle- and bone-strengthening activities. Although current science is not complete, it appears that, as with adults, the total amount of physical activity is more important for achieving health benefits than is any one component (frequency, intensity, or duration) or specific mix of activities (aerobic, muscle strengthening, bone strengthening). Even so, bone-strengthening activities remain especially important for children and young adolescents because the greatest gains in bone mass occur during the years just before and during puberty. In addition, the majority of peak bone mass is obtained by the end of adolescence.

This chapter provides physical activity guidance for children and adolescents aged 6 to 17 and focuses on physical activity beyond baseline activity.

Parents and other adults who work with or care for youth should be familiar with the guidelines in this chapter. These adults should be aware that, as children become adolescents, they typically reduce their physical activity. Adults play an important role in providing age-appropriate opportunities for physical activity. In doing so, they help lay an important foundation for life-long, health-promoting physical activity. Adults need to encourage active play in children and encourage sustained and structured activity as children grow older.

Key Guidelines for Children and Adolescents

- Children and adolescents should do 60 minutes (one hour) or more of physical activity daily.

  - **Aerobic:** Most of the 60 or more minutes a day should be either moderate- or vigorous-intensity aerobic physical activity and should include vigorous-intensity physical activity at least three days a week.

  - **Muscle-strengthening:** As part of their 60 or more minutes of daily physical activity, children and adolescents should include muscle-strengthening physical activity on at least three days of the week.

  - **Bone-strengthening:** As part of their 60 or more minutes of daily physical activity, children and adolescents should include bone-strengthening physical activity on at least three days of the week.

- It is important to encourage young people to participate in physical activities that are appropriate for their age, that are enjoyable, and that offer variety.

Explaining the Guidelines

Types of Activity

The Guidelines for children and adolescents focus on three types of activity: aerobic, muscle strengthening, and bone strengthening. Each type has important health benefits.

- **Aerobic activities** are those in which young people rhythmically move their large muscles. Running, hopping, skipping, jumping rope, swimming, dancing, and bicycling are all examples of aerobic activities. Aerobic activities increase cardiorespiratory fitness. Children often do activities in short bursts, which may not technically be aerobic activities. However, this document will also use the term aerobic to refer to these brief activities.

- **Muscle-strengthening activities** make muscles do more work than usual during activities of daily life. This is called "overload," and it strengthens the muscles. Muscle-strengthening activities can be unstructured and part of play, such as playing on playground equipment, climbing trees, and playing tug-of-war. Or these activities can be structured, such as lifting weights or working with resistance bands.

- **Bone-strengthening activities** produce a force on the bones that promotes bone growth and strength. This force is commonly produced by impact with the ground. Running, jumping rope, basketball, tennis, and hopscotch are all examples of bone-strengthening activities. As these examples illustrate, bone-strengthening activities can also be aerobic and muscle strengthening.

How Age Influences Physical Activity in Children and Adolescents

Children and adolescents should meet the guidelines by doing activity that is appropriate for their age. Their natural patterns of movement differ from those of adults. For example, children are naturally active in an intermittent way, particularly when they do unstructured active play. During recess and in their free play and games, children use basic aerobic and bone-strengthening activities, such as running, hopping, skipping, and jumping, to develop movement patterns and skills. They alternate brief periods of moderate- and vigorous-intensity physical activity with brief periods of rest. Any episode of moderate- or vigorous-intensity physical activity, however brief, counts toward the guidelines.

Children also commonly increase muscle strength through unstructured activities that involve lifting or moving their body weight or working against resistance. Children don't usually do or need formal muscle-strengthening programs, such as lifting weights.

Regular physical activity in children and adolescents promotes a healthy body weight and body composition.

As children grow into adolescents, their patterns of physical activity change. They are able to play organized games and sports and are able to sustain longer periods of activity. But they still commonly do intermittent activity, and no period of moderate- or vigorous-intensity activity is too short to count toward the guidelines.

Adolescents may meet the guidelines by doing free play, structured programs, or both. Structured exercise programs can include aerobic activities, such as playing a sport, and muscle-strengthening activities, such as lifting weights, working with resistance bands, or using body weight for resistance (such as push-ups, pull-ups, and sit-ups). Muscle-strengthening activities count if they involve a moderate to high level of effort and work the major muscle groups of the body: legs, hips, back, abdomen, chest, shoulders, and arms.

Levels of Intensity for Aerobic Activity

Children and adolescents can meet the guidelines by doing a combination of moderate- and vigorous-intensity aerobic physical activities or by doing only vigorous-intensity aerobic physical activities.

Youth should not do only moderate-intensity activity. It's important to include vigorous-intensity activities because they cause more improvement in cardiorespiratory fitness.

Table 10.1. Examples of Moderate- and Vigorous-Intensity Aerobic Physical Activities and Muscle- and Bone-Strengthening Activities for Children and Adolescents

Type of Physical Activity: **Moderate-intensity aerobic**

Age Group Children	Age Group Adults
Active recreation, such as hiking, skateboarding, rollerblading	Active recreation, such as canoeing, hiking, skateboarding, rollerblading
Bicycle riding	Bicycle riding (stationary or road bike)
Brisk walking	Brisk walking
	Housework and yard work, such as sweeping or pushing a lawn mower
	Games that require catching and throwing, such as baseball and softball

Type of Physical Activity: **Vigorous-intensity aerobic**

Age Group Children	Age Group Adults
Active games involving running and chasing, such as tag	Active games involving running and chasing, such as flag football
Bicycle riding	Bicycle riding
Jumping rope	Jumping rope
Martial arts, such as karate	Martial arts, such as karate
Running	Running
Sports such as soccer, ice or field hockey, basketball, swimming, tennis	Sports such as soccer, ice or field hockey, basketball, swimming, tennis

The intensity of aerobic physical activity can be defined on either an absolute or a relative scale. Either scale can be used to monitor the intensity of aerobic physical activity:

- **Absolute intensity** is based on the rate of energy expenditure during the activity, without taking into account a person's cardiorespiratory fitness.

- **Relative intensity** uses a person's level of cardiorespiratory fitness to assess level of effort.

Relative intensity describes a person's level of effort relative to his or her fitness. As a rule of thumb, on a scale of 0 to 10, where sitting is 0 and the highest level of effort possible is 10, moderate-intensity activity is a 5 or 6. Young people doing moderate-intensity activity will notice

Table 10.1. Continued

Type of Physical Activity: **Vigorous-intensity aerobic,** continued

Cross-country skiing	Vigorous dancing
	Cross-country skiing

Type of Physical Activity: **Muscle-strengthening**

Age Group Children	Age Group Adults
Games such as tug-of-war	Games such as tug-of-war
Modified push-ups (with knees on the floor)	Push-ups and pull-ups
Resistance exercises using body weight or resistance bands	Resistance exercises with exercise bands, weight machines, hand-held weights
Rope or tree climbing	Climbing wall
Sit-ups (curl-ups or crunches)	Sit-ups (curl-ups or crunches)
Swinging on playground equipment/bars	

Type of Physical Activity: **Bone-strengthening**

Age Group Children	Age Group Adults
Hopping, skipping, jumping	Hopping, skipping, jumping
Jumping rope	Jumping rope
Running	Running
Sports such as gymnastics, basketball, volleyball, tennis	Sports such as gymnastics, basketball, volleyball, tennis
Games such as hopscotch	

Note: Some activities, such as bicycling, can be moderate or vigorous intensity, depending upon level of effort.

that their hearts are beating faster than normal and they are breathing harder than normal. Vigorous-intensity activity is at a level of 7 or 8. Youth doing vigorous-intensity activity will feel their heart beating much faster than normal, and they will breathe much harder than normal.

When adults supervise children, they generally can't ascertain a child's heart or breathing rate. But they can observe whether a child is doing an activity which, based on absolute energy expenditure, is considered to be either moderate or vigorous. For example, a child walking briskly to school is doing moderate-intensity activity. A child running on the playground is doing vigorous-intensity activity. Table 10.1 includes examples of activities classified by absolute intensity. It shows that the same activity can be moderate or vigorous intensity, depending on factors such as speed (for example, bicycling slowly or fast).

Physical Activity and Healthy Weight

Regular physical activity in children and adolescents promotes a healthy body weight and body composition.

Exercise training in overweight or obese youth can improve body composition by reducing overall levels of fatness as well as abdominal fatness. Research studies report that fatness can be reduced by regular physical activity of moderate to vigorous intensity three to five times a week, for 30 to 60 minutes.

Meeting the Guidelines

American youth vary in their physical activity participation. Some don't participate at all, others participate in enough activity to meet the guidelines, and some exceed the guidelines.

Children and adolescents can meet the Physical Activity Guidelines and become regularly physically active in many ways.

One practical strategy to promote activity in youth is to replace inactivity with activity whenever possible. For example, where appropriate and safe, young people should walk or bicycle to school instead of riding in a car. Rather than just watching sporting events on television, young people should participate in age-appropriate sports or games.

- Children and adolescents who do not meet the guidelines should slowly increase their activity in small steps and in ways that they enjoy. A gradual increase in the number of days and the time spent being active will help reduce the risk of injury.

- Children and adolescents who meet the guidelines should continue being active on a daily basis and, if appropriate, become even more active. Evidence suggests that even more than 60 minutes of activity every day may provide additional health benefits.

- Children and adolescents who exceed the guidelines should maintain their activity level and vary the kinds of activities they do to reduce the risk of overtraining or injury.

Children and adolescents with disabilities are more likely to be inactive than those without disabilities. Youth with disabilities should work with their health care provider to understand the types and amounts of physical activity appropriate for them. When possible, children and adolescents with disabilities should meet the guidelines. When young people are not able to participate in appropriate physical activities to meet the guidelines, they should be as active as possible and avoid being inactive.

Section 10.5

Physical Fitness Education in Schools

This section excerpted from "School Health Policies and Programs Study 2006: Physical Education" and "School Health Policies and Programs Study 2006: Physical Activity," Centers for Disease Control and Prevention (www .cdc.gov), 2006.

Physical Education

- 69.3% of elementary schools, 83.9% of middle schools, and 95.2% of high schools required physical education.

- Among schools that required physical education, 20.8% of elementary schools, 22.7% of middle schools, and 30.9% of high schools allowed students to be exempted from physical education requirements for at least one of the following reasons: high physical competency test score, participation in community service activities, participation in community sports activities, and participation in school activities other than sports (e.g., band or chorus).

- 3.8% of elementary schools, 7.9% of middle schools, and 2.1% of high schools provided daily physical education or its equivalent

(150 minutes per week in elementary schools; 225 minutes per week in middle schools and high schools) for the entire school year (36 weeks) for students in all grades in the school.

- 13.7% of elementary schools, 15.2% of middle schools, and 3.0% of high schools provided physical education at least three days per week or its equivalent for the entire school year for students in all grades in the school.

- 68.1% of schools that required physical education taught dodgeball or bombardment, and more than half of elementary schools that required physical education taught king of the hill or steal the flag, elimination tag, and duck duck goose.

- The percentage of states that required or encouraged districts or schools to follow standards or guidelines based on the National Standards for Physical Education increased from 59.2% in 2000 to 76.0% in 2006.[1]

Table 10.2. Percentage of Schools in Which Teachers Used Criteria in at Least One Required Physical Education Class or Course to Assess Student Performance in Physical Education

Criterion	Schools
Level of participation	95.8
Student attitude	89.3
Attendance	56.9
Improvement in movement skills test scores	53.7
Final scores on movement skills tests	49.3
Physical fitness test scores	45.9
Demonstration of self-management skills	39.7
Participation in physical activity outside of physical education	11.8

- Among the 78.3% of schools that required physical education, 36.0% had a maximum allowable student-to-teacher ratio for required physical education. The median maximum allowable ratio among these schools was 29.6 students per teacher.

- The percentage of states that prohibited schools from using physical activity to punish students for bad behavior in physical education increased from 2.1% in 2000 to 16.0% in 2006, and the percentage of states that actively discouraged schools from this practice also increased, from 25.5% in 2000 to 56.0% in 2006.

Table 10.3. Percentage of States and Districts That Provided Funding for Staff Development or Offered Staff Development to Those Who Teach Physical Education during the Two Years Preceding the Study, 2000 and 2006

Topic	States 2000	States 2006	Districts 2000	Districts 2006
Administering or using fitness tests	30.6	61.2	49.8	62.5
Assessing or evaluating student performance in physical education	54.0	71.4	48.0	62.2
Encouraging family involvement in physical activity	24.5	59.2	28.0	51.0
Methods to increase the amount of class time students are physically active	28.0	55.1	32.6	54.3

- In 25.6% of middle and high schools, teachers in at least one required physical education class or course required students to develop individualized physical activity plans.

- During the two years preceding the study, the percentage of states that provided funding for staff development or offered staff development to those who teach physical education on using technology such as computers or video cameras for physical education increased from 40.0% in 2000 to 55.1% in 2006.

- 84.2% of districts required newly hired elementary school physical education teachers to be certified, licensed, or endorsed by the state to teach physical education, 86.5% had this requirement at the middle school level, and 92.6% at the high school level.

- In 80.1% of elementary schools, physical education was taught only by a physical education teacher or specialist, and in 73.3% of middle schools and 66.3% of high schools, physical education was taught only by a physical education teacher.

The following were true during the two years preceding the study:

- 77.6% of states and 90.9% of districts provided funding for staff development or offered staff development to those who teach physical education on at least one physical education topic.

- 87.7% of physical education classes or courses had a teacher who received staff development on at least one physical education topic.

Physical Activity

The following occurred during the two years preceding the study:

- The percentage of states that provided funding for staff development or offered staff development on physical activity and fitness to those who teach health education increased from 68.8% in 2000 to 82.4% in 2006.[1]

- The percentage of districts that provided funding for staff development or offered staff development on physical activity and fitness to those who teach health education increased from 43.3% in 2000 to 75.3% in 2006.

Table 10.4. Percentage of Schools in Which Teachers Taught* Physical Activity Topics as Part of Required Instruction, by School Level

Topic	Elementary	Middle	High
Decreasing sedentary activities (e.g., TV watching)	72.7	71.5	75.6
Health-related fitness (i.e., cardiovascular endurance, muscular endurance, muscular strength, flexibility, and body composition)	63.8	72.0	76.2
Physical, psychological, or social benefits of physical activity	72.1	70.3	78.0

* In at least one elementary school class or in at least one required health education course in middle schools or high schools.

- 96.8% of elementary schools provided regularly scheduled recess for students in at least one grade. Among these schools, students were scheduled to have recess an average of 4.9 days per week for an average of 30.2 minutes per day.

- 79.1% of elementary schools provided daily recess for students in all grades in the school.

- 48.4% of schools offered intramural activities or physical activity clubs to students, and 22.9% of these schools provided transportation home for students participating in these activities or clubs.

- The percentage of schools with intramural activities or physical activity clubs that required students to pay a fee for these activities increased from 23.0% in 2000 to 35.0% in 2006.

- 77.0% of middle schools and 91.3% of high schools offered students opportunities to participate in at least one interscholastic sport, and 29.1% of these schools provided transportation home for participating students.

Table 10.5. Percentage of Schools That Offered Selected Intramural Activities or Physical Activity Clubs and Interscholastic Sports, by School Level

Activity, Club, or Sport	Elementary	Middle	High
Intramural Activity or Physical Activity Club			
Baseball, softball, or whiffleball	27.7	28.0	22.2
Basketball	38.3	42.4	37.2
Dance	15.0	16.2	13.6
Frisbee, Frisbee golf, or ultimate Frisbee	10.8	15.9	14.5
Jump rope	22.9	19.1	16.2
Running or jogging	28.6	29.0	24.1
Soccer	28.6	27.7	18.8
Volleyball	24.6	35.5	27.4
Walking	20.0	19.2	20.4
Interscholastic Sport			
Baseball	NA	35.7	79.6
Basketball	NA	76.4	90.9
Bowling	NA	3.0	17.2
Cheerleading or competitive spirits	NA	50.9	77.3
Cross-country	NA	38.9	68.4
Fast pitch or slow pitch softball	NA	45.2	77.9
Football	NA	53.0	71.0
Ice hockey	NA	2.4	14.3
Track and field	NA	52.1	73.2
Volleyball	NA	57.3	71.4
Wrestling	NA	28.7	49.6

NA = not asked.

- Outside of school hours or when school was not in session, children and adolescents used the school's physical activity or athletic facilities for community-sponsored sports teams in 68.9% of schools, for supervised "open-gym" or "free-play" in 40.3% of schools, and for community-sponsored classes or lessons (e.g., tennis or gymnastics) in 33.3% of schools.

103

- The percentage of school health services coordinators who served as study respondents who received staff development on physical activity and fitness counseling during the two years preceding the study increased from 29.4% in 2000 to 48.6% in 2006.

1. Selected changes between 2000 and 2006 are included if they met at least two of three criteria (p<0.01 from a t-test, a difference greater than 10 percentage points, or an increase by at least a factor of two or decrease by at least half). Variables are not included if they did not meet these criteria or if no comparable variable existed in both survey years.

Chapter 11

Physical Fitness and Teenagers

Chapter Contents

Section 11.1

Statistics on Physical Activity in Teenagers

"Physical Activity and the Health of Young People," Centers for Disease Control and Prevention (www.cdc.gov), October 28, 2008.

Benefits of Regular Physical Activity

- Helps build and maintain healthy bones and muscles.[1]

- Helps reduce the risk of developing obesity and chronic diseases such as diabetes and cardiovascular disease.[1]

- Reduces feelings of depression and anxiety and promotes psychological well-being.[1]

Long-Term Consequences of Physical Inactivity

- Overweight and obesity, influenced by physical inactivity and poor diet, are significantly associated with an increased risk of diabetes, high blood pressure, high cholesterol, asthma, arthritis, and poor health status.[2]

- Physical inactivity increases the risk of dying prematurely, dying of heart disease, and developing diabetes, colon cancer, and high blood pressure.[1]

Obesity among Youth

- The prevalence of obesity among children aged 6–11 more than doubled in the past 20 years, going from 6.5% in 1980 to 17.0% in 2006. The rate among adolescents aged 12–19 more than tripled, increasing from 5.0% to 17.6%.[3]

- Children and adolescents who are overweight are more likely to be overweight or obese as adults;[4] one study showed that children who became obese by age eight were more severely obese as adults.[5]

Participation in Physical Activity by Young People

- During the seven days preceding the survey, 77% of children aged 9–13 reported participating in free-time physical activity.[6]

- Thirty-five percent of high school students had participated in at least 60 minutes per day of physical activity on five or more of the seven days preceding the survey.[7]

- Twenty-five percent of high school students did not participate in 60 or more minutes of any kind of physical activity that increased their heart rate or made them breathe hard some of the time on at least one day during the seven days before the survey (i.e., did not participate in 60 or more minutes of physical activity on any day).[7]

- Participation in physical activity declines as children get older.[7]

Table 11.1. Percentage of High School Students Participating in Physical Activity and Physical Education, by Sex, 2007[7]

Type of Activity	Girls	Boys
At least 60 minutes/day of physical activity[a]	25.6%	43.7%
Attended physical education class daily[b]	27.3%	33.2%

a. Any kind of physical activity that increased heart rate and made them breathe hard some of the time for at least 60 minutes per day on five or more of the seven days preceding the survey.

b. Attended physical education classes five days in an average week when they were in school.

Participation in Physical Education Classes

- Over half (54%) of high school students (62% of 9th grade students but only 41% of 12th grade students) attended physical education classes in 2007.[7]

- The percentage of high school students who attended physical education classes daily decreased from 42% in 1991 to 25% in 1995 and has remained stable at that level until 2007 (30%). In 2007, 40% of 9th grade students but only 24% of 12th grade students attended physical education class daily.[7]

- Among the 54% of students who attended physical education classes, 84% actually exercised or played sports for 20 minutes or longer during an average class.[7]

References

1. U.S. Department of Health and Human Services. *Physical activity guidelines advisory committee report.* Washington, DC: U.S. Department of Health and Human Services, 2008.

2. Mokdad AH, Ford ES, Bowman BA, et al. Prevalence of obesity, diabetes, and obesity-related health risk factors, 2001. *Journal of the American Medical Association* 2003;289(1):76–79.

3. Ogden CL, Carroll MD, Flegal KM. High Body Mass Index for Age among U.S. Children and Adolescents, 2003–2006. *JAMA.* 2008;299(20):2401–2405.

4. Ferraro KF, Thorpe RJ Jr, Wilkinson JA. The life course of severe obesity: Does childhood overweight matter? *Journal of Gerontology* 2003;58B(2):S110–S119.

5. Freedman DS, Khan LK, Dietz WH, Srinivasan SR, Berenson GS. Relationship of childhood obesity to coronary heart disease risk factors in adulthood: The Bogalusa Study. *Pediatrics* 2001;108(3):712–718.

6. CDC. Physical activity levels among children aged 9–13 years—United States, 2002. *Morbidity and Mortality Weekly Report* August 22, 2003; 52(SS-33):785–788.

7. CDC. Youth Risk Behavior Surveillance—United States, 2007. *Morbidity and Mortality Weekly Report* 2008;57(No.SS-4).

Section 11.2

Teenagers and Physical Fitness

Kids who enjoy sports and exercise tend to stay active throughout their lives.

Immediate benefits include maintaining a healthy weight, feeling more energetic, and promoting a better outlook. Participating in team and individual sports can boost self-confidence, provide opportunities for social interaction, and offer a chance to have fun. And regular physical activity can help prevent heart disease, diabetes, and other medical problems later in life.

Fitness in the Teen Years

It's recommended that teens get at least one hour of physical activity on most, preferably all, days of the week. Yet physical activity tends to decline during the teen years. Many teens drop out of organized sports and participation in daily physical education classes is a thing of the past.

But given the opportunity and interest, teens can reap health benefits from almost any activity they enjoy, from skateboarding, inline skating, yoga, swimming, dancing, or kicking a footbag in the driveway. Weight training, under supervision of a qualified adult, can improve strength and help prevent sports injuries.

Teens can work physical activity into everyday routines, such as walking to school, doing chores, or finding an active part-time job. They can be camp counselors, babysitters, or assistant coaches for young sports teams, jobs that come with a chance to be active.

Motivating Teens to Be Active

Teens face many new social and academic pressures in addition to dealing with emotional and physical changes. Studies show that teens on average spend more than six hours a day on various media, including watching TV, listening to music, surfing online, and playing video games. It's not surprising that teens can't seem to find the time to exercise and many parents can't motivate them to be active.

Parents should try to give teens control over how they decide to be physically active. Teens are defining themselves as individuals and want the power to make their own decisions, so they're reluctant to do yet another thing they're told to do. Emphasize that it's not what they do; they just need to be physically active regularly.

Once they get started, many teens enjoy the feeling of well-being, reduced stress, and increased strength and energy they get from exercise, and then might gravitate to exercise without nudging from a parent.

To keep teens motivated the activities have to be fun. Support your teen's choices by providing equipment, transportation, and companionship. Peers can play an influential role in teens' lives, so create opportunities for them to be active with their friends.

Help your teen stay active by finding an exercise regimen that fits with his or her schedule. Your teen may not have time to play a team sport at school or in a local league, but many gyms offer teen memberships, and kids may be able to squeeze in a visit before or after school. Your teen might also feel more comfortable doing home exercise videos. If transportation is an obstacle, try coordinating your teen's exercise schedule with your own.

And all teens should limit the time spent in sedentary activities, including watching TV and using the computer.

When to Speak with Your Doctor

If you're concerned about your teen's fitness, speak with your doctor. Teens who are overweight or very sedentary may need to start slowly and the doctor may be able to recommend programs or help you devise a fitness plan.

A teen with a chronic health condition or disability should not be excluded from fitness activities. Some activities may need to be modified or adapted, and some may be too risky. Consult your doctor about which activities are safe.

And some teens may overdo it when it comes to fitness. Young athletes, particularly those involved in gymnastics, wrestling, or dance, may face pressures to lose weight. If your teen refuses to eat certain food groups (such as fats), becomes overly concerned with body image, appears to be exercising compulsively, or experiences a sudden change in weight, talk with your doctor.

Another dangerous issue is the use of steroids, particularly in sports where size and strength are valued. Talk with your doctor if you suspect your teen is using steroids or other performance-enhancing substances.

Finally, speak with your doctor if your teen complains of pain during sports and exercise.

Fitness for Everyone

Everyone can benefit from being physically fit. Staying fit can help improve self-esteem and decrease the risk of serious illnesses (such as heart disease and stroke) later in life. In addition, regular physical activity can help teens learn to meet physical and emotional challenges they face every day.

Help your teen commit to fitness by being a positive role model and exercising regularly, too. For fitness activities you can enjoy together, try bike rides, hitting a tennis ball around, going to a local swimming pool, or even playing games like capture the flag and touch football. Not only are you working together to reach your fitness goals, it's a great opportunity to stay connected with your teen.

Section 11.3

Teenagers Exercising Far Less than Younger Kids

"Teens Exercising Far Less than Kids," July 2008, reprinted with permission from www.kidshealth.org. Copyright © 2008 The Nemours Foundation. This information was provided by KidsHealth, one of the largest resources online for medically reviewed health information written for parents, kids, and teens. For more articles like this one, visit www.KidsHealth.org, or www.TeensHealth.org.

Young kids are naturally compelled to be active—they run, jump, tumble, and climb their way through the day without even realizing they're wracking up countless hours of healthy exercise.

But as kids get older their social and school calendars usually become busier. Plus, they're often increasingly more interested in a veritable buffet of technologies—social networking sites, video games, wireless texting, instant messaging, TV, DVDs—that often keep them plopped down in one very sedentary spot.

So, it's no surprise that kids' fitness time starts to plummet in adolescence. But a new study reveals just how drastically different activity levels among school-aged kids vs. teens really are.

From 2000–2006, researchers recorded the movements of more than 1,000 kids using a special device (called an accelerometer) attached to their belts for one week a year (at ages 9, 11, 12, and 15).

Turns out, not even a third of 15-year-olds are getting the recommended bare minimum amount of physical activity during the week (at least an hour of "moderate-to-vigorous" exercise per day). And a mere 17% got that much on weekends.

But just six years younger, at age 9, kids were active for about three hours a day during both the week and weekends. And at age 11 almost all of the kids were meeting the suggested activity levels just fine.

So, when did their habits start changing? At about age 13, girls generally stopped getting enough exercise during the week, whereas boys stayed active for a little longer—until just before 15. But weekend exercise went downhill even sooner for both sexes—about 12½ for girls and roughly 13½ for boys.

What This Means to You

As with most things health related, kids usually can't make the connection between how what they do now can have a huge effect on their health later. They tend to live in the here and now, not in the "what will be." So, they often don't grasp that too little exercise during their childhood or teen years can mean not just putting on a few too many pounds today, but also becoming at risk for obesity, diabetes, and other serious, life-threatening conditions like heart disease and stroke down the road.

But getting older kids and teens, who are often preoccupied with other pursuits, moving can be tough. So, let them feel like they have some control over their own physical activity, instead of it feeling like something dreadful they're being forced to do. Involve them in picking out gear—be it equipment they can use or cool workout duds they can wear.

And let them choose how they want to be active. Emphasize that it's not what they do—just that they need to do something physically active on a regular basis, preferably most days of the week.

Especially on the weekends and during school breaks, when their social calendars and requests to relax more may prevail, try to get them to squeeze some physical activities into their schedule.

On top of conventional sports and pumping iron in the gym suggest alternative, less structured activities like:

- outdoor activities (hiking, road or mountain biking, rock climbing, horseback riding, Ultimate Frisbee, skiing, snowboarding);

- classes (yoga, Pilates, kickboxing, fencing, gymnastics, martial arts like tai chi, dance);

- water sports and activities (swimming, surfing, wakeboarding, canoeing, kayaking, rowing, sailing, water skiing, windsurfing);

- "extreme" sports (skateboarding, inline skating, BMX biking).

Find out if your local gym or YMCA offers teen memberships, which may make older kids feel more like they have ownership of their membership and when and how they opt to work out.

If your kids aren't getting enough exercise because they're so attached to their technologies, as many preteens and teens are, encourage them to use some of their gadgets to make exercise more enjoyable:

- Buy some digital tunes for their MP3 players for their walking, running, or working-out pleasure.

- Pick up video games that require simulating activities like dancing or tennis.

- Turn them on to TV and DVD workouts they can do in the privacy of their own room. Find some that incorporate kids their own age, too.

Or, have your kids earn their cell phone, TV, computer, or video game privileges with every hour they spend exercising. And make sure to put the kibosh on too much screen time—no more than two hours of quality content per day.

But if your kids aren't taking to the thought of moving more than their thumbs for texting or gaming, you might need to take the bull by the horns and organize some regular family fitness fun time. Sure, they may resist and resent it at first. But, chances are, they'll probably eventually learn to enjoy—and maybe even look forward to that together time—even if they may never admit it.

Source: "Moderate-to-Vigorous Physical Activity From Ages 9 to 15 Years," *Journal of the American Medical Association (JAMA)*, July 16, 2008.

Chapter 12

Promoting Physical Activity in Children and Teenagers

Chapter Contents

Section 12.1

Motivating Children and Teenagers to Be Active

Keeping Kids Active

Anyone who's seen kids on a playground knows that most are naturally physically active and love to move around. But what might not be apparent is that climbing to the top of a slide or swinging from the monkey bars can help lead kids to a lifetime of being active.

As they get older, it can be a challenge for kids to get enough daily activity. Reasons include increasing demands of school, a feeling among some kids that they aren't good at sports, a lack of active role models, and busy working families.

And even if kids have the time and the desire to be active, parents may not feel comfortable letting them freely roam the neighborhood as kids once did. So their opportunities might be limited.

Despite these barriers, parents can instill a love of activity and help kids fit it into their everyday routines. Doing so can establish healthy patterns that will last into adulthood.

Watch for Changing Interests

As time passes, your child may lose interest in old favorites, such as soccer. The trick is to help your child continue to be active, even if league play falls by the wayside. Staying active and keeping fit are the goals, so help find a replacement activity or activities that your child enjoys.

Benefits of Being Active

When kids are active, their bodies can do the things they want and need them to do. Why? Because regular exercise provides these benefits:

- Strong muscles and bones
- Weight control
- Decreased risk of developing type 2 diabetes
- Better sleep
- A better outlook on life

Healthy, physically active kids also are more likely to be academically motivated, alert, and successful. And physical competence builds self-esteem at every age.

What Motivates Kids?

So there's a lot to gain from regular physical activity, but how do you encourage kids to do it? The three keys are:

1. choosing the right activities for a child's age (if you don't, the child may be bored or frustrated);

2. giving kids plenty of opportunity to be active (kids need parents to make activity easy by providing equipment and taking them to playgrounds and other active spots);

3. keeping the focus on fun (kids won't do something they don't enjoy).

When kids enjoy an activity, they want to do more of it. Practicing a skill—whether it's swimming or riding a tricycle—improves their abilities and helps them feel accomplished, especially when the effort is noticed and praised. These good feelings often make kids want to continue the activity and even try others.

Age-Appropriate Activities

The best way for kids to get physical activity is by incorporating physical activity into their daily routine. Toddlers to teens need at least 60 minutes on most (preferably all) days. This can include free play at home, active time at school, and participation in classes or organized sports.

Here's Some Age-Based Advice

Preschoolers: Preschoolers need play and exercise that helps them continue to develop important motor skills—kicking or throwing a ball, playing tag or follow the leader, hopping on one foot, riding a bike, freeze dancing, or running obstacle courses.

Although some sports leagues may be open to kids as young as four, organized and team sports are not recommended until they're a little older. Preschoolers can't understand complex rules and often lack the attention span, skills, and coordination needed to play sports. Instead of learning to play a sport, they should work on fundamental skills.

School-age: With school-age kids spending more time on sedentary pursuits like watching TV and playing computer games, the challenge for parents is to help them find physical activities they enjoy and feel successful doing. These can range from traditional sports like baseball and basketball to Scouting, biking, camping, hiking, and other outdoor pursuits.

As kids learn basic skills and simple rules in the early school-age years, there might only be a few athletic standouts. As kids get older, differences in ability and personality become more apparent. Commitment and interest level often go along with ability, which is why it's important to find an activity that's right for your child. Schedules start getting busy during these years, but don't forget to set aside some time for free play.

Teenagers: Teens have many choices when it comes to being active—from school sports to after-school interests, such as yoga or skateboarding. It's important to remember that physical activity must be planned and often has to be sandwiched between various responsibilities and commitments.

Do what you can to make it easy for your teen to exercise by providing transportation and the necessary gear or equipment (including workout clothes). In some cases, the right clothes and shoes might help a shy teen feel comfortable biking or going to the gym.

Kids' Fitness Personalities

In addition to a child's age, it's important to consider his or her fitness personality. Personality traits, genetics, and athletic ability combine to influence kids' attitudes toward participation in sports and other physical activities, particularly as they get older.

Which of these three types best describes your child?

1. **The nonathlete:** This child may lack athletic ability, interest in physical activity, or both.

2. **The casual athlete:** This child is interested in being active but isn't a star player and is at risk of getting discouraged in a competitive athletic environment.

3. **The athlete:** This child has athletic ability, is committed to a sport or activity, and is likely to ramp up practice time and intensity of competition.

If you understand the concepts of temperament and fitness types, you'll be better able to help your kids find the right activities and get enough exercise—and find enjoyment in physical activity. Some kids want to pursue excellence in a sport, while others may be perfectly happy and fit as casual participants.

The athlete, for instance, will want to be on the basketball team, while the casual athlete may just enjoy shooting hoops in the playground or on the driveway. The nonathlete is likely to need a parent's help and encouragement to get and stay physically active. That's why it's important to encourage kids to remain active even through they aren't top performers.

Whatever their fitness personality, all kids can be physically fit. A parent's positive attitude will help a child who's reluctant to exercise.

Be active yourself and support your kids' interests. If you start this early enough, they'll come to regard activity as a normal—and fun—part of your family's everyday routine.

Section 12.2

Fitness for Kids Who Don't Like Sports

Team sports can boost kids' self-esteem, coordination, and general fitness and help them learn how to work with other kids and adults.

But some kids aren't natural athletes and they may tell you—directly or indirectly—that they just don't like sports. What then?

Why Some Kids Don't Like Teams

Not every child has to join a team, and with enough other activities, kids can be fit without them. But try to find out why your child isn't interested. You might be able to help address deeper concerns or steer your child toward something else.

Tell your child that you'd like to work on a solution together. This might mean making changes and sticking with the team sport or finding a new activity to try.

Here are some reasons why sports might be a turnoff for kids:

Still Developing Basic Skills

Though many sports programs are available for preschoolers, it's not until about age six or seven that most kids have the physical skills, the attention span, and the ability to grasp the rules needed to play organized sports.

Kids who haven't had much practice in a specific sport might need time to reliably perform necessary skills such as kicking a soccer ball on the run or hitting a baseball thrown from the pitcher's mound. Trying and failing, especially in a game situation, might frustrate them or make them nervous.

What you can do: Practice with your child at home. Whether it's shooting baskets, playing catch, or going for a jog together, you'll give your child an opportunity to build skills and fitness in a safe environment. Your child can try—and, possibly, fail—new things without the self-consciousness of being around peers. And you're also getting a good dose of quality together time.

Coach or League Is Too Competitive

A kid who's already a reluctant athlete might feel extra nervous when the coach barks out orders or the league focuses heavily on winning.

What you can do: Investigate sports programs before signing your child up for one. Talk with coaches and other parents about the philosophy. Some athletic associations, like the YMCA, have noncompetitive leagues. In some programs, they don't even keep score.

As kids get older, they can handle more competitive aspects such as keeping score and keeping track of wins and losses for the season. Some kids may be motivated by competitive play, but most aren't ready for the increased pressure until they're 11 or 12 years old. Remember that even in more competitive leagues, the atmosphere should remain positive and supportive for all the participants.

Stage Fright

Kids who aren't natural athletes or are a little shy might be uncomfortable with the pressure of being on a team. More self-conscious kids also might worry about letting their parents, coaches, or teammates down. This is especially true if a child is still working on basic skills and if the league is very competitive.

What you can do: Keep your expectations realistic—most kids don't become Olympic medalists or get sports scholarships. Let your child know the goal is to be fit and have fun. If the coach or league doesn't agree, it's probably time to look for something new.

Still Shopping for a Sport

Some kids haven't found the right sport. Maybe a child who doesn't have the hand-eye coordination for baseball has the drive and the build to be a swimmer, a runner, or a cyclist. The idea of an individual sport also can be more appealing to some kids who like to go it alone.

What you can do: Be open to your child's interests in other sports or activities. That can be tough if, for instance, you just loved basketball and wanted to continue the legacy. But by exploring other options, you give your child a chance to get invested in something he or she truly enjoys.

Other Barriers

Different kids mature at different rates, so expect a wide range of heights, weights, and athletic abilities among kids of the same age group. A child who's much bigger or smaller than other kids of the same age—or less coordinated or not as strong—may feel self-conscious and uncomfortable competing with them.

Kids also might be afraid of getting injured or worried that they can't keep up. Kids who are overweight might be reluctant to participate in a sport, for example, while a child with asthma might feel more comfortable with sports that require short outputs of energy, like baseball, football, gymnastics, golf, and shorter track and field events.

What you can do: Give some honest thought to your child's strengths, abilities, and temperament and find an activity that might be a good match. Some kids are afraid of the ball, so they don't like softball or volleyball but may enjoy an activity like running. If your child is overweight, he or she might lack the endurance to run, but might enjoy a sport like swimming. A child who's too small for the basketball team may enjoy gymnastics or wrestling.

Remember that some kids will prefer sports that focus on individual performance rather than teamwork. The goal is to prevent your child from feeling frustrated, wanting to quit, and being turned off from sports and physical activity altogether.

Try to address your child's concerns. By being understanding and providing a supportive environment, you'll help foster success in whatever activity your child chooses.

Smart Start

Before beginning any sport or fitness program, it's a good idea for your child to have a physical examination from the doctor. Kids with undiagnosed medical conditions, vision or hearing problems, or other disorders may have difficulty participating in certain activities.

Fitness Outside of Team Sports

Even kids who once said they hated sports might learn to like team sports as their skills improve or they find the right sport or a league. But even if team sports never thrill your child, there's plenty a kid can do to get the recommended 60 minutes or more of physical activity each day.

Free play can be very important for kids who don't play a team sport. What's free play? It's the activity kids get when they're left to their own devices, like shooting hoops, riding bikes, playing whiffleball, playing tag, jumping rope, or dancing.

Kids might also enjoy individual sports or other organized activities that can boost fitness, such as:

- swimming;
- dance classes;
- cycling;
- skateboarding;
- golf;
- fencing;
- martial arts;
- ultimate Frisbee;

- horseback riding;
- inline skating;
- cheerleading;
- hiking;
- tennis;
- gymnastics;
- yoga and other fitness classes;
- running.

Supporting Your Kid's Choices

Even if the going's tough, work with your child to find something active that he or she likes. Try to remain open-minded. Maybe your child is interested in an activity that is not offered at school. If your daughter wants to try flag football or ice hockey, for example, help her find a local league or talk to school officials about starting up a new team.

You'll need to be patient if your child has difficulty choosing and sticking to an activity. It often takes several tries before kids find one that feels like the right fit. But when something clicks, you'll be glad you invested the time and effort. For your child, it's one big step toward developing active habits that can last a lifetime.

Section 12.3

Tips on Promoting Physical Fitness for Girls

This section excerpted from "Tips on Getting Girls Active," © 2008 Women's Sports Foundation. All rights reserved. Reprinted with permission. The complete text of this document including references is available at www .womenssportsfoundation.org.

You've heard many of the reasons girls should be active. We know that if a girl does not participate in sports by the age of 10, there is only a 10% likelihood she will be participating at age 25. Research suggests that physical activity is an effective tool for reducing the symptoms of stress and depression among girls. Sports help girls develop leadership and teamwork skills. Girls who participate in sports have higher self-esteem and pride in themselves.

So how do you get the girls in your life to get on the path to being physically active and reaping all of these rewards? These tips will give you all the information you need to introduce physical activity to a girl and make a critical difference in her life.

Change Attitudes about Physical Fitness

At an early age, young women are programmed to shy away from sports and activity because they are afraid of being perceived as unfeminine or are afraid of failure or being teased. Here are some tips on how to turn those attitudes around:

"I'm not an athlete." Many inactive girls think that the world of physical activity is black and white: you are either a jock or not. Some girls believe that unless you are going to go all out or if you're just not a "natural," there is no use in being active. The label of jock can be perceived as unfeminine or possibly just a clique that they don't want to belong to. Girls need to be reminded that it's ok to work up a sweat, get your heart pumping, and challenge your body.

What you can do: Encourage her. Tell her that you don't have to be a hard-core athlete to get up and move (and follow this advice yourself!). There doesn't have to be competition involved to be physically active.

Also, reinforce that no one is ever born an athlete. Even champions had to start at the beginning and learn how to play their sports.

"I'm afraid of getting teased." This is such a vulnerable age, and girls are very sensitive to peer-group influence. "Fitting in" becomes a primary goal so girls don't want to try anything new that steps outside of the world they already know and are comfortable in. This is especially true of girls' participation in sports or even just their school's PE program. Girls fear that stepping into a game might make them a target of ridicule.

What you can do: Understand and identify with her fears and talk to her about them. Girls want to fit in and be accepted. Sports can be all about belonging—being part of the group—with team names, uniforms, and cheers. Most of us remember how nervous we were about our junior high and high school PE [physical education] classes. Many of us also have funny stories to tell about embarrassing things that did happen and how we got over them. Ask her what her worst fear is. Maybe she's nervous about wearing the gym uniform or having to climb ropes in front of her classmates. One she identifies the worst-case scenario, you can discuss how you would deal with this and take away some of her fears. Or share something that happened to you and let her know it really wasn't a big deal.

"I don't know anything about sports." A girl may worry that her lack of knowledge about sports or physical fitness will make her look dumb when she attempts to play. She also may not know what sports are available to girls. Even if she does know, she might not feel confident or capable enough to be proactive and sign up on her own.

What you can do: Teach her the skills to be successful. Start to watch different sports together so she can understand the rules and how different games are played. Learn the sports lingo. Go to a local girls' sporting match so she can see that girls just like her can master the skills needed to play the game. Experiment with different sports until she finds one that comes easily for her. If she has good hand-eye coordination, maybe softball or tennis is her game. In trying different sports, she may be surprised by how great she is at a sport she never thought she could master. You also don't want to rule out sports just because she may not be the perfect physical match for it. For example, she could be on the shorter side and end up loving basketball.

For other activity suggestions, visit the GoGirlGo! Sports Matchmaker (at www.gogirlgo.com). There's an interactive survey you can do together or she can do on her own that allows her to express her interests and preferences and gives suggestions for sport and activities that meet her profile.

Once she has chosen a few activities she's interested in, call the office of that sport's national governing body (for example: USA Basketball) to have them give you local program contact information. Many girls' organizations have sports and physical activities—the YWCA [Young Women's Christian Association], PAL [Police Athletic League], community recreation centers, local park and recreation department, the Girl Scouts, etc. Ask the PE teacher or counselor at school. Look in the local papers, check the Internet at the library, or look in the yellow pages of your phone book for specific activities. Check out local hospitals and rehabilitation centers for programs for disabled girls. These programs are usually affordable and some even offer scholarships for some girls.

As you investigate local programs together, consider these general tips in what you should look for in an activity program:

- **Small group environment.** A group with 15–20 girls and two adult leaders is ideal for girls to learn together and develop a strong sense of belonging. Look for programs that have at least one adult leader for every 10 girls to ensure each girl will get individual attention.

- **Safe and nurturing all-girl environments.** Co-ed physical activity environments are problematic for inactive girls because they contain opposite sex and same sex teasing about the skill level and body of inactive girls and other pressures characteristic of co-ed group dynamics. When girls are concentrating on what boys think, a cultural requirement for teen girls, they don't take care of themselves.

- **Fun and supportive place.** Does it look like fun? Are the girls all participating? Is it a caring, supportive and positive environment? Are girls allowed to express themselves, participate in decision-making, and develop relationships with other girls? The program shouldn't be about winning and losing. Beginners need a friendly social environment where they will learn skills together in a fun way.

Keep It Fun!

Debby Burgard runs a nonprofit organization called The Body Positive based in Berkeley, California, that works to help teens and children with body image issues. She believes that fears about embarrassment (that we discussed earlier) can get in the way of embracing being active. "Most people have negative experiences in junior high PE class or at their gyms that get in the way of them believing they can have fun exercising," Burgard said.

The best way to combat this is to move in ways your body and personality type enjoy. You may envision yourself as a hard-core athlete, but have a mellow personality more suited to yoga. Overall, it's important to try to make every encounter that a girl has with activity a positive one. Here are some easy tips on keeping it fun:

1. **Take her to girls' and women's sports events.** Introduce her to a heroine! At the very least, she will see that girls who engage in sports and physical activity are applauded and admired. Look in the local papers, high school websites, and community center bulletin boards.

2. **Take advantage of the seasons.** Each season try a weather-appropriate sport. For example, tackle snowboarding, snowshoeing, or skiing in the winter; volleyball and swimming in the summer; softball and track in the spring; and soccer, cross-country, or basketball in the fall. This will also make certain sports feel routine and natural so that when next year rolls around, the girl equates the fall as soccer season and is anticipating signing up for a league.

3. **Rate the neighborhood!** Pick a different walking route each time. What's the prettiest house, the best mailbox, the prettiest flowers? Include bouts of power walking (big steps, pumping your arms, going as fast as you can), go from phone pole to phone pole or hydrant to hydrant. And then slow down to laugh, rest, and recover.

4. **Vary the environment.** Instead of running around a track or playing soccer on a soccer field, take your activities to the beach or a local park. Or take in a local arts festival and take a couple laps around it, checking out the booths and talent. Go to a different park every week. Discover the public walking trails. Hike and explore.

5. **Get the scoop on women athletes.** There are plenty of biographies and films on women sports heroes like Billie Jean King, Mia Hamm, and the Williams sisters. Check out the local bookstore or library and read these books together. Then discuss the obstacles these women had to overcome and how they did it. These inspirational stories will also show

girls that even the most talented athletes had to start somewhere and learn from the bottom up. View a list of girls' sports books (www.womenssportsfoundation.org/cgi-bin/iowa/issues/family/article.html?record=945) or a list of sports movies for girls (www.womenssportsfoundation.org/cgi-bin/iowa/issues/family/article.html?record=989).

6. **Make a sports scrapbook.** Collect pictures of females doing physical activities. Look for teen and women's magazines. Make sure she is signed up to be a GoGirlGo! Club member so she gets SportsTalk (it's free!—just request your girl activation kit from www.wsfecomm.com/shop/wsfproductlist.aspx?CategoryID=15&selection=7).

7. **Give gifts of sports equipment and apparel.** Look for cool stuff in teen magazines and give her the gift with a copy of the magazine page. Gifts of sports equipment can tell her that you think she can.

8. **Try an activity that you aren't equipped for.** Take advantage of local sports equipment rental outfits to help equip you for trying a new sport. Rent a canoe, skis, snowboards, or bicycles and discover a sport you never tried before.

9. **Mandatory daily physical education.** There is no better guarantee that a girl will be physically active every day than a mandatory daily physical education requirement in her school. School curriculum can be affected by the action of local school boards. Contact your school board and get others to do the same.

Buddy Up: The Importance of Teamwork

The most important thing you can do to inspire a girl is to make everything a team effort. A girl is more likely to be active if her parent, guardian, or other key adult in her life is active. Let her see you working out, sweating, and making physical activity part of your life. Be a real-life hero as she sees you jogging that extra lap, attempting that three-point shot, striking that yoga pose. There are a number of ways you can emphasize that you are in this together:

1. **Keep activity logs.** This is a great way to track progress. Have fun picking out a cool diary or journal and then keep track of your physical activity experiences: What you did, for how long, and how intense it was. Also record your feelings

about what you liked and didn't like about the experience. This will help to plan and schedule the next activity and help you get to know one another.

2. **Do an activity bracelet.** Charm bracelets, whether they are the traditional ones with charms or the new "Italian" bracelets with tiles, are hot right now. Start an activity bracelet that includes balls and activity charms that commemorate the activities you tried and did together.

3. **Take a class together.** Look for a class that interests both of you, like yoga, Pilates, or tae kwon do. You can also do it at home by renting or buying a video.

4. **Show her your moves.** Teach her to enjoy the activities that you enjoy now or did as a child. Recruit some rope turners and try double-dutch. Or show her your old dance moves to some retro music. She'll admire you for having the guts to try something you haven't enjoyed in years.

Chapter 13

Physical Fitness and Adults

Chapter Contents

Section 13.1

Fitness Guidelines for Adults

This section excerpted from "Chapter 4. Active Adults," *Physical Activity Guidelines for Americans*, U.S. Department of Health and Human Services (www.hhs.gov), October 16, 2008.

Adults who are physically active are healthier and less likely to develop many chronic diseases than adults who are inactive. They also have better fitness, including a healthier body size and composition. These benefits are gained by men and women and people of all races and ethnicities who have been studied.

Adults gain most of these health benefits when they do the equivalent of at least 150 minutes of moderate intensity aerobic physical activity (2 hours and 30 minutes) each week. Adults gain additional and more extensive health and fitness benefits with even more physical activity. Muscle-strengthening activities also provide health benefits and are an important part of an adult's overall physical activity plan.

This section provides guidance for most men and women aged 18 to 64 years and focuses on physical activity beyond baseline activity (the usual light or sedentary activities of daily living).

The guidelines for adults focus on two types of activity: aerobic and muscle strengthening. Each type provides important health benefits.

Aerobic Activity

Aerobic activities, also called endurance activities, are physical activities in which people move their large muscles in a rhythmic manner for a sustained period. Running, brisk walking, bicycling, playing basketball, dancing, and swimming are all examples of aerobic activities. Aerobic activity makes a person's heart beat more rapidly to meet the demands of the body's movement. Over time, regular aerobic activity makes the heart and cardiovascular system stronger and fitter.

The purpose of the aerobic activity does not affect whether it counts toward meeting the guidelines. For example, physically active occupations can count toward meeting the guidelines, as can active transportation choices (walking or bicycling). All types of aerobic activities can count as long as they are of sufficient intensity and duration. Time spent in muscle strengthening activities does not count toward the aerobic activity guidelines.

When putting the guidelines into action, it's important to consider the total amount of activity, as well as how often to be active, for how long, and at what intensity.

Key Guidelines for Adults

- All adults should avoid inactivity. Some physical activity is better than none, and adults who participate in any amount of physical activity gain some health benefits.

- For substantial health benefits, adults should do at least 150 minutes (2 hours and 30 minutes) a week of moderate-intensity, or 75 minutes (1 hour and 15 minutes) a week of vigorous-intensity aerobic physical activity, or an equivalent combination of moderate- and vigorous-intensity aerobic activity. Aerobic activity should be performed in episodes of at least 10 minutes, and preferably, it should be spread throughout the week.

- For additional and more extensive health benefits, adults should increase their aerobic physical activity to 300 minutes (5 hours) a week of moderate-intensity, or 150 minutes a week of vigorous-intensity aerobic physical activity, or an equivalent combination of moderate- and vigorous-intensity activity. Additional health benefits are gained by engaging in physical activity beyond this amount.

- Adults should also do muscle-strengthening activities that are moderate or high intensity and involve all major muscle groups on two or more days a week, as these activities provide additional health benefits.

How Much Total Activity a Week?

When adults do the equivalent of 150 minutes of moderate-intensity aerobic activity each week, the benefits are substantial. These benefits include lower risk of premature death, coronary heart disease, stroke, hypertension, type 2 diabetes, and depression.

Not all health benefits of physical activity occur at 150 minutes a week. As a person moves from 150 minutes a week toward 300 minutes (5 hours) a week, he or she gains additional health benefits. Additional benefits include lower risk of colon and breast cancer and prevention of unhealthy weight gain.

Also, as a person moves from 150 minutes a week toward 300 minutes a week, the benefits that occur at 150 minutes a week become more extensive. For example, a person who does 300 minutes a week has an even lower risk of heart disease or diabetes than a person who does 150 minutes a week.

The benefits continue to increase when a person does more than the equivalent of 300 minutes a week of moderate-intensity aerobic activity. For example, a person who does 420 minutes (7 hours) a week has an even lower risk of premature death than a person who does 150 to 300 minutes a week. Current science does not allow identifying an upper limit of total activity above which there are no additional health benefits.

How Many Days a Week and for How Long?

Aerobic physical activity should preferably be spread throughout the week. Research studies consistently show that activity performed on at least three days a week produces health benefits. Spreading physical activity across at least three days a week may help to reduce the risk of injury and avoid excessive fatigue.

Both moderate- and vigorous-intensity aerobic activity should be performed in episodes of at least 10 minutes. Episodes of this duration are known to improve cardiovascular fitness and some risk factors for heart disease and type 2 diabetes.

How Intense?

The guidelines for adults focus on two levels of intensity: moderate-intensity activity and vigorous-intensity activity. To meet the guidelines, adults can do either moderate-intensity or vigorous-intensity aerobic activities, or a combination of both. It takes less time to get the same benefit from vigorous-intensity activities as from moderate-intensity activities. A general rule of thumb is that 2 minutes of moderate-intensity activity counts the same as 1 minute of vigorous-intensity activity. For example, 30 minutes of moderate-intensity activity a week is roughly the same as 15 minutes of vigorous-intensity activity.

There are two ways to track the intensity of aerobic activity: absolute intensity and relative intensity.

- Absolute intensity is the amount of energy expended per minute of activity. The energy expenditure of light-intensity activity, for example, is 1.1 to 2.9 times the amount of energy expended when a person is at rest. Moderate-intensity activities expend

3.0 to 5.9 times the amount of energy expended at rest. The energy expenditure of vigorous-intensity activities is 6.0 or more times the energy expended at rest.

- Relative intensity is the level of effort required to do an activity. Less fit people generally require a higher level of effort than fitter people to do the same activity. Relative intensity can be estimated using a scale of 0 to 10, where sitting is 0 and the highest level of effort possible is 10. Moderate intensity activity is a 5 or 6. Vigorous-intensity activity is a 7 or 8.

The guidelines for adults refer to absolute intensity because most studies demonstrating lower risks of clinical events (for example, premature death, cardiovascular disease, type 2 diabetes, cancer) have focused on measuring absolute intensity. That is, the guidelines are based on the absolute amount of energy expended in physical activity that is associated with health benefits.

When using relative intensity, people pay attention to how physical activity affects their heart rate and breathing. As a rule of thumb, a person doing moderate-intensity aerobic activity can talk, but not sing, during the activity. A person doing vigorous-intensity activity cannot say more than a few words without pausing for a breath.

Examples of Moderate-Intensity Aerobic Activities

- Walking briskly (3 miles per hour or faster, but not race walking)
- Water aerobics
- Bicycling slower than 10 miles per hour
- Tennis (doubles)
- Ballroom dancing
- General gardening

Examples of Vigorous-Intensity Aerobic Activities

- Race walking, jogging, or running
- Swimming laps
- Tennis (singles)
- Aerobic dancing
- Bicycling 10 miles per hour or faster
- Jumping rope

- Heavy gardening (continuous digging or hoeing, with heart rate increases)

- Hiking uphill or with a heavy backpack

Muscle-Strengthening Activity

Muscle-strengthening activities provide additional benefits not found with aerobic activity. The benefits of muscle-strengthening activity include increased bone strength and muscular fitness. Muscle-strengthening activities can also help maintain muscle mass during a program of weight loss.

Muscle-strengthening activities make muscles do more work than they are accustomed to doing. That is, they overload the muscles. Resistance training, including weight training, is a familiar example of muscle-strengthening activity. Other examples include working with resistance bands, doing calisthenics that use body weight for resistance (such as push-ups, pull-ups, and sit-ups), carrying heavy loads, and heavy gardening (such as digging or hoeing).

Muscle-strengthening activities count if they involve a moderate to high level of intensity or effort and work the major muscle groups of the body: the legs, hips, back, chest, abdomen, shoulders, and arms. Muscle strengthening activities for all the major muscle groups should be done at least two days a week.

No specific amount of time is recommended for muscle strengthening, but muscle-strengthening exercises should be performed to the point at which it would be difficult to do another repetition without help. When resistance training is used to enhance muscle strength, one set of 8 to 12 repetitions of each exercise is effective, although two or three sets may be more effective. Development of muscle strength and endurance is progressive over time. Increases in the amount of weight or the days a week of exercising will result in stronger muscles.

Meeting the Guidelines

Adults have many options for becoming physically active, increasing their physical activity, and staying active throughout their lives. In deciding how to meet the guidelines, adults should think about how much physical activity they're already doing and how physically fit they are. Personal health and fitness goals are also important to consider.

In general, healthy men and women who plan prudent increases in their weekly amounts of physical activity do not need to consult a health care provider before becoming active.

Inactive adults: Inactive adults or those who don't yet do 150 minutes of physical activity a week should work gradually toward this goal. The initial amount of activity should be at a light or moderate intensity, for short periods of time, with the sessions spread throughout the week. The good news is that "some is better than none."

People gain some health benefits even when they do as little as 60 minutes a week of moderate-intensity aerobic physical activity.

To reduce risk of injury, it is important to increase the amount of physical activity gradually over a period of weeks to months. For example, an inactive person could start with a walking program consisting of 5 minutes of slow walking several times each day, five to six days a week. The length of time could then gradually be increased to 10 minutes per session, three times a day, and the walking speed could be increased slowly.

Muscle-strengthening activities should also be gradually increased over time. Initially, these activities can be done just one day a week starting at a light or moderate level of effort. Over time, the number of days a week can be increased to two, and then possibly to more than two. Each week, the level of effort (intensity) can be increased slightly until it becomes moderate to high.

Active adults: Adults who are already active and meet the minimum guidelines can gain additional and more extensive health and fitness benefits by increasing physical activity above this amount. Most American adults should increase their aerobic activity to exceed the minimum level and move toward 300 minutes a week. Adults should also do muscle-strengthening activities on at least two days each week.

One time-efficient way to achieve greater fitness and health goals is to substitute vigorous-intensity aerobic activity for some moderate-intensity activity. Using the 2-to-1 rule of thumb, doing 150 minutes of vigorous-intensity aerobic activity a week provides about the same benefits as 300 minutes of moderate-intensity activity.

Adults are encouraged to do a variety of activities, as variety probably reduces risk of injury caused by doing too much of one kind of activity (this is called an overuse injury).

Highly active adults: Adults who are highly active should maintain their activity level. These adults are also encouraged to do a variety of activities.

Ways to get the equivalent of 150 minutes (2 hours and 30 minutes) of moderate-intensity aerobic physical activity a week plus muscle-strengthening activities:

137

- Thirty minutes of brisk walking (moderate intensity) on five days, exercising with resistance bands (muscle strengthening) on two days

- Twenty-five minutes of running (vigorous intensity) on three days, lifting weights on two days (muscle strengthening)

- Thirty minutes of brisk walking on two days, 60 minutes (1 hour) of social dancing (moderate intensity) on one evening, 30 minutes of mowing the lawn (moderate intensity) on one afternoon, heavy gardening (muscle strengthening) on two days

- Thirty minutes of an aerobic dance class on one morning (vigorous intensity), 30 minutes of running on one day (vigorous intensity), 30 minutes of brisk walking on one day (moderate intensity), calisthenics (such as sit-ups, push-ups) on three days (muscle strengthening)

Section 13.2

Daily Exercise Dramatically Lowers Men's Death Rates

"Daily Exercise Dramatically Lowers Men's Death Rates,"
reprinted with permission from www.americanheart.org.
© 2008 American Heart Association, Inc.

Increased exercise capacity reduces the risk of death in African-American and Caucasian men, researchers reported in *Circulation: Journal of the American Heart Association*.

The government-supported Veterans Affairs study included 15,660 participants and is the largest known to assess the link between fitness and mortality.

"It is important to emphasize that it takes relatively moderate levels of physical activity—like brisk walking—to attain the associated health benefits. Certainly, one does not need to be a marathon runner. This is the message that we need to convey to the public," said Peter Kokkinos, PhD, lead author of the study and director of the Exercise

Testing and Research Lab in the cardiology department at the Veterans Affairs Medical Center in Washington, DC.

Professor Kokkinos and colleagues investigated exercise capacity as an independent predictor of overall mortality for African American men (6,749) and Caucasian men (8,911) and also examined whether racial differences in exercise capacity influence the risk of death. Veterans were tested by a standardized treadmill test to assess exercise capacity between May 1983 and December 2006 at Veterans Affairs medical centers in Washington, DC, and Palo Alto, California. The men were encouraged to exercise until fatigued unless they developed symptoms or other indicators of ischemia. These individuals were then followed for an average of 7.5 years and death rates were recorded.

Researchers classified the subjects into fitness categories based on their treadmill performance, expressed as peak metabolic equivalents (METs) achieved. Technically, a MET is equivalent to oxygen consumption of 3.5 milliliters per kilograms of body weight per minute. One MET represents the amount of oxygen the person uses at rest. Anything above one MET represents work. The higher the MET level achieved, the more fit the individual.

Based on this concept, the researchers divided the participants into four categories:

- 3,170 men were "low fit," achieving less than 5 METs

- 5,153 men were "moderately fit," achieving 5 to 7 METs

- 5,075 were "highly fit," achieving 7.1 to 10 METs

- 2,261 were "very highly fit," achieving more than 10 METs

The study found that "highly fit" men had half the risk of death compared to "low fit" men. Men who achieved "very highly fit" levels had a 70% lower risk of death compared to those in the "low fit" category. For every 1-MET increase in exercise capacity (fitness), the risk for death from all causes was 13% for both African Americans and Caucasians.

Kokkinos said, "These findings are important for several reasons: First, we were able to quantify the health benefits per unit increase in exercise capacity. Second, this is the first study to provide information on physical activity and mortality in African Americans, information lacking until now. Keep in mind that death rates in African Americans are much higher when compared with Caucasians, in part because race and income negatively influence access to healthcare."

"The Veterans Affairs' health system is unique in that it ensures equal access to care regardless of a patient's financial status," he added.

"Thus, it provides us with a unique opportunity to assess the impact of exercise or physical activity on death without the influence of health-care differences."

According to Kokkinos, most middle-age and older individuals can attain fitness levels with a brisk walk, 30 minutes per day, five to six days each week. "I do not advocate that everyone can start with 30 minutes of physical activity. In fact, 30 minutes may be too much for some people. If this is the case, split the routine into 10–15 minutes in the morning and another 10–15 minutes in the evening. The benefits will be similar if the exercise volume accumulated is similar," he said.

"Our findings show that the risk of death is cut in half with an exercise capacity that can easily be achieved by a brisk walk of about 30 minutes per session five to six days per week," he added. "Physicians should encourage individuals to initiate and maintain a physically active lifestyle, which is likely to improve fitness and lower the risk of death. Individuals should also discuss exercise with their physician before embarking on an exercise program."

Co-authors are: Jonathan Myers, PhD; John Peter Kokkinos; Andreas Pittaras, MD; Puneet Narayan, MD; Athanasios Manolis, MD; Pamela Karasik, MD; Michael Greenberg, MD; Vasilios Papademetriou, MD; and Steven Singh, MD.

American Heart Association editor's note: Start! is the American Heart Association's national movement that calls on all Americans and their employers to create a culture of physical activity and health through walking. Recently, the Army National Guard Readiness Center in Arlington, Virginia, was named a Start! Fit Friendly workplace—part of the alliance between the American Heart Association and the Army National Guard. For more information about Start! visit heart.org/start.

Section 13.3

Women, Physical Fitness, and Heart Health

Reprinted with permission of the American College of Sports Medicine, "Women's Heart Health and a Physically Active Lifestyle," November 1999, www.acsm.org. Reviewed by David A. Cooke, MD, FACP, May 2010.

Women and Coronary Artery Disease: The Facts

Coronary heart disease (CHD) is the leading cause of death in women and men, but more women than men die each year of CHD. The overall risk of heart attack in women is close to that of men a decade younger, but with increasing age, the risk of heart attack becomes similar in men and women. Of great concern is the fact that death rate due to CHD in women ages 35–74 years is 74% higher in black than in white women. Despite these statistics, clinicians and the public often cite breast cancer and osteoporosis as the greatest health risks for women over 50 years. These misconceptions regarding women's heart health are startling, considering that the lifetime risk of death from CHD among postmenopausal women is approximately 31% compared to 2.8% for hip fracture and breast cancer alike.

Once women manifest CHD, they have more adverse clinical outcomes than men do. Women are twice as likely as men to die within the first year after a heart attack, and nearly 63% of the women who die suddenly from CHD have had no previous symptoms. Women who undergo coronary artery bypass graft surgery are almost twice as likely to die as a result of the procedure, have less relief from their symptoms, and more often require another operation than men. These data as well as the nearly eight-year life span advantage of women compared to men underscore the importance of preventive cardiac care for women of all ages. The primary CHD risk factors of abnormal blood lipids and lipoproteins (dyslipidemia), high blood pressure, physical inactivity, overweight, and diabetes mellitus (DM) are of particular importance in women.

Unique Coronary Risk Factor Concerns for Women

While CHD deaths have declined in both women and men over the past 20 years, the rate of decline is less in women compared to men. This phenomenon is partly attributable to a greater clustering of coronary risk factors associated with metabolic syndrome (MS) among older women than men and may explain the elimination of the "female advantage" as women age. The diseases and conditions of MS include obesity, especially about the abdomen, high blood pressure, dyslipidemia, and impaired glucose utilization. Metabolic syndrome often leads to CHD and Type 2 DM.

More than 50% of women 20 years of age and older are overweight or obese compared to 60% of men. Of more concern is the fact that more than 65% of black and Mexican-American women are overweight or obese. Older women are at greater risk for weight gain and abdominal fat accumulation, a major component of MS. Physical inactivity has been implicated as a major contributor to overall and abdominal obesity. High blood pressure affects about 52% of women over 40 years of age, and nearly three out of four women over 75 are similarly affected. It is more common among black than white women and is thought to contribute to their higher rate of CHD death. While there has been some controversy, it appears that drug treatment of high blood pressure offers benefit. These observations again speak to the importance of preventive cardiac care for women of all ages. Recently, a constellation of blood lipid and lipoprotein abnormalities has been linked with MS and CH, and is called "atherogenic dyslipidemia." These abnormalities consist of slightly to moderately elevated low-density lipoprotein cholesterol (LDL) and triglycerides with a predominance of smaller, more dense and atherogenic LDL, and low levels of high-density lipoprotein cholesterol (HDL).

After age 65, low HDL and elevated triglycerides appear to be stronger risk factors for CHD compared to men. The age-related increases in LDL and total cholesterol are greater among women than men, as is the shift to smaller, more dense and atherogenic LDL particles. More than 40% of women over 55 years of age have elevated cholesterol levels.

No other cardiac risk factor so significantly erases the female advantage of acquiring CHD disease than does DM, which affects 8% of all women over age 20 and is more prevalent among black, Hispanic, and Native American women. A woman with DM is from three to seven times at greater risk of a coronary event than is a woman without DM. This is in contrast to a two-to-threefold increase in CHD risk in men with DM. DM doubles the risk of a second heart attack in women but not in men. Moreover, 80% of women with DM will die from some form of cardiovascular disease. Type 2 DM affects more women than men. Women's heart health is clearly related to the state of their metabolic health, particularly as they age.

Physical Activity and Women's Heart Health

Of the unique cardiac risk factor concerns among women addressed in this section, physical inactivity is the most prevalent. More than 60% of women do not meet current recommendations for physical activity, with more than 25% of women doing no regular physical activity. Sedentary behavior increases with age and is greatest among minorities and those of lower socioeconomic status.

Physical inactivity is a major independent risk factor for CHD, in part due to its unfavorable influence on the diseases and conditions of MS. An inverse, dose-response relationship between physical activity or physical fitness and deaths due to cardiovascular disease has been demonstrated in many studies. Women and men who are sedentary have a higher rate of non-fatal myocardial infarction, stroke, peripheral vascular disease, high blood pressure, and Type 2 DM. In addition, blood-clotting factors, blood triglycerides, LDL, body mass index or body weight, and smoking prevalence are higher and HDL cholesterol lower with decreasing levels of physical activity. Controlled trials of exercise training have resulted in reductions in total cholesterol, triglycerides, LDL, systolic and diastolic blood pressure, body fat, and blood-clotting factors and increased HDL cholesterol, fibrinolytic ("clot-busting") factors, and insulin sensitivity. Although limited data are available, women appear to derive benefit similar to men from being physically active.

Conclusions

CHD is a major health threat to women. Consequently, it is vital to increase the awareness of women, health, and fitness professionals about this fact. Preventive strategies have the potential to significantly lower the risk of CHD in both women and men. Increasing physical activity is the lifestyle change most likely to have far-reaching consequences in the primary and secondary prevention of CHD. Physical activity has been shown to favorably alter the MS and related CHD risk factors including dyslipidemia, obesity, Type 2 DM, and high blood pressure. Further, for women and men with CHD, improved risk factor profiles are likely to result in improved survival and enhanced quality of life. In view of these facts, the American College of Sports Medicine strongly endorses physical activity as a means to improve heart health among women of all ages.

Section 13.4

Physical Activity for Pregnant and Postpartum Women

This section excerpted from "Chapter 7. Additional Considerations for Some Adults," *Physical Activity Guidelines for Americans*, U.S. Department of Health and Human Services (www.hhs.gov), October 16, 2008.

Physical activity during pregnancy benefits a woman's overall health. For example, moderate-intensity physical activity by healthy women during pregnancy maintains or increases cardiorespiratory fitness.

Strong scientific evidence shows that the risks of moderate-intensity activity done by healthy women during pregnancy are very low and do not increase risk of low birth weight, preterm delivery, or early pregnancy loss. Some evidence suggests that physical activity reduces the risk of pregnancy complications, such as preeclampsia and gestational diabetes, and reduces the length of labor, but this evidence is not conclusive.

During a normal postpartum period, regular physical activity continues to benefit a woman's overall health. Studies show that moderate-intensity physical activity during the period following the birth of a child increases a woman's cardiorespiratory fitness and improves her mood. Such activity does not appear to have adverse effects on breast milk volume, breast milk composition, or infant growth.

Physical activity also helps women achieve and maintain a healthy weight during the postpartum period, and when combined with caloric restriction, helps promote weight loss.

Key Guidelines for Women during Pregnancy and the Postpartum Period

- Healthy women who are not already highly active or doing vigorous-intensity activity should get at least 150 minutes (2 hours and 30 minutes) of moderate-intensity aerobic activity per week during pregnancy and the postpartum period. Preferably, this activity should be spread throughout the week.

- Pregnant women who habitually engage in vigorous-intensity aerobic activity or are highly active can continue physical activity during pregnancy and the postpartum period, provided that they remain healthy and discuss with their health care provider how and when activity should be adjusted over time.

Women who are pregnant should be under the care of a health care provider with whom they can discuss how to adjust amounts of physical activity during pregnancy and the postpartum period. Unless a woman has medical reasons to avoid physical activity during pregnancy, she can begin or continue moderate-intensity aerobic physical activity during her pregnancy and after the baby is born.

When beginning physical activity during pregnancy, women should increase the amount gradually over time. The effects of vigorous-intensity aerobic activity during pregnancy have not been studied carefully, so there is no basis for recommending that women should begin vigorous-intensity activity during pregnancy.

Women who habitually do vigorous-intensity activity or high amounts of activity or strength training should continue to be physically active during pregnancy and after giving birth. They generally do not need to drastically reduce their activity levels, provided that they remain healthy and discuss with their health care provider how to adjust activity levels during this time.

During pregnancy, women should avoid doing exercises involving lying on their back after the first trimester of pregnancy. They should also avoid doing activities that increase the risk of falling or abdominal trauma, including contact or collision sports, such as horseback riding, downhill skiing, soccer, and basketball.

Section 13.5

Research Shows Overweight Women Improve Quality of Life through Exercise

"Overweight, Obese Women Improve Quality of Life with
10 to 30 Minutes of Exercise," reprinted with permission from
www.americanheart.org. © 2008 American Heart Association, Inc.

Sedentary, overweight, or obese women can improve their quality of life by exercising as little as 10 to 30 minutes a day, researchers reported at the American Heart Association's Conference on Nutrition, Physical Activity, and Metabolism.

The Dose Response to Exercise in postmenopausal Women (DREW) study, first reported in 2007, was the largest randomized, controlled trial examining the role of exercise in postmenopausal women. These secondary results focus on quality of life among 430 women divided into four groups: three groups exercising at various levels and one control group that did not exercise.

"While the women who participated in the highest exercise group saw the greatest improvements in most quality of life scales, the women in the lowest exercise group also saw improvements," said Angela Thompson, MSPH, co-author of the study and research associate at Pennington Biomedical Research Center in Baton Rouge, Louisiana. "The public health message is tremendous, because it provides further support for the notion that even if someone cannot exercise an hour or more daily, getting out and exercising 10 to 30 minutes per day is beneficial, too."

All participants in the exercise groups reported a statistically significant improvement in social functioning compared to those in the control group of women who didn't exercise. However, women who participated in more exercise, from 135 to 150 minutes a week, also showed significant improvements in general health, vitality, and mental health.

The women who exercised more also improved in physical functioning, role limitations in work or other activities due to physical problems, and role limitations due to emotional problems, the researchers said. None of the women reported a statistically significant improvement in pain.

After exercising six months, the women improved almost 7% in physical function and general health, 16.6% in vitality, 11.5% in performing work or other activities, 11.6% in emotional health, and more than 5% in social functioning.

"This has not been shown in a large controlled study before," said Timothy S. Church, MD, principal investigator and research director at Pennington Biomedical Research Center. "This is the first large controlled study of postmenopausal women to look at the effect of exercise training on the quality of life. It shows that exercise gives you energy and makes you feel better."

This study included 430 sedentary women, average age 57, who were overweight or obese. Researchers randomly assigned women to one of three exercise groups, including those expending about 4 kilocalories per kilogram (kcal/kg) of energy each week amounting to 70 minutes a week; 8 kcal/kg/week amounting to 135 minutes per week; or 12 kcal/kg/week amounting to 190 minutes a week. Most of the exercise was divided into three or four sessions a week. When not in organized exercise, these women were fitted with pedometers. A fourth group had no planned exercise and served as controls.

Researchers measured quality of life before and after the six-month exercise intervention with the Medical Outcomes Study Short-Form 36 Health Status Survey. The scores were adjusted for ethnicity, age, employment status, smoking, antidepressant use, and marital status.

To determine physical health, women were asked about physical functioning such as what types of physical activities they participated in from carrying groceries to climbing stairs to walking a mile; limitations in physical activity; pain; and their own assessment of their health.

Researchers determined mental health by having the women do a self-assessment of vitality, social time, ability to accomplish what they set out to do, and whether they were nervous, down in the dumps, peaceful, or happy.

Though the women in the study were overweight or obese, sedentary, and postmenopausal, they were fairly healthy and reported a fairly high quality of life at baseline.

"At baseline the average vitality and role emotional scores for these women were lower than for the U.S. population," Thompson said. "At follow-up, the average vitality and role emotional scores were higher than the average U.S. population."

The data showed a positive association between six months of exercise and changes in quality of life.

"This association was strongest among the group who received the highest dose of exercise, which was 150% of the National Institute of

Health's Consensus Development recommended physical activity dose," Thompson said. "Some of the women did lose weight over the course of the study but the self-reported improvement in quality of life was not dependent on weight loss."

Many of the women grew up when females didn't participate in sports and most had never been physically active before. The research program included a team to teach the women how to exercise.

"Walking a little bit every day will help tremendously," Thompson said. "Walk with your mother, a neighbor, or friend. A little physical activity will improve your quality of life."

Researchers also advised older women to join gyms that have specific sections for women or that are targeted at women.

"Physical activity not only provides a better quality of life but better balance, stronger bones, and confidence in walking," Church said. "Start exercising for small amounts of time and then gradually work up to 150 minutes a week. A little is better than nothing."

Church and Thompson's co-author is Steven N. Blair, PED.

The National Institutes of Health funded the study.

Statements and conclusions of abstract authors that are presented at American Heart Association/American Stroke Association scientific meetings are solely those of the abstract authors and do not necessarily reflect association policy or position. The associations make no representation or warranty as to their accuracy or reliability.

Section 13.6

Statistics and Research on Women and Physical Activity

This compilation of facts is a representative sample of the data that exists in women's sports as of the publication date. If a reference appears old (i.e., 1975, 1985), it generally means that either there has been so much research on the topic that researchers see no need to replicate the studies or that the Foundation has found no more recent credible studies on the topic.

Benefits of Participation

- Of those students attending NCAA Division I schools, female athletes post the highest graduation rates, followed by female students in general, male students, and male athletes. (*NCAA Research Related to Graduation Rates of Division I Student-Athletes, 1984-2000.* NCAA, 2007).

- Of the female student-athletes who entered NCAA Division I programs on scholarship in 1998, 71% graduated within six years of enrollment. This is 8% higher than the overall rate for female students (63%) and 16% higher than the overall rate for male student-athletes (55%). (*2005 Graduation-Rates Report for NCAA Division I Schools.* NCAA, 2005.)

- Both white female athletes (68%) and female athletes of color who are on scholarship (55%) graduated at higher rates than their counterparts in the general student population (54% and 42%, respectively). (Butler, J. & Lopiano, D. (2003). *The Women's Sports Foundation Report: Title IX and Race in Intercollegiate Sport.* Women's Sports Foundation.)

- Eleven (69%) of the 2003 women's Sweet 16 Division I basketball teams had student-athlete graduation rates that were equal to or higher than the school's overall student-athlete graduation rates. Among the men's programs, three (19%) Sweet 16 teams had student-athlete graduation rates that were higher than the school's overall student-athlete graduation rates. (*Keeping Score When It Counts: Graduation Rates for 2003 NCAA Division I Women's Basketball Championship.* Institute for Diversity and Ethics in Sport, 2003.)

- According to an Oxygen/Markle Pulse poll, 56% of women agree with the statement that seeing successful female athletes makes them feel proud to be a woman. (*Marketing to Women*, March 2001.)

- According to a study of 2,993 women, older women who exercise tend to be motivated toward physical activity by expectations of benefit to their health and longevity. Inactive women tend not to have the self-confidence, skill, and experience with physical activity that active women do. ("Motivation for exercise studied." *Melpomene Journal*, Fall 1997.)

- In a study of 17,000 Medicare beneficiaries, researchers found that the average, non-overweight female costs the program $6,224 per year, but overweight and obese patients cost Medicare $7,653 and $9,612 each year, respectively. (*Journal of the American Medical Association* as cited in "Overweight in youth adulthood and middle age increases health care costs after age 65." Robert Wood Johnson Foundation newsletter, Dec. 2004.)

- In 2003, the estimated total national cost of physical inactivity was $251.11 billion, while the estimated total national cost for excess weight was $256.57 billion. These numbers include the cost of medical care, worker's compensation, and productivity losses. An estimated $31 billion could be saved per year with a 5% reduction of physically inactive and overweight adults. If no changes are made by 2008 the estimated cost per year will reach $708 billion. (Chenoweth, D. & Leutzinger, J. (2006). "The Economic Cost of Physical Inactivity and Excess Weight in American Adults." *Journal of Physical Activity and Health*.)

- A Harvard study that followed 72,488 nurses for eight years concluded that the more a woman exercises, the lower odds she will suffer a stroke. (*Journal of the American Medical Association* as cited in "Physically active women reduce risk of stroke: Walking is step in right direction." *Harvard University Gazette*, June 15, 2000.)

- High school sports participation may help prevent osteoporosis (loss of bone mass). Bone density has been shown to be an important factor in preventing osteoporosis from occurring in the first place. Purdue University researchers found that of minimally active women aged 18–31, those who had participated in high school sports had a significantly greater bone density than those who had not. (Teegarden, D., et al. (1996). "Previous physical activity relates to bone mineral measures in young women." *Medicine and Science in Sports and Exercise.*)

- Researchers from Penn State say exercise may be more important than calcium consumption for young women to ensure proper bone health as they get older. They studied 81 young women, aged 12 to 16, beginning in 1990. When the girls reached 18, the researchers found no relationship between calcium consumption and bone mineral density. However, there was a strong link between physical activity and bone mineral density (BMD). The researchers found that consistent activity, rather than fitness or exercise intensity, was the best predictor of healthy levels of BMD. (*Pediatrics Fitness Bulletin*, Aug. 2000.)

- Women who exercise vigorously while trying to quit smoking are twice as likely to kick the habit than wannabe ex-smokers who don't work out regularly. Researchers also found that women who worked out as they tried to quit gained only about half the weight of those who did not exercise. (*Archives of Internal Medicine* as cited in "Exercise helps women quit smoking." *New York Times*, June 14, 1999.)

- Half of all girls who participate in some kind of sport experience had higher than average levels of self-esteem and less depression. (Colton, M. & Gore, S. (1991). "Risk, Resiliency, and Resistance: Current Research on Adolescent Girls." Ms. Foundation for Women.)

- Research suggests that girls who participate in sports are more likely to experience academic success and graduate from high school than those who do not play sports. (Sabo, D., Melnick, M. & Vanfossen (1989). *Women's Sports Foundation Report: Minorities in Sports*. Women's Sports Foundation.)

- Sports participation is associated with less risk for body dissatisfaction and disordered eating among adolescent girls. It is also associated higher self-esteem. (Tiggemann, M. (2001). "The impact of adolescent girls' life concerns and leisure activities on

151

body dissatisfaction, disordered eating, and self-esteem." *The Journal of Genetic Psychology*.)

- The 2002 National Youth Survey of Civic Engagement showed that young women who participated in sports were more likely to be engaged in volunteering, be registered to vote, feel comfortable making a public statement, follow the news, and boycott than young women who had not participated in sports. (Lopez, M.H. & Moore, K. (2006). *Participation in Sports and Civic Engagement.* The Center for Information and Research on Civic Learning and Engagement.)

- Exercise has been shown to improve cardiovascular fitness, muscle strength, body composition, fatigue, anxiety, depression, self-esteem, happiness, and several components of quality of life (physical, functional, and emotional) in cancer survivors. (Brown, J.K., et al. (2003). "Nutrition and physical activity during and after cancer treatment: An American Cancer Society guide for informed choices." *CA: A Cancer Journal for Clinicians*.)

- Teenage female athletes are less likely to use marijuana, cocaine, or "other" illicit drugs (such as LSD, PCP, speed, or heroin), less likely to be suicidal, less likely to smoke, and more likely to have positive body images than female non-athletes. (Miller, K, Sabo, D.F., Melnick, M.J., Farrell, M.P. & Barnes, G.M. (2000). *The Women's Sports Foundation Report: Health Risks and the Teen Athlete.* Women's Sports Foundation.)

- Being both physically active and a team sports participant is associated with a lower prevalence of sexual risk-taking behaviors for teen girls. (Kulig, K., Brener, N. & McManus, T. (2003). "Sexual activity and substance use among adolescents by category of physical activity plus team sport participation." *Pediatrics and Adolescent Medicine*.)

- Teenage female athletes are less than half as likely to get pregnant as female non-athletes (5% and 11%, respectively), more likely to report that they had never had sexual intercourse than female non-athletes (54% and 41%, respectively), and more likely to experience their first sexual intercourse later in adolescence than female non-athletes. (Sabo, D., Miller, K., Farrell, M., Barnes, G. & Melnick, M. (1998). *The Women's Sports Foundation Report: Sport and Teen Pregnancy.* Women's Sports Foundation.)

- Women who practice the same well-designed strength training programs as men do benefit from bone and soft-tissue modeling, increased lean body mass, decreased fat, and enhanced self-confidence. (Ebben, W.P. & Jensen, R.L. (1998). "Strength training for women: Debunking myths that block opportunity." *The Physician and Sportsmedicine*.)

- According to one study, elderly women recovering from heart attacks derive many benefits from exercise training, including decreased obesity, better quality of life, and lower anxiety. (Lavie, C.J. & Milani, R.V. (1997). "Effects of cardiac rehabilitation, exercise training, and weight reduction on exercise capacity, coronary risk factors, behavioral characteristics, and quality of life in obese coronary patients." *American Journal of Cardiology*.)

- A 10-year follow-up study of 96 post-menopausal women who had started a walking-for-exercise program in an earlier study and 100 post-menopausal women who hadn't started an exercise walking program suggests that making walking part of your exercise plan may increase your overall activity level, which in turn may increase health benefits you reap. Women who walked for exercise were more likely to report participating in other sports and types of exercise, rated their health better, and had lower rates of chronic disease than women who had not started a regular routine. (Periera, M.A., et al. (1998). "A randomized walking trial in postmenopausal women: Effects on physical activity and health 10 years later." *Archives of Internal Medicine*.)

- In a study of 1,224 Finnish men and women over the age of 65, the most frequently cited motives for participating in exercise activities were health promotion (80%), social reasons (40–50%), psychological reasons (30%), personal satisfaction (15–40%), and referral by health care provider (5–19%). The most commonly cited barriers to participation were lack of interest (26–28%), poor health (19–38%), feeling no need to participate (4–9%), and distance to exercise facilities (5%). There were no gender differences in either motives or barriers cited. (Hirvensalo, M., Lampinen, P. & Rantanen, T., (1998). "Physical exercise in old age: An eight-year follow-up study on involvement, motives, and obstacles among persons age 65–84." *Journal of Aging and Physical Activity*.)

- Daily physical education in primary school appears to have a significant long-term positive effect on exercise habits in women. They are more active as they age. ("Daily primary school physical education: Effects on physical activity during adult life." *Medicine & Science in Sports and Exercise*, 1999.)

- The potential for some girls to derive positive experiences from physical activity and sport is marred by lack of opportunity, gender stereotyping, and homophobia. (*Physical Activity & Sport in the Lives of Girls.* President's Council on Physical Fitness and Sports, 1997.)

- In a 1997 study of collegiate women athletes and non-athletes, athletes reported having more physically active parents than non-athletes. (Miller, J.L. & Levy, G.D. (1996). "Gender role conflict, gender-typed characteristics, self-concepts, and sport socialization in female athletes and non athletes." *Sex Roles.*)

- Exercise and sport participation can be used as a therapeutic and preventive intervention for enhancing the physical and mental health of adolescent females. It also can enhance mental health by offering them positive feelings about body image, improved self-esteem, tangible experiences of competency and success, and increased self-confidence. (*Physical Activity & Sport in the Lives of Girls.* President's Council on Physical Fitness and Sports, 1997.)

- With enough strength training, women can lift, carry, and march as well as men, according to Army researchers. They say 78% of female volunteers they tested could qualify for Army jobs considered very heavy, involving the occasional lifting of 100 pounds, after six months of training 90 minutes, five days a week. (*Morning Call*, Jan. 30, 1996.)

- Women who exercise weigh less; have lower levels of blood sugar, cholesterol, and triglycerides; and have lower blood pressure than non-exercising women. They also report being happier, believe they have more energy, and felt they were in excellent health more often than non-exercising women. Exercisers also miss fewer days of work. (Glanz, K., Sorensen, G. & Farmer, A. (1996). "The health impact of worksite nutrition and cholesterol intervention programs." *American Journal of Health Promotion.*)

- Postmenopausal women who engaged in the equivalent of 75 to 180 minutes a week of brisk walking had 18% less risk of developing breast cancer than inactive women. (McTiernan, A., et al. (2003). "Recreational physical activity and the risk of breast cancer in postmenopausal women." *Journal of the American Medical Association,* 2003.)

- A 15-year follow-up of close to 4,000 female athletes and non-athletes revealed that the less active women had a higher prevalence of breast cancer than the more active women. (Wyshak, G. & Frisch, R.E. (2000). "Breast cancer among former college athletes compared to non-athletes: A 15-year follow-up." *British Journal of Cancer.*)

- One to three hours of exercise a week over a woman's reproductive lifetime (the teens to about age 40) may bring a 20–30% reduction in the risk of breast cancer, and four or more hours of exercise a week can reduce the risk almost 60%. (Bernstein, L., Henderson, B.E., Hanish, R., Sullivan-Halley, J. & Ross, R.K. (1994). "Physical exercise and reduced risk of breast cancer in young women." *Journal of the National Cancer Institute.*)

- According to the Nurses Health Study, by exercising one to three hours a week, women recovering from breast cancer reduced their risk of dying from the disease by one-quarter. By exercising three to eight hours a week, the risk is cut in half. (Holmes, M.D., Chen, W.Y., Feskanich, D. & Colditz, G.A. (2005). "Physical activity and survival after breast cancer diagnosis." *Journal of the American Medical Association.*)

Fitness

- In the United States, physical inactivity and unhealthy eating contribute to obesity, cancer, cardiovascular disease, and diabetes, which are responsible for at least 300,000 deaths each year. (*Physical Activity and Good Nutrition: Essential Elements to Prevent Chronic Diseases and Obesity, 2002.* Centers for Disease Control and Prevention, 2002.)

- Between 2001–2004, 30% of men and 34% of women 20–74 years of age were obese (age adjusted). The prevalence of obesity among women differed significantly by racial and ethnic group. In 2001–2004, one-half of non-Hispanic black women were obese compared with nearly one-third of non-Hispanic white women. In contrast, the prevalence of obesity among men was similar by race and ethnicity. ("Health, United States, 2006, With Chartbook on Trends in the Health of Americans." Centers for Disease Control and Prevention, 2006.)

- The overall cost of health care in the United States doubled between 1993 and 2004, and in 2004, health care spending topped $1.9 trillion, or 16% of the nation's economic output —the largest share on record. (Center for Medicare and Medicaid Services, 2006.)

- There is no federal law that requires physical education to be provided to students in the American education system, nor any incentives for offering physical education programs. (*Shape of the Nation Report*. National Association for Sport & Physical Activity, 2006.)

- About 17% of U.S. children between the ages of 2 and 19 were overweight in 2003–2004 compared to 14% in 1999–2000. (*National Health and Nutrition Examination Survey*. Centers for Disease Control and Prevention, 2006.)

- Between 1999 and 2004, there was a significant increase in the prevalence of overweightness among girls in the United States (13.8% in 1999 to 16.0% in 2004). Among boys there was an increase from 14.0% in 1999 to 18.2% in 2004. The prevalence of obesity among men also increased significantly from 27.5% to 31.1%, while there was no significant change in the prevalence of obesity among women (33.4% in 1999 to 33.2% in 2004). (*National Health and Nutrition Examination Survey*. Centers for Disease Control and Prevention, 2006.)

- A decade-long research study showed that 80% of obese nine-year-old girls were entering puberty. Additionally, 58% of overweight girls were entering puberty compared to just 40% of normal-weight nine-year-olds. Early development in girls has been linked to more risk-taking behaviors such as using alcohol and drugs and to a higher prevalence of depression and scholastic problems. (Lee, J.M., Appugliese, D., Kaciroti, N., Corwyn, R.F., Bradley, R.H. & Lumeng, J.C. (2007). "Weight status in young girls and the onset of puberty." *Pediatrics*.)

- In 2005, 99% of U.S. public elementary schools had some scheduled physical education. However, the frequency of scheduled activity varies. Between 17% and 22% of students had physical education every day; about half had one or two days each week. The average amount of time spent at recess and physical education was about 221 minutes/week for first graders and 214 minutes per week for sixth graders. (*Calories In, Calories Out: Food and Exercise in Public Elementary Schools*. U.S. Department of Education, 2005.)

- Illinois and Massachusetts are the only states that mandate physical education for school children in all grades K–12. Over 70% of states (36) mandate physical education for elementary school students, 65% of states (33) mandate it for middle/junior high school students, and 83% of states (42) mandate it for high school students. (*Shape of the Nation Report*. National Association for Sport and Physical Education, 2006).

- A recent study found that the number of overweight girls decreased 10% in schools that gave first-graders an hour more per week devoted to physical activity than the same students had previously received in kindergarten. Based on the results of this study, researchers believe that the prevalence of obesity and overweightness among girls could be reduced by 43% if kindergarteners were given at least five hours of physical education time per week. (Datar, A. & Sturm, R. (2004). "Physical education in elementary school and body mass index: Evidence from the early childhood longitudinal study." Rand Corporation.)

- Among 7- to 12-year-old children, 98% have at least one risk factor for heart disease, including high blood pressure, high cholesterol, and excess body fat. Between 1979–1999, annual hospital costs for treating obesity-related diseases in children rose from $35 million to $127 million. (*Sports Trend*, April 2000; Wang G. & Dietz W. (2002). "Economic burden of obesity in youths aged 6 to 17 years: 1979-1999." *Pediatrics*.)

- Increased weight gain in girls during their transition from childhood to adulthood may be caused by a decline in physical activity. A University of New Mexico study followed the level of physical activity, body mass index (BMI), skinfold thickness, and eating habits of more than 2,200 girls over a course of 10 years. It was found that the girls' participation in physical activity declined while their rate of overweightness and obesity doubled. The authors suggested that increasing physical activity equivalent to 2.5 hours of brisk walking per week could potentially prevent weight gain. (Kimm, S.Y.S., et al. (2005). "Relation between the changes in physical activity and body-mass index during adolescence: A multicentre longitudinal study." *The Lancet*.)

- A 2006 research study found that adolescent girls living in close proximity to public parks (within a half-mile) are more physically active than girls who do not have such easy access to public parks. (Cohen, D. A., et al. (2006). "Public parks and physical activity among adolescent girls." *Pediatrics*.)

- A Centers for Disease Control and Prevention survey of high school students in 2003 found that 59.3% of females described themselves as trying to lose weight. In an effort to lose weight or to keep from gaining weight, 18.3% of the girls had gone longer than 24 hours without food. In the 30 days before the survey, 11.3% of the female students had taken diet pills, powders, or liquids without a doctor's consent to lose weight or keep from gaining weight. In the 30 days preceding distribution of the survey, 8.4% of the female students had vomited or used laxatives to lose weight (*Youth Risk Behavior Surveillance—United States, 2003*. Centers for Disease Control and Prevention, 2004.)

• Scientists found an association between lower levels of parental education and activity decline in white girls of all ages and in older black girls (ages 13–17). Higher body mass index (a measure of body weight adjusted for height) predicted a decline in activity among both racial groups. (Kimm, S.Y.S., et al. (2002). "Decline in physical activity in black girls and white girls during adolescence." *The New England Journal of Medicine*.)

• The American College of Sports Medicine recommends exercising 200–300 minutes each week for effective weight loss and the prevention of weight regain (for example, 40–60 minutes, five days per week). At the same time, individuals seeking to lose weight should reduce their overall calorie intake by 500–1,000 calories and reduce fat intake to less than 30% of total calories (*Exercise Tips for Weight Loss*. Hospital for Special Surgery, Aug., 2004.)

• More than 60% of adults in the United States are overweight or obese. More than 50% of American women are overweight or obese. Among women in their 20s with severe obesity, the decrease in life expectancy is eight years for whites and five years for African Americans. For any degree of overweightness, younger adults risked losing more years of life than older adults. (Berger, L. (June 22, 2003). "The 10 percent solution: Losing a little brings big gains." *New York Times*; Fintaine, K.R., Redden, D.T., Wang, C., Westfall, A.O. & Allison, D.B. (2003). "Years of life lost due to obesity." *Journal of the American Medical Association*.)

• More than 60% of adult women do not do the recommended amount of physical activity (30 minutes of moderate activity daily). More than 25% of women are not active at all. In 2000, just under 30% of women and men ages 45–64 were inactive. For ages 65–74 about 35% of women and 30% of men were inactive. For ages 75 and over about 35% of women were inactive and more than 40% of men were inactive. (*Surgeon General's Report on Physical Activity and Health, 1999; Physical Inactivity for U.S. Men and Women*. Centers for Disease Control & Prevention, 2000.)

Chapter 14

Fitness for Mid-Life and Older Persons

Chapter Contents

Section 14.1

Exercise Program for Mid-Life Persons

This section excerpted from "Pep Up Your Life: A Fitness Book for Mid-Life and Older Persons," U.S. Department of Health and Human Services, The President's Council on Physical Fitness and Sports (www.fitness.gov), April 23, 2008.

The exciting news from recent scientific studies is that exercise benefits everyone—regardless of age. Exercise can help you take charge of your health and maintain the level of fitness necessary for an active, independent lifestyle.

Many people think that as we age, we tend to slow down and do less; that physical decline is an inevitable consequence of aging. For the most part, this is not true. According to the President's Council on Physical Fitness and Sports, much of the physical frailty attributed to aging is actually the result of inactivity, disease, or poor nutrition. But the good news is—many problems can be helped or even reversed by improving lifestyle behaviors. One of the major benefits of regular physical activity is protection against coronary heart disease. Physical activity also provides some protection against other chronic diseases such as adult-onset diabetes, arthritis, hypertension, certain cancers, osteoporosis, and depression. In addition, research has proven that exercise can ease tension and reduce the amount of stress you feel.

To put it simply—exercise is one of the best things you can do for your health. The exercise program in this chapter is a daily routine that takes 20 to 30 minutes. Performing each exercise properly is as important as spending enough time on them.

You are what you eat: No matter what your age, a balanced, nutritious diet is essential to good health. Older adults need to eat a balanced diet with foods from all the food groups. Eating a variety of foods helps ensure adequate levels of vitamins and minerals in the body. The U.S. Dietary Guidelines also recommend that adults reduce the fat, saturated fat, cholesterol, sodium, and sugar in the foods they eat.

Some adults find they have problems being overweight as they age. This is generally due to overeating and inactivity. If you are overweight, the best way to lose body fat is to eat fewer calories, especially from saturated fats, and to participate in aerobic exercises.

Sleep and rest: Sleep and rest are great rejuvenators. As you grow older, your sleep patterns and need for sleep may change. Be sure to include rest periods in your daily exercise program, especially if you sleep fewer than eight hours each night. Exercise can help relieve problems with insomnia too. Mild exercise a few hours before bed, or during the day, helps many people get a restful night's sleep.

Balance and agility: Balance and agility are important capabilities often taken for granted. Regular exercise can help to maintain or restore them. Older adults can sometimes lose their sense of balance, particularly if they wear bifocal or trifocal glasses. A well-maintained sense of balance can help make up for the dizziness sometimes caused by vision changes. In addition, when muscles are not toned, the resulting weakness and unsteadiness can contribute to falls. Thus, it is important to maintain or restore physical agility through exercise, which can help avoid the risk of injury from falls and accidents.

Preparing to exercise: No matter at what age you begin to exercise, or how long you may have been inactive, proper exercise will always improve your physical condition. The exercises in this chapter can be done by people who have been inactive for some time. Programs to improve flexibility, strength, and endurance are arranged in three levels of difficulty. It is important to begin any exercise program slowly and build up gradually. Remember, it may take several months to attain the minimal levels of physical fitness identified in Level I activities. Some people will take less time, others more.

Before beginning an exercise program, have a physical examination and discuss the program with your doctor. In addition, if your mobility is limited as a result of a chronic or disabling condition, be sure to review these exercises with your doctor. Keep in mind your level of ability and endurance so that you don't risk discomfort or injury. If you experience pain while exercising, stop that particular movement and ask your doctor about it on your next visit.

Stick with it, and you will see results!

Warming up: Preparing the body for exercise is important for people at any age and all fitness levels. A warm-up period should begin with slow, rhythmic activities such as walking or jogging in place.

Gradually increase the intensity until your pulse rate, respiration rate, and body temperature are elevated, which is usually about the time that you break a light sweat. It also is advisable to do some easy stretching exercises before moving on to the strength and endurance activities.

161

Effective exercising: Once you begin your daily exercise routine, keep these points in mind to get the best results:

- Always drink water before, during, and after your exercise session.

- Make exercising a part of your daily routine. You may want to set a regular time to exercise each day and invite a friend to join you.

- Start gradually, about 5 to 10 minutes at first.

- Increase the amount of exercise each day, up to about 30 to 60 minutes.

- Breathe deeply and evenly during and between exercises. Don't hold your breath.

- Rest whenever it is necessary.

- Keep a daily written record of your progress.

- Exercise to lively music, TV, or with friends for added enjoyment.

Cool down: If you have been participating in vigorous physical activity, it is extremely important not to stop suddenly. Abrupt stopping interferes with the return of the blood to the heart and may result in dizziness or fainting. Simply reduce the intensity of the exercise gradually and end with a few slow stretches from the section on stretching.

Exercising from a wheelchair: A number of the exercises in this chapter can be performed from a chair or a wheelchair. They are identified with the symbol: (o).

Flexibility

Exercises in this category will help you maintain your range of motion. Through the normal aging process, muscles tend to lose elasticity and tissues around the joints thicken. Exercise can delay this process by stretching muscles to prevent them from becoming short and tight. It also helps slow down the development of arthritis, one of the most common and painful diseases associated with advancing age.

In addition to performing flexibility exercises, you should try to bend, move, and stretch every day to keep joints flexible and muscles elastic. Avoid reliance on push buttons and conveniences that take away the need for personal motion. And, compliment this program with such recreational activities as dancing, yoga, swimming golfing, gardening, and housework.

Be sure to begin each workout with deep breathing and continue deep breathing at intervals throughout the session. You should work up to a total of 50 deep breaths per workout.

Flexibility Level I

Finger Stretching: to maintain finger dexterity. With the palm of the right hand facing down, gently force fingers back toward forearm, using left hand for leverage; then place left hand on top and push fingers down. Suggested repetitions: five each hand. (o)

Hand Rotation: to maintain wrist flexibility and range of motion. Grasp right wrist with left hand. Keep right palm facing down. Slowly rotate hand five times each clockwise and counter-clockwise. Suggested repetitions: five each hand. (o)

Ankle and Foot Circling: to improve flexibility and range of motion of ankles. Cross right leg over opposite knee, rotate foot slowly, making large complete circles. Ten rotations to the right, 10 to the left, each leg. (o)

Neck Extension: to improve flexibility and range motion of neck. Sit up comfortably. Bend head forward until chin touches chest. You may want to stretch forward by simply jutting your chin out. Return to starting position and slowly rotate head to left. Return to starting position and slowly rotate head to right. Return to starting position. Suggested repetitions: five. (o)

Single Knee Pull: to stretch lower back and back of leg. Lie on back, hands at sides. Pull one leg to chest, grasp with both arms and hold for five counts. Repeat with opposite leg. Suggested repetitions: three to five.

Simulated Crawl Stroke/Back Stroke/Breast Stroke: to stretch shoulder girdle. Stand with feet shoulder-width apart, arms at sides, relaxed. Bend knees and alternately swing right and left arms backward ... upward ... and forward as if swimming. Suggested repetitions: six to eight movements on each stroke. (o)

Reach: to stretch shoulder girdle and rib cage. Take deep breath, extend arms overhead. If standing, rise on toes while reaching. Exhale slowly, lowering arms. Can be done in a seated position. Suggested repetitions: six to eight. (o)

Backstretch: to improve the flexibility of the lower back. Sit up straight. Bend far forward and straighten up. Repeat, clasping hands on left knee. Repeat clasping hands on right knee. Exhale while bending forward. Suggested repetitions: four to six over each knee. (o)

Chain Breaker: to stretch chest muscles. Stand erect, feet about six inches apart. Tighten leg muscles, tighten stomach by drawing it in, with hips forward, extend chest, bring arms up with clenched fists chest high, take deep breath, let it out slowly. Slowly pull arms back as far as possible keeping elbows chest high. Suggested repetitions: 8–10. (o)

Flexibility Level II

Double Knee Pull: to stretch lower back and buttocks. Lie on back, hands at sides. Pull legs to chest, lock arms around legs, pull buttocks slightly off ground. Hold for 10 to 15 counts. Suggested repetitions: three to five.

Seated Pike Stretch: to stretch lower back and hamstrings. Sit on floor, with legs forward, knees together. Exhale and stretch forward, slowly sliding hands down to ankles. Stretch only as far as is comfortable and use your hands for support. Hold for five to eight counts. Don't bounce; inhale deeply. Repetitions: three to four.

Chest Stretch: to stretch muscles in chest and shoulders. Stand arm-length distant from a doorway opening. Raise one arm shoulder height with slight bend in elbow. Place hand against door jamb and turn upper body away so that the muscles in chest and shoulders are stretched. Suggested repetitions: three to four each arm.

Seated Stretch: to stretch lower back and hamstrings. Sit on floor one leg extended to your side and one leg bent comfortably in front of your body. Supporting your body weight with your hands and keeping your back straight, lean forward until you feel a comfortable leg and hamstring. Hold the stretch for a few seconds, exhaling. Switch sides. Suggested repetitions: three to five each side.

Flexibility Level III

Sitting Stretch: to increase flexibility of lower back and hamstrings. Sit on floor with legs extended as far apart as is comfortable. Exhale and stretch forward slowly, sliding your hands down your legs. Reach as far as is comfortable and hold for five to eight counts. Suggested repetitions: three to four.

Achilles Stretch: to stretch calf muscles on back leg (Achilles tendon). Stand facing wall two to three feet away. Extend arms, lean into wall. Move left leg forward one-half step, right leg backward one-half step or more. Lower right heel to floor. Lean hips forward, stretching the calf muscles in the right leg. Hold 5 to 10 counts. Breathe normally. Reverse leg position and repeat. Suggested repetitions: three to six each leg.

Modified Seal: to stretch abdominal wall, chest, and front of neck. Lie on the floor with arms extended, stomach down, feet extended, with toes pointed. While exhaling, slowly lift head and push up until arms are bent at right angles, with back arching gently. Keep hips on the floor. Keeping arms bent, hold for 5 to 10 counts. Return to starting position, inhaling deeply. Suggested repetitions: four to six.

Half Bow: to stretch the top of the thigh and groin area. Lie on left side. Hold ankle of right foot with right hand just above toes. Slightly arch back. Hold 5 to 10 counts. Suggested repetitions: three to five.

Strength

Exercises designed to build strength can help prevent premature loss of muscle tissue and can improve muscle strength, size, and endurance at any age. The benefits of strength exercises also include improving reaction time, reducing the rate of muscle atrophy, increasing work capacity, and helping prevent back problems and injury.

The following program of muscle conditioning exercises for the whole body has been designed specifically for older adults. Calisthenics work muscles against resistance, enabling them to grow and maintain muscle tone. In addition to the strength exercises suggested in this section, other physical activities that are essentially recreational can provide benefits to help maintain muscle integrity. Such activities include bicycling and swimming,

Strength Level I

Finger Squeeze: to strengthen the hands. Extend arms in front at shoulder height, palms down. Squeeze fingers slowly, then release. Suggested repetitions: five. Turn palms up, squeeze fingers, release. Suggested repetitions: five. Extend arms in front, shake fingers. Suggested repetitions: five.

Touch Shoulders: to increase flexibility of the shoulders and elbows and tone the upper arm; can be done in a seated position. Touch shoulders with hands, extend arms out straight. Bring arms back to starting position. Suggested repetitions: 10–15.

Leg Extensions: to tone the upper leg muscles. Sit upright. Lift 1eft leg off the floor and extend it fully. Lower it very slowly. Suggested repetitions: 10–15 each leg. (o)

Back Leg Swing: to firm the buttocks and strengthen the lower back. Stand up, holding on to the back of a chair. Keep your back and hips in line with the chair as you do the exercise. Extend one leg back, foot pointed toward the floor. Keeping the knee straight, lift the leg backward approximately four inches and concentrate on squeezing the muscles in the buttocks with each lift. Make sure you keep your back straight as you raise your legs. Return to starting position. Suggested repetitions: 10 each leg.

Quarter Squat: to tone and strengthen lower leg muscles. Stand erect behind a chair, hands on chair back for balance. Bend knees, then rise to an upright position. Be careful not to let knees go beyond your toes. Suggested repetitions: 8–12.

Heel Raises: to strengthen the calf muscles and ankles. Stand erect, holding a chair for balance if needed, hands on hips, feet together. Raise body on toes. Return to starting position. Suggested repetitions: 10.

Knee Lift: to strengthen hip flexors and lower abdomen. Stand erect. Raise left knee to chest or as far upward as possible while back remains straight. Return to starting position. Repeat with right leg. Suggested repetitions: five each leg.

Head and Shoulder Curl: to firm stomach muscles. Lie on the floor, knees bent, arms at sides, head bent slightly forward. Reach forward with arms extended until fingertips touch your knees. Hold for five counts. Return to starting position. Suggested repetitions: 10.

Strength Level II

Arm Curl: to strengthen arm muscles. Use a weighted object such as a book or a can of vegetables or small dumbbell. Stand or sit erect with arms at side, holding weighted object. Bend your arm, raising the weight. Lower it. Can be done seated. Suggested repetitions: 10–15 each arm. (o)

Arm Extension: to tone muscles in the back of the arm. Sit or stand erect with arms at sides, holding a weighted object of less than five pounds overhead. Slowly bend arm until head, then slowly extend arm overhead again. The arm curl and arm extension can be done separately or together. Can be done seated. (o)

Modified Knee Push-Up: to strengthen upper back, chest, and back of arms. Start on bent knees, hands on floor and slightly forward of shoulders. Lower body until chin touches floor. Return to start. Suggested repetitions: 5–10.

Calf Raise: to strengthen lower leg and ankle. Stand erect, hands on hip or on back of chair for balance. Spread feet 6 to 12 inches. Slowly raise body up to toes, lifting heels. Return to starting position. Breathe normally. Suggested repetitions: 10–15.

Alternate Leg Lunges: to strengthen upper thighs and inside legs. Also stretches back of leg. Take a comfortable stance with hands on hips. Step forward 18 to 24 inches with right leg. Keep left heel on floor. Shove off right leg and resume standing position. Suggested repetitions: 5–10 each leg.

Modified Sit-Up: to improve abdominal strength. Lie on back, feet on the floor with fingertips behind your ears. Look straight up at the ceiling and lift head and shoulders off floor. Suggested repetitions: 10.

Side-Lying Leg Lift: to strengthen and tone outside of thigh and hip muscles. Lie on right side, legs extended. Raise leg four to five inches. Lower to starting position. Suggested repetitions: 10 on each side.

Strength: Level III

In Level III strength exercise, lightweight resistance equipment, such as the dumbbell, is introduced to overload the muscles. While equipment of this kind is low in cost and desirable, a number of substitutes can be used. These include a bucket of soil, a heavy household item such as an iron, a can of food, a stone, or a brick.

Seated Alternate Dumbbell Curls: to strengthen biceps of upper arms. Sit comfortably on a flat bench with arms at side. Hold a pair of dumbbells with an underhand grip so that palms face up. Bending left elbow, raise dumbbell until left arm is fully flexed. Lower left dumbbell while raising right dumbbell from the elbow until right arm is fully flexed. Breathe normally. Suggested repetitions: two sets of 8–10 each arm. (o)

Dumbbell Fly: to strengthen chest muscles and improve lateral range of motion in shoulder girdle. Lie on your back on a flat bench or floor if bench is not available. Grasp dumbbells in each hand over chest. Inhale and lower dumbbell to side with elbow slightly bent. Raise dumbbell in an arc to the starting position while exhaling. Suggested repetitions: 8–12.

167

Alternate Dumbbell Shrug: to strengthen muscles in shoulders, upper back, and neck. Stand comfortably with dumbbells in each hand. Elevate shoulders as high as possible, rolling them first backward and then down to the starting position. Exhale as you lower the shoulders. Suggested repetitions: 10 forward, 5 backward. (o)

One Arm Dumbbell Extension: to strengthen triceps (back of arm) and improve range of motion. Bring weight up to shoulder and lift overhead. Slowly lower it behind the back as far as is comfortable. Extend arm to original position. Inhale on the way down, exhale on the way up. Suggested repetitions: 8–12 on each arm. (o)

Dumbbell Calf Raise: to strengthen calf muscle and improve range of motion of ankle joint. Stand with feet shoulder-width apart, weights in each hand, toes on a two-by-four-inch block (preferred but not necessary). Raise up on toes lifting heels as high as possible. Slowly lower heels to starting position. Breathe normally. Suggested repetitions: five with heels straight back, five with heels turned out, five with heels turned in.

Dumbbell Half Squats: to strengthen thigh muscles in front. Stand with feet shoulder-width apart and heels on a two-by-four-inch block (not necessary, but preferred). Holding weights in each hand, slowly descend to a comfortable position where the tops of the thighs are about at a 45-degree angle to the floor. There is no benefit to a deeper squat. Inhale on the way down. Stand up slowly, keeping knees slightly bent. Exhale on the way up. Suggested repetitions: 10–12.

Modified Sit-Up: to improve abdominal strength. Lie on back, feet on the floor, with fingertips behind your ears. Look straight up at ceiling and lift head and shoulders off floor. Suggested repetitions: 12–15.

Section 14.2

Exercise for Menopause-Aged Women

"Exercise Recommendations for Menopause-Aged Women," by Chris
Eschbach, PhD. Reprinted with permission of the American College of
Sports Medicine, ACSM Fit Society® Page, Fall 2009, pp 1–2.

The symptoms of menopause are numerous, and they can affect the
quality of life of women moving through this stage. The good news is
that exercise can often help reduce menopause-related symptoms.

Menopause is the term commonly used to refer to the period of time
both before and after a woman's last menstrual period. Technically,
menopause is a woman's last menstrual period, while the time period
immediately prior to menopause is referred to as "peri-menopause" and
the time following menopause is referred to as "post-menopause."

This process of changing hormone levels can last for more than
10 years and women may experience widely varying hormone levels,
specifically estrogen, progesterone, follicle stimulating hormone, and
luteinizing hormone. These hormones alone, and in combination, are
responsible for a wide range of processes within the body. The changes
that occur during this stage of life may result in disruptions to normal
daily living. These disruptions may include hot flashes, sleep disruption, weight gain, loss of libido, short-term memory impairment or a
lack of focus, increased anxiety, fatigue, depression and drastic mood
swings, joint/muscle aches and pains, irregular periods, heavy bleeding,
dry eyes, vaginal changes, hair loss, osteoporosis, and cardiovascular
disease—most of which can be lessened with an effective exercise program. It is important to note that not all women experience the same
changes or with similar intensity, which is one reason why menopause
can be quite frustrating for many women.

Research has demonstrated the positive effects of exercise and
physical activity on reducing menopausal symptoms. Interestingly,
the positive changes do not seem to be brought on by "correction" of
hormonal concentration but rather from the acute effects of exercise
and the long-term positive adaptations that result from exercise training. The positive outcomes resulting from regular exercise and/or physical
activity programs include increased cardiovascular fitness, improvements

in body composition, decreased anxiety and depression, and enhanced feelings of well-being. Additionally, exercise and/or physical activity have, in some cases, been shown to decrease feelings of fatigue and chronic muscle pain, improve quality and duration of sleep, and increase or minimize loss of bone density.

The exercise recommendations for women in either peri- or post-menopause are very similar to those recommended for all women. Starting an exercise program can be a difficult task, especially during a time when hormonal fluctuations result in a variety of physiological and psychological changes. The key is to remember that the main goal is to boost your health and minimize any symptoms brought about by natural body changes. It is important to choose activities that you enjoy.

Any cardiovascular activity (brisk walking, cycling, water aerobics, mowing the lawn) that causes you to elevate your heart rate and break a sweat while still able to carry on a conversation is adequate for meeting the ACSM [American College of Sports Medicine]-recommended 30 minutes a day, five days a week (or 150 minutes per week). Even short bouts of exercise lasting at least 10 minutes can be accumulated toward the 30-minutes-per-day goal. In addition to cardiovascular exercise, twice-a-week bouts of strength training with at least eight exercises of 8 to 12 repetitions working the whole body can result in positive outcomes.

For both cardiovascular and strength training exercises, remember to increase the amount of exercise gradually, starting with realistic amounts and moving toward achieving the minimum recommendations. Exceeding the minimum recommendations further reduces the risk of inactivity-related chronic disease and may be helpful in minimizing symptoms of menopause.

Special consideration should be given for those women who are especially affected by hot flashes. Research has shown that a relaxation-based method with paced respiration significantly reduces objectively measured hot flash occurrence. With this in mind, programs that encourage focused relaxation and breathing, such as yoga, may be beneficial for reducing hot flashes. While the benefits of cardiovascular activity are numerous, researchers have not consistently found positive effects specific to hot flashes, although it may work for some women.

It is important to consult your physician on a regular schedule as peri-menopause approaches and work with him or her to balance the changing needs of your body. Be sure to use exercise to help manage complications brought about by this life change.

Chapter 15

Physical Fitness and the Elderly

Chapter Contents

Section 15.1

Fitness Guidelines for the Elderly

This section excerpted from "Chapter 5. Active Older Adults," *Physical Activity Guidelines for Americans*, U.S. Department of Health and Human Services (www.hhs.gov), October 16, 2008.

Regular physical activity is essential for healthy aging. Adults aged 65 years and older gain substantial health benefits from regular physical activity, and these benefits continue to occur throughout their lives. Promoting physical activity for older adults is especially important because this population is the least physically active of any age group.

Older adults are a varied group. Most, but not all, have one or more chronic conditions, and these conditions vary in type and severity. All have experienced a loss of physical fitness with age, some more than others. This diversity means that some older adults can run several miles, while others struggle to walk several blocks.

This chapter provides guidance about physical activity for adults aged 65 years and older. The chapter focuses on physical activity beyond baseline activity. The guidelines seek to help older adults select types and amounts of physical activity appropriate for their abilities. The guidelines for older adults are also appropriate for adults younger than age 65 who have chronic conditions and those with a low level of fitness.

For adults aged 65 and older who are fit and have no limiting chronic conditions, the guidance in this chapter is essentially the same as that for active adults [see Chapter 13 Section 1, "Fitness Guidelines for Adults"].

Explaining the Guidelines

Like the guidelines for other adults, those for older adults mainly focus on two types of activity: aerobic and muscle strengthening. In addition, these guidelines discuss the addition of balance training for older adults at risk of falls. Each type provides important health benefits.

People doing aerobic activities move large muscles in a rhythmic manner for a sustained period. Brisk walking, jogging, biking, dancing, and swimming are all examples of aerobic activities. This type of activity is also called endurance activity.

Aerobic activity makes a person's heart beat more rapidly to meet the demands of the body's movement. Over time, regular aerobic activity makes the heart and cardiovascular system stronger and fitter.

When putting the guidelines into action, it's important to consider the total amount of activity, as well as how often to be active, for how long, and at what intensity.

Key Guidelines for Older Adults

The following guidelines are the same for adults and older adults:

- All older adults should avoid inactivity. Some physical activity is better than none, and older adults who participate in any amount of physical activity gain some health benefits.

- For substantial health benefits, older adults should do at least 150 minutes (2 hours and 30 minutes) a week of moderate-intensity, or 75 minutes (1 hour and 15 minutes) a week of vigorous-intensity aerobic physical activity, or an equivalent combination of moderate- and vigorous-intensity aerobic activity. Aerobic activity should be performed in episodes of at least 10 minutes and preferably should be spread throughout the week.

- For additional and more extensive health benefits, older adults should increase their aerobic physical activity to 300 minutes (5 hours) a week of moderate-intensity, or 150 minutes a week of vigorous-intensity aerobic physical activity, or an equivalent combination of moderate- and vigorous-intensity activity. Additional health benefits are gained by engaging in physical activity beyond this amount.

- Older adults should also do muscle-strengthening activities that are moderate or high intensity and involve all major muscle groups on two or more days a week, as these activities provide additional health benefits.

The following guidelines are just for older adults:

- When older adults cannot do 150 minutes of moderate-intensity aerobic activity a week because of chronic conditions, they should be as physically active as their abilities and conditions allow.

- Older adults should do exercises that maintain or improve balance if they are at risk of falling.

- Older adults should determine their level of effort for physical activity relative to their level of fitness.

- Older adults with chronic conditions should understand whether and how their conditions affect their ability to do regular physical activity safely.

How Much Total Activity a Week?

Older adults should aim to do at least 150 minutes (2 hours and 30 minutes) of moderate-intensity physical activity a week, or an equivalent amount (75 minutes or 1 hour and 15 minutes) of vigorous-intensity activity. Older adults can also do an equivalent amount of activity by combining moderate- and vigorous-intensity activity. As is true for younger people, greater amounts of physical activity provide additional and more extensive health benefits to people aged 65 years and older.

No matter what its purpose—walking the dog, taking a dance or exercise class, or bicycling to the store—aerobic activity of all types counts toward the guidelines.

How Many Days a Week and for How Long?

Aerobic physical activity should be spread throughout the week. Research studies consistently show that activity performed on at least three days a week produces health benefits. Spreading physical activity across at least three days a week may help to reduce the risk of injury and avoid excessive fatigue.

Episodes of aerobic activity count toward meeting the guidelines if they last at least 10 minutes and are performed at moderate or vigorous intensity. These episodes can be divided throughout the day or week. For example, a person who takes a brisk 15-minute walk twice a day on every day of the week would easily meet the minimum guidelines for aerobic activity.

How Intense?

Older adults can meet the guidelines by doing relatively moderate-intensity activity, relatively vigorous-intensity activity, or a combination of both. Time spent in light activity (such as light housework) and sedentary activities (such as watching TV) does not count.

The relative intensity of aerobic activity is related to a person's level of cardiorespiratory fitness.

174

Table 15.1. Examples of Aerobic and Muscle-Strengthening Activities for Older Adults

Aerobic	Muscle-Strengthening
Walking	Exercises using exercise bands, weight machines, hand-held weights
Dancing	Calisthenic exercises (body weight provides resistance to movement)
Swimming	Digging, lifting, and carrying as part of gardening
Water aerobics	Carrying groceries
Jogging	Some yoga exercises
Aerobic exercise classes	Some tai chi exercises
Bicycle riding (stationary or on a path)	
Some activities of gardening, such as raking and pushing a lawn mower	
Tennis	
Golf (without a cart)	

- Moderate-intensity activity requires a medium level of effort. On a scale of 0 to 10, where sitting is 0 and the greatest effort possible is 10, moderate-intensity activity is a 5 or 6 and produces noticeable increases in breathing rate and heart rate.

- Vigorous-intensity activity is a 7 or 8 on this scale and produces large increases in a person's breathing and heart rate.

A general rule of thumb is that two minutes of moderate-intensity activity count the same as one minute of vigorous-intensity activity. For example, 30 minutes of moderate-intensity activity a week is roughly same as 15 minutes of vigorous-intensity activity.

Muscle-Strengthening Activities

At least two days a week, older adults should do muscle-strengthening activities that involve all the major muscle groups. These are the muscles of the legs, hips, chest, back, abdomen, shoulders, and arms. Muscle-strengthening activities make muscles do more work than they are accustomed to during activities of daily life. Examples of muscle-strengthening activities include lifting weights, working with resistance bands, doing calisthenics using body weight for resistance (such as push-ups, pull-ups, and sit-ups), climbing stairs, carrying heavy loads, and heavy gardening.

Muscle-strengthening activities count if they involve a moderate to high level of intensity, or effort, and work the major muscle groups of the body. Whatever the reason, any muscle-strengthening activity counts toward meeting the guidelines. For example, muscle-strengthening activity done as part of a therapy or rehabilitation program can count.

No specific amount of time is recommended for muscle strengthening, but muscle-strengthening exercises should be performed to the point at which it would be difficult to do another repetition without help. When resistance training is used to enhance muscle strength, one set of 8 to 12 repetitions of each exercise is effective, although two or three sets may be more effective. Development of muscle strength and endurance is progressive over time. This means that gradual increases in the amount of weight or the days per week of exercise will result in stronger muscles.

Balance Activities for Older Adults at Risk of Falls

Older adults are at increased risk of falls if they have had falls in the recent past or have trouble walking. In older adults at increased risk of falls, strong evidence shows that regular physical activity is safe and reduces the risk of falls. Reduction in falls is seen for participants in programs that include balance and moderate-intensity muscle-strengthening activities for 90 minutes (1 hour and 30 minutes) a week plus moderate-intensity walking for about 1 hour a week. Preferably, older adults at risk of falls should do balance training three or more days a week and do standardized exercises from a program demonstrated to reduce falls. Examples of these exercises include backward walking, sideways walking, heel walking, toe walking, and standing from a sitting position. The exercises can increase in difficulty by progressing from holding onto a stable support (like furniture) while doing the exercises to doing them without support. It's not known whether different combinations of type, amount, or frequency of activity can reduce falls to a greater degree. Tai chi exercises also may help prevent falls.

Meeting the Guidelines

Older adults have many ways to live an active lifestyle that meets the guidelines. Many factors influence decisions to be active, such as personal goals, current physical activity habits, and health and safety considerations.

176

Healthy older adults generally do not need to consult a health care provider before becoming physically active. However, health care providers can help people attain and maintain regular physical activity by providing advice on appropriate types of activities and ways to progress at a safe and steady pace.

Adults with chronic conditions should talk with their health care provider to determine whether their conditions limit their ability to do regular physical activity in any way. Such a conversation should also help people learn about appropriate types and amounts of physical activity.

Inactive older adults: Older adults should increase their amount of physical activity gradually. It can take months for those with a low level of fitness to gradually meet their activity goals. To reduce injury risk, inactive or insufficiently active adults should avoid vigorous aerobic activity at first. Rather, they should gradually increase the number of days a week and duration of moderate-intensity aerobic activity. Adults with a very low level of fitness can start out with episodes of activity less than 10 minutes and slowly increase the minutes of light-intensity aerobic activity, such as light-intensity walking.

Older adults who are inactive or who don't yet meet the guidelines should aim for at least 150 minutes a week of relatively moderate-intensity physical activity. Getting at least 30 minutes of relatively moderate-intensity physical activity on five or more days each week is a reasonable way to meet these guidelines. Doing muscle-strengthening activity on two or three nonconsecutive days each week is also an acceptable and appropriate goal for many older adults.

Active older adults: Older adults who are already active and meet the guidelines can gain additional and more extensive health benefits by moving beyond the 150 minutes a week minimum to 300 or more minutes a week of relatively moderate-intensity aerobic activity. Muscle-strengthening activities should also be done at least two days a week.

Older adults with chronic conditions: Older adults who have chronic conditions that prevent them from doing the equivalent of 150 minutes of moderate-intensity aerobic activity a week should set physical activity goals that meet their abilities. They should talk with their health care provider about setting physical activity goals. They should avoid an inactive lifestyle. Even 60 minutes (one hour) a week of moderate-intensity aerobic activity provides some health benefits.

Special Considerations

Doing a variety of activities, including walking: Older adults have many ways to live an active lifestyle that meets the guidelines. In working toward meeting the guidelines, older adults are encouraged to do a variety of activities. This approach can make activity more enjoyable and may reduce the risk of overuse injury.

Older adults also should strongly consider walking as one good way to get aerobic activity. Many studies show that walking has health benefits, and it has a low risk of injury. It can be done year-round and in many settings.

Physical activity for older adults who have functional limitations: When a person has lost some ability to do a task of everyday life, such as climbing stairs, the person has a functional limitation. In older adults with existing functional limitations, scientific evidence indicates that regular physical activity is safe and helps improve functional ability.

Resuming activity after an illness or injury: Older adults may have to take a break from regular physical activity because of illness or injury, such as the flu or a muscle strain. If these interruptions occur, older adults should resume activity at a lower level and gradually work back up to their former level of activity.

Flexibility, warm-up, and cool-down: Older adults should maintain the flexibility necessary for regular physical activity and activities of daily life. When done properly, stretching activities increase flexibility. Although these activities alone have no known health benefits and have not been demonstrated to reduce risk of activity-related injuries, they are an appropriate component of a physical activity program. However, time spent doing flexibility activities by themselves does not count toward meeting aerobic or muscle-strengthening guidelines.

Research studies of effective exercise programs typically include warm-up and cool-down activities. Warm-up and cool-down activities before and after physical activity can also be included as part of a personal program. A warm-up before moderate- or vigorous-intensity aerobic activity allows a gradual increase in heart rate and breathing at the start of the episode of activity. A cool-down after activity allows a gradual decrease at the end of the episode. Time spent doing warm-up and cool-down may count toward meeting the aerobic activity guidelines if the activity is at least moderate intensity (for example, walking briskly to warm-up for a jog). A warm-up for muscle-strengthening activity commonly involves doing exercises with less weight than during the strengthening activity.

Section 15.2

Balance Exercises for Older Adults

This section excerpted from "Chapter 4. Sample Exercises—Strength/Balance Exercises," *Exercise and Physical Activity: Your Everyday Guide from the National Institute on Aging*, National Institute on Aging (www.nia.nih .gov), January 31, 2008.

Each year, U.S. hospitals have 300,000 admissions for broken hips, and falling is often the cause of those fractures. Balance exercises can help you stay independent by helping you avoid the disability—often permanent—that may result from falling.

There is a lot of overlap between strength and balance exercises; very often, one exercise serves both purposes. Lower-body exercises for strength also are balance exercises. They include plantar flexion, hip flexion, hip extension, knee flexion, and side leg raise.

These exercises can improve your balance even more if you add the following modifications. Note that these exercises instruct you to hold onto a table or chair for balance. Hold onto the table with only one hand. As you progress, try holding on with only one fingertip. Next, try these exercises without holding on at all. If you are very steady on your feet, move on to doing the exercises using no hands, with your eyes closed. Have someone stand close by if you are unsteady.

Plantar Flexion

1. Stand straight; hold onto a table or chair for balance.
2. Slowly stand on tiptoe, as high as possible.
3. Hold position for one second.
4. Slowly lower heels all the way back down. Pause.
5. Repeat 8 to 15 times.
6. Rest; then do another set of 8 to 15 repetitions.
7. Add modifications as you progress.

179

Knee Flexion

1. Stand straight; hold onto a table or chair for balance.

2. Slowly bend knee as far as possible, so foot lifts up behind you.

3. Hold position for one second.

4. Slowly lower foot all the way back down. Pause.

5. Repeat with other leg.

6. Alternate legs until you have done 8 to 15 repetitions with each leg.

7. Rest; then do another set of 8 to 15 alternating repetitions.

8. Add modifications as you progress.

Hip Flexion

1. Stand straight; hold onto a table or chair for balance.

2. Slowly bend one knee toward chest, without bending waist or hips.

3. Hold position for one second.

4. Slowly lower leg all the way down. Pause.

5. Repeat with other leg.

6. Alternate legs until you have done 8 to 15 repetitions with each leg.

7. Rest; then do another set of 8 to 15 alternating repetitions.

8. Add modifications as you progress.

Hip Extension

1. Stand 12 to 18 inches from a table or chair, feet slightly apart.

2. Bend forward at hips at about 45-degree angle; hold onto a table or chair for balance.

3. Slowly lift one leg straight backward without bending your knee, pointing your toes, or bending your upper body any farther forward.

4. Hold position for one second.

5. Slowly lower leg. Pause.

6. Repeat with other leg.

7. Alternate legs until you have done 8 to 15 repetitions with each leg.

8. Rest; then do another set of 8 to 15 alternating repetitions.

9. Add modifications as you progress.

Side Leg Raise

1. Stand straight, directly behind table or chair, feet slightly apart.

2. Hold onto table or chair for balance.

3. Slowly lift one leg to side 6–12 inches out to side. Keep your back and both legs straight. Don't point your toes outward; keep them facing forward.

4. Hold position for one second.

5. Slowly lower leg all the way down. Pause.

6. Repeat with other leg.

7. Alternate legs until you have done 8 to 15 repetitions with each leg.

8. Rest; then do another set of 8 to 15 alternating repetitions.

9. Add modifications as you progress.

Anytime/Anywhere

These types of exercises also improve your balance. You can do them almost anytime, anywhere, and as often as you like, as long as you have something sturdy nearby to hold onto if you become unsteady.

- Walk heel-to-toe. Position your heel just in front of the toes of the opposite foot each time you take a step. Your heel and toes should touch or almost touch.

- Stand on one foot (for example, while waiting in line at the grocery store or at the bus stop). Alternate feet.

- Stand up and sit down without using your hands.

Chapter 16

Encouraging Physical Fitness through the Community Environment

Community Design and Physical Activity

Urban planning and transportation researchers have been studying how community design affects travel behavior for several decades. They found people walked more when they lived in areas with two characteristics: mixed land use, in which homes, shops, and services are intermingled; and connected streets with frequent intersections and short blocks that provide direct routes for pedestrians. This general pattern of development is very common in older parts of the United States and around the world in places built before cars became the dominant mode of transportation. Such communities are referred to as "walkable," meaning it is convenient to walk to several destinations. Sometimes other concepts are included in walkability, such as high residential density (often required to support neighborhood shops), sidewalks lining all streets, and buildings built right up to the sidewalk rather than having parking lots between the building and the street. The alternative low-walkable development pattern is seen mainly in communities built since the 1950s and is commonly referred to as the suburbs or sprawl. These places were designed to facilitate automobile travel. It is not possible for most people in the suburbs to walk for daily errands, and street patterns are disconnected, with many winding streets, long blocks, and cul-de-sacs.

This section excerpted from "Physical Activity and the Built Environment," President's Council on Physical Fitness and Sports (www.fitness.gov), December 2006. The full document, including references, is available at www.fitness.gov/ publications/digests/december2006digest.pdf.

Studies of Adults

Reviews of numerous studies in the urban planning literature consistently show people walk and cycle more for transportation in high-walkable neighborhoods than in low-walkable areas. A typical difference of one walking trip per week translates into 30–60 more minutes of physical activity, and this difference should persist as long as the person lives in the same type of neighborhood. Mixed land use, street connectivity, and residential density are consistently supported as correlates of active travel, while presence of sidewalks has inconsistent results.

For the health field, a key question is whether walkability is related to total physical activity. Studies using objective accelerometer-based measures of physical activity demonstrate total physical activity is substantially higher among people living in high-walkable, compared to low-walkable, communities. These findings generally are supported whether built environments are measured by self-report, observational audits, or using Geographic Information System (GIS) software. However, findings are emerging that people's perceptions of the environment may not match the objective data. Thus, both are important to measure.

Studies on physical activity and community design were reviewed by panels from the Transportation Research Board and Institute of Medicine and Task Force for Community Preventive Services. Both groups concluded there is a consistent association between land use patterns and physical activity. Thus, land use is now accepted as an important issue for physical activity and public health. These groups recommended policy changes in zoning, development regulations, and transportation investments that would encourage development of more walkable communities.

Most studies focused on travel behavior or overall physical activity. More recent studies have compared different domains of activity, for example, walking for transportation versus recreation, and found specific community design attributes are related to each. This is an important research area because these studies can identify how to design communities that support several types of physical activity.

Several limitations to this literature have been identified. Because virtually all the studies are cross-sectional, there is the potential for self-selection bias in which results can be explained by physically active people choosing to live in neighborhoods where they can walk or bike to nearby destinations. Prospective studies that can follow people who move to different types of neighborhoods are needed. Another limitation is that most studies have been conducted on homogeneous samples or have not analyzed whether associations generalize across subgroups defined by sex, income, and race/ethnicity. Some studies have found built environment and physical activity were related in whites but not African Americans, which could be explained by lower levels of perceived safety in low-income neighborhoods that could prevent residents from taking advantage of walkable neighborhoods. Other studies have found gender differences. An emerging finding is that psychosocial variables, such as attitudes, self-efficacy, and social support, explain much more variance in physical activity than does community design. One way to put this finding in perspective is that altering the built environment is likely to affect everyone living there on a relatively permanent basis, so even a small effect on an individual's behavior is multiplied across people and time.

Studies of Youth

Krizek proposed a model of the relevance of community design for youth physical activity. Though youth have different issues, such as commuting to school, access to play areas, and role of parents, many of the walkability associations with physical activity are presumed to be the same for youth and adults. Two studies using GIS measures of walkability and accelerometer measures of physical activity supported the relevance of walkability for adolescents. In one study, a walkability index explained about the same amount of variance as sex and ethnicity. However, a finding that higher street connectivity was related to lower activity levels in girls suggests that young people may use cul-de-sacs and suburban streets as play areas. Thus, street connectivity could encourage walking for transportation while discouraging play.

Active commuting to school can contribute to overall physical activity, and there appears to be a connection with community design. Kerr and colleagues found active commuting was higher in high-walkable neighborhoods, but this effect was seen for higher-income children only. Braza et al. reported more active commuting to school in high-density neighborhoods, but no relation to street connectivity. Ewing and colleagues found more active commuting when sidewalks were present, but no association with density and land use mix. A significant effect of sidewalks was replicated by Fulton et al. McMillan confirmed high active commuting in walkable neighborhoods but found other contributors, such as perceived safety, traffic, and attitudes. Timperio and colleagues reported the surprising finding that higher street connectivity was associated with less active commuting.

The few studies of community design and youth physical activity generally support a positive association of walkability indicators with both walking to school and total physical activity. There is some evidence that poorly connected streets with less traffic could provide youth with places to play and may encourage active commuting to school. Many studies of youth benefit from objective measures of physical activity. An important research priority is to examine how community design attributes may operate both similarly and differently for youth and adults.

Studies of Older Adults

Though it is likely the principles of walkability support walking for transportation among seniors, there are additional specific age-related issues in considering how to design activity-friendly communities. The design of the environment must take into account the declining acuity of senses. Impaired hearing and vision need to be compensated for by louder crossing signals and increased lighting. Changes in gait and balance mean that hazards such as uneven sidewalks and high curbs need to be eliminated. Loss of stamina suggests more resting places are required. Interviews with seniors revealed having access to services was important so they could walk and take care of daily activities, thus maintaining their independence. Frequent crosswalks with sufficient crossing time were a priority. Interviewees in one study indicated their choice of walking routes was influenced by length of route, sidewalk quality, people along the route, traffic, signaled crosswalks, safety from crime, and scenery.

A few quantitative studies illustrate the potential for the built environment to support older adults' physical activity. In a Canadian study, physical activity was related to presence of hills, biking and walking trails, street lights, recreation facilities, seeing other people, and unattended dogs. Li and colleagues found density, street connectivity, and safety were related to walking. Patterson and Chapman reported women over 70 years old living in neighborhoods with mixed services and good pedestrian access to services walked more. Studies using pedometers as objective measures of physical activity provide more convincing results. Older women living within a 20-minute walk of a park, trail, or store had more total steps than those with no destinations, and there was a direct relation between number of nearby destinations and number of steps. In older overweight women, predominance of older homes (representing more pedestrian-friendly neighborhoods) and access to destinations were related to more walking.

Maintaining independence is a major goal for seniors, and one study showed living in a mixed use neighborhood was associated with better ability to perform daily activities. The evidence linking community design and walkability factors with older adults' physical activity is limited, but results are consistent. Additional work is needed to document the specific design factors that are particularly important in creating activity-friendly communities for seniors.

Recreation Environments and Physical Activity

Researchers in the health, behavioral science, and leisure science fields have studied the relation of recreation environments and leisure-time physical activity for many years, but until recently the literature was very small. The main concept is that easy access to parks, trails, health clubs, and other places for physical activity could stimulate their use.

Studies of Adults

Humpel and colleagues reviewed the health literature on the environment and physical activity recently and found only 19 studies. Only access to recreation facilities, access to opportunities (such as activity programs), and aesthetic factors were consistently associated with higher levels of physical activity. Godbey and colleagues summarized findings of leisure science research related to active living. Parks are commonly used for a variety of physical activities, with walking being the most common. Distance to recreation facilities is strongly related to their use, and degree of naturalness was positively related to park use. Lee and Vernez-Moudon incorporated an urban planning and transportation perspective in their review of correlates of recreational physical activity. They pointed out neighborhood sidewalks are a common place for recreational walks, so sidewalks may be important for both recreational and transportation physical activity. Trails can also be used for transportation and recreation purposes.

Recent studies have confirmed and expanded early results. Access to parks and trails is consistently related to activity levels, with few exceptions. The evidence is growing on the importance of aesthetics of recreation facilities and neighborhoods in general for walking, running, and total leisure-time physical activity. Presence and quality of sidewalks is emerging as an important correlate of leisure walking and physical activity. It is important to identify specific characteristics of recreation facilities that are strongly related to physical activity, because these findings can be translated into policies and design guidelines. Giles-Corti et al. identified people were very likely to walk in parks when they were nearby, large, and had a variety of attractive features. Lindsey and colleagues reported the most used urban trails were in densely populated neighborhoods with mixed land uses and convenient parking.

It is clear that having easy access to parks and trails is associated with more walking and physical activity among adults. Sidewalks also play a crucial role in supporting physical activity. It appears people are more likely to use these facilities if they are aesthetically pleasing. Important research priorities are developing a better understanding of how to build and equip parks and trails so they attract more people for regular physical activity.

Studies of Youth

In addition to their own yards, the main places where children are physically active seem to be the neighborhood streets and sidewalks, parks, and school grounds. So it is not surprising an early review found proximity to recreation facilities and opportunities such as programs were consistent correlates of physical activity in children and adolescents. Recent studies mainly have confirmed these early findings, but some studies report significance only in some groups or no significant associations. There is new evidence that proximity to schools and their activity facilities is related to physical activity. New studies extended adult findings by showing aesthetics of recreation facilities and neighborhoods are related to youth physical activity.

There is consistent evidence that children and adolescents with recreation facilities near their homes are more likely to be active than those with few facilities. One study showed quality of facilities was more important than simple proximity so examining the role of quality and amenities at public recreation facilities is a priority. Because youth of different ages vary widely in common types of activity and use different equipment and supplies, it is important to learn how to design and equip parks and other recreation facilities so they serve youth of all ages.

Studies of Older Adults

Older adults are likely to use parks for physical activity, but they also use sidewalks for walking and may rely on senior centers for activity programs. There are enough studies of recreation environments and physical activity in older adults to indicate this is a promising area. For example, Payne and colleagues reported older adults who visited local parks were more active and had better mental health than those who did not use parks. Li and colleagues found proximity to parks, perceptions of safety, and number of nearby recreation facilities were related to walking in seniors. They built on this study by following participants over one year to examine possible reasons for the commonly seen decline in physical activity. They found that over a 12-month period, walking decreased less in older adults who lived in neighborhoods with safe walking environments and access to recreation facilities. Older adults may benefit from access to places where they can feel safe being active. Because easy access to shopping malls was associated with more walking, providing access to facilities that serve these same functions could be an effective intervention. Research on built environments and physical activity among seniors is just beginning.

Disparities in Recreation Environments

It is not clear whether all sociodemographic groups benefit equally from having access to recreation facilities, because this question rarely has been examined. However, the findings appear contradictory. Reed and colleagues found presence of sidewalks was related to physical activity only in whites, not in African Americans. In a study by Wilson et al., access to trails was related to physical activity in low socioeconomic status (SES) participants, but not among the high SES. Additional studies are needed to understand whether recreation facility/physical activity associations generalize across population subgroups. There are physical activity disparities in youth, with lower income and racial/ethnic minority youth usually having lower activity levels, and a national study showed recreational environments may help explain the disparities. Thus, it is of great interest to determine whether there are disparities in access to recreation facilities which could affect physical activity of all age groups. In self-report studies, lower-income adults perceive less access to recreation facilities. It is surprising that two studies reported high income participants had better access to free-for-use facilities such as public parks, but not pay-for-use facilities such as health clubs and dance studios. In a large national study using GIS-based measures, Gordon-Larsen and colleagues found less access to both free and pay facilities in low-education and high-minority areas. Another national study replicated the finding of fewer private recreation facilities in low-income and high-minority communities.

The evidence indicates that low-income and racial/ethnic minority populations have less access to recreation facilities. Thus, recreation policies and investments need to ensure low-income communities have equal access to recreation facilities. Disadvantaged communities need better access to public parks and trails, because pay-for-use facilities are generally not available to them.

Importance of the Social Environment

Though this section focuses on the built environment, an ecological perspective would indicate that built and social environments are likely to act together to influence physical activity. Of the many social environment issues that could be relevant to physical activity, built environment researchers have been most interested in safety. Perceived or objective danger from crime or traffic hazards could negate benefits of activity-friendly built environments if people are too afraid to walk on the streets, go to the park, or allow their children to play outdoors.

A 2002 review concluded the data on safety and physical activity are inconsistent. However, many of the measures of safety are crude, and many do not distinguish among safety related to crime or traffic. There are enough significant findings to justify further study of safety. Several recent studies of youth report significant associations of physical activity with crime safety or traffic safety, though some do not support an association. Among adults, African Americans perceive their neighborhoods as less safe than whites, so safety concerns could contribute to disparities in physical activity. A finding that safety was related to walking in whites but not in African Americans needs to be replicated. In the adult literature, most recent studies show an association of crime and physical activity. Because there are built environment strategies for reducing both the actual and perceived risk of crime, safety variables should continue to be included in built environment/physical activity studies.

Conclusion

Knowledge about the built environment and physical activity is growing rapidly, and efforts already are being made to use research findings to guide policy changes. The built environment is a direct reflection of policies, and creating more activity-friendly environments will involve collaboration among multiple government departments and sectors of society outside government. Government agencies dealing with zoning, planning, transportation, building codes, education, and recreation are directly responsible for the built environment variables described throughout this section. Industries dealing with construction of buildings and roads, real estate, recreation, and health have important stakes in the built environment, so they need to be engaged in efforts to change policies. Because physical activity is a significant determinant of health and health care costs, there is a strong rationale for adopting and implementing policies to create built environments that make it convenient, safe, and attractive for people of all ages and circumstances to be physically active.

Part Three

Start Moving

Chapter 17

Ways to Add Physical Activity to Your Life

Chapter Contents

Section 17.1

Get Active

This section excerpted from "Be Active Your Way: A Guide for Adults," *Physical Activity Guidelines for Americans*, U.S. Department of Health and Human Services (www.hhs.gov), October 16, 2008.

Getting Started

Thinking about adding physical activity to your life, but not sure how to get started? Sometimes taking the first step is the hardest part.

If you have not been active in some time, start at a comfortable level and add a little more activity as you go along. Some people find that getting active with a friend makes it easier to get started.

Is something holding you back?

Think about reasons why you have not been physically active. Then try to come up with some ways to get past what is keeping you from getting active. Have you said to yourself ...?

I haven't been active in a very long time. Solution: Choose something you like to do. Many people find walking helps them get started. Before you know it, you will be doing more each day.

I don't have the time. Solution: Start with 10-minute chunks of time a couple of days a week. Walk during a break. Dance in the living room to your favorite music. It all adds up.

It costs too much. Solution: You don't have to join a health club or buy fancy equipment to be active. Play tag with your kids. Walk briskly with your dog for 10 minutes or more.

What can physical activity do for you?

You may have heard the good things you can gain from regular physical activity. The following are benefits you can gain from active living:

- Be healthier

- Increase my chances of living longer
- Feel better about myself
- Have less chance of becoming depressed
- Sleep better at night
- Help me look good
- Be in shape
- Get around better
- Have stronger muscles and bones
- Help me stay at or get to a healthy weight
- Be with friends or meet new people
- Enjoy myself and have fun

When you are not physically active, you are more likely to experience the following health consequences:

- Get heart disease
- Get type 2 diabetes
- Have high blood pressure
- Have high blood cholesterol
- Have a stroke

Start by doing what you can, and then look for ways to do more. If you have not been active for a while, start out slowly. After several weeks or months, build up your activities—do them longer and more often.

Walking is one way to add physical activity to your life. When you first start, walk 10 minutes a day on a few days during the first couple of weeks. Add more time and days. Walk a little longer. Try 15 minutes instead of 10 minutes. Then walk on more days a week.

Pick up the pace. Once this is easy to do, try walking faster. Keep up your brisk walking for a couple of months. You might want to add biking on the weekends for variety.

How much physical activity do you need each week?

Aerobic

- Adults should get at least 2 hours and 30 minutes each week of aerobic physical activity that requires moderate effort.

- You need to do this type of activity for at least 10 minutes at a time.

Strengthening

- Adults should also do strengthening activities at least two days a week.
- Strengthening activities include push-ups, sit-ups, and lifting weights.

Do It Your Way

- Pick an activity you like and one that fits into your life.
- Find the time that works best for you.
- Be active with friends and family. Having a support network can help you keep up with your program.
- There are many ways to build the right amount of activity into your life. Every little bit adds up and doing something is better than doing nothing.

Moderate-Level Activities

- Biking slowly
- Canoeing
- Dancing
- General gardening (raking, trimming shrubs)
- Tennis (doubles)
- Using your manual wheelchair
- Using hand cyclers—also called arm ergometers
- Walking briskly
- Water aerobics

Making Physical Activity a Part of Your Life

Congratulations! You are doing some regular physical activity each week and are ready to do more. You may be feeling the benefits of getting active, such as having fun with friends, sleeping better, and getting toned. Are you looking for ways to do more activities at a moderate level?

Here are two examples for adding more activity:

1. You can do more by being active longer each time. Walking for 30 minutes, three times a week? Go longer—walk for 50 minutes, three times a week.

2. You can do more by being active more often. Are you biking lightly three days a week for 25 minutes each time? Increase the number of days you bike. Work up to riding six days a week for 25 minutes each time.

If you have not been this active in the past, work your way up. In time, replace some moderate activities with vigorous activities that take more effort.

Activities for Stronger Muscles and Bones

Adults should do activities to strengthen muscles and bones at least two days a week. Choose activities that work all the different parts of the body—your legs, hips, back, chest, stomach, shoulders, and arms. Exercises for each muscle group should be repeated 8 to 12 times per session. Try some of these activities a couple of days a week:

- Heavy gardening (digging, shoveling)
- Lifting weights
- Push-ups on the floor or against the wall
- Sit-ups
- Working with resistance bands (long, wide rubber strips that stretch)

Some people like resistance bands because they find them easy to use and put away when they are done. Others prefer weights; you can use common grocery items, such as bags of rice, vegetable or soup cans, or bottled water.

For Best Success

- Team up with a friend. It will keep you motivated and be more fun.
- Pick activities that you like to do.
- Track your time and progress. It helps you stay on course.
- Add in more strength-building activities over time. For example, you can do sit-ups or push-ups.

Planning Your Activity for the Week

Physical activity experts say that spreading aerobic activity out over at least three days a week is best. Also, do each activity for at least 10 minutes at a time. There are many ways to fit in 2 hours and 30 minutes a week. For example, you can do 30 minutes of aerobic activity each day for five days. On the other two days, do activities to keep your muscles strong. Find ways that work well for you.

Other Ways to Add Physical Activity to Your Life

- Join a fitness group.
- Talk to your health care provider about good activities to try.
- Speak to the worksite wellness coordinator at your job.
- Visit www.healthfinder.gov and type "activity" in the search box.

Keeping It Up, Stepping It Up

Already doing 2 hours and 30 minutes a week of aerobic physical activity? Good for you! Do you want to gain even more health benefits from physical activity? Slowly add more time to your weekly routine.

Strive to double your weekly activity time. Work to be active five or more hours each week. This activity level can lower your chances of getting breast and colon cancer.

Adding More Effort

Instead of doing only moderate-level activities, replace some with vigorous aerobic activities that will make your heart beat even faster. Adding vigorous activities provides benefits in less activity time. In general, 15 minutes of vigorous activity provides the same benefits as 30 minutes of moderate activity.

Have you been walking for 30 minutes five days a week? On two days, try jogging instead of walking for 15 minutes each time. Keep on walking for 30 minutes on the other three days.

Would you like to have stronger muscles? If you have been doing strengthening activities two days a week, try adding an extra day.

You can do all moderate activities, all vigorous activities, or some of each. You should always start with moderate activities and then add vigorous activities little by little.

To mix it up, you can try 30 minutes of biking fast to and from your job three days a week. Then play softball for 60 minutes one day.

Then lift weights for two days. You've mixed vigorous aerobic activity (biking fast) with moderate aerobic activity (softball) and activities for stronger muscles (weights).

Vigorous-Level Activities

- Aerobic dance
- Basketball
- Fast dancing
- Jumping rope
- Martial arts (such as karate)
- Race walking, jogging, or running
- Riding a bike on hills or riding faster
- Soccer
- Swimming fast or swimming laps
- Tennis (singles)

You can choose moderate or vigorous activities, or a mix of both each week. You should do at least 2 hours and 30 minutes each week of aerobic physical activity at a moderate level or you should do at least 1 hour and 15 minutes each week of aerobic physical activity at a vigorous level.

You can replace some or all of your moderate activity with vigorous activity. With vigorous activities, you get similar health benefits in half the time it takes you with moderate ones.

Strive to double your weekly activity time. Work to be active five or more hours each week for even more health benefits.

For Everyone: Staying Safe and Avoiding Injury

Physical activity is generally safe for everyone. People who are physically fit have less chance of injury than those who are not fit. The health benefits you gain from being active are far greater than the chances of getting hurt. Being inactive is definitely not good for your health.

Here are some things you can do to stay safe while you are active:

- If you haven't been active in a while, start slowly and build up.
- Learn about the types and amounts of activity that are right for you.

- Choose activities that are appropriate for your fitness level.

- Build up the time you spend before switching to activities that take more effort.

- Use the right safety gear and sports equipment.

- Choose a safe place to do your activity.

- See a health care provider if you have a health problem.

Section 17.2

Exercise Opportunities in Your Daily Life

"Physical Activity in Your Daily Life," reprinted with permission from www.americanheart.org. © 2010 American Heart Association, Inc.

At Home

It's convenient, comfortable, and safe to work out at home. It allows your children to see you being active, which sets a good example for them. You can combine exercise with other activities, such as watching TV. If you buy exercise equipment, it's a one-time expense and other family members can use it. It's easy to have short bouts of activity several times a day. Try these tips:

- Do housework yourself instead of hiring someone else to do it.

- Work in the garden or mow the grass. Using a riding mower doesn't count! Rake leaves, prune, dig, and pick up trash.

- Go out for a short walk before breakfast, after dinner, or both! Start with 5–10 minutes and work up to 30 minutes.

- Walk or bike to the corner store instead of driving.

- When walking, pick up the pace from leisurely to brisk. Choose a hilly route. When watching TV, sit up instead of lying on the sofa. Better yet, spend a few minutes pedaling on your stationary bicycle while watching TV. Throw away your video remote control. Instead of asking someone to bring you a drink, get up off the couch and get it yourself.

- Stand up while talking on the telephone.

- Walk the dog.

- Park farther away at the shopping mall and walk the extra distance. Wear your walking shoes and sneak in an extra lap or two around the mall.

- Stretch to reach items in high places and squat or bend to look at items at floor level.

- Keep exercise equipment repaired and use it!

At the Office

Most of us have sedentary jobs. Work takes up a significant part of the day. What can you do to increase your physical activity during the work day? Why not...:

- Brainstorm project ideas with a co-worker while taking a walk.

- Stand while talking on the telephone.

- Walk down the hall to speak with someone rather than using the telephone.

- Take the stairs instead of the elevator. Or get off a few floors early and take the stairs the rest of the way.

- Walk while waiting for the plane at the airport.

- Stay at hotels with fitness centers or swimming pools and use them while on business trips.

- Take along a jump rope in your suitcase when you travel. Jump and do calisthenics in your hotel room.

- Participate in or start a recreation league at your company.

- Form a sports team to raise money for charity events.

- Join a fitness center or Y near your job. Work out before or after work to avoid rush-hour traffic, or drop by for a noon workout.

- Schedule exercise time on your business calendar and treat it as any other important appointment.

- Get off the bus a few blocks early and walk the rest of the way to work or home.

- Walk around your building for a break during the work day or during lunch.

At Play

Play and recreation are important for good health. Look for opportunities such as these to be active and have fun at the same time:

- Plan family outings and vacations that include physical activity (hiking, backpacking, swimming, etc.).

- See the sights in new cities by walking, jogging, or bicycling.

- Make a date with a friend to enjoy your favorite physical activities. Do them regularly.

- Play your favorite music while exercising, something that motivates you.

- Dance with someone or by yourself. Take dancing lessons. Hit the dance floor on fast numbers instead of slow ones.

- Join a recreational club that emphasizes physical activity.

- At the beach, sit and watch the waves instead of lying flat. Better yet, get up and walk, run, or fly a kite.

- When golfing, walk instead of using a cart.

- Play singles tennis or racquetball instead of doubles.

- At a picnic, join in on badminton instead of croquet.

- At the lake, rent a rowboat instead of a canoe.

Chapter 18

Make a Fitness
Plan and Stick with It

Chapter Contents

Section 18.1

Making Exercise Fun through a Personal Fitness Plan

"The Benefits of Exercise: How to Get Moving and Supercharge Your Life," by Sarah Kovatch, MFA, and Melinda Smith, MA © 2010 Helpguide.org. All rights reserved. Reprinted with permission. Helpguide provides a detailed list of references and resources for this article, including links to related Helpguide topics and information from other websites. For a complete list of these resources, including information about exercise options and maintaining motivation, go to http://www.helpguide.org/life/exercise.htm.

If you are even thinking about ways to fit exercise into your bursting-at-the-seams schedule, you are on the right track. Research indicates that modest amounts of exercise—even just 15 minutes a day—helps ease depression, enhances self-image, relieves stress, and much more. That's right, exercise makes you happy, and you don't have to be a gym rat to do it. By making "start slow" and "have fun" your mottos, you'll be well on your way to using physical activity as a tool to make you feel better every day.

The Life-Changing Benefits of Exercise

Consider "No Pain, No Gain" the old fashioned way of thinking about exercise. Current health studies prove that exercise doesn't have to hurt to be incredibly effective. Research indicates that even short low-impact intervals of exercise act as a powerful tool to supercharge your health. If you have time for a 15-minute walk with the dog, your body will thank you in many ways.

How Exercise Boosts Your Energy, Mood, and Brainpower

- **Relieves stress and anxiety.** A 20-minute bike ride won't sweep away life's troubles, but exercising regularly helps you take charge of anxiety and reduce stress. How so? Aerobic exercise releases hormones that relieve stress and give a sense of well-being.

- **Alleviates depression.** Did you know that exercise treats mild to moderate depression as effectively as anti-depression medicine? Experts believe that physical activity increases serotonin, a brain chemical that fights negative thoughts and depression.

- **Boosts mood.** Exercise also releases endorphins, powerful chemicals in our brain that energize our spirits and simply make us feel good.

- **Sharpens brainpower.** The same endorphins that make us feel better also help us concentrate and feel mentally sharp for our tasks at hand.

- **Improves self-esteem.** Regular activity is an investment in your mind, body, and soul. When it becomes habit, it can help foster a stronger sense of self-worth since you take the time to take care of yourself.

- **Energy gain.** Want less fatigue, improved sleep, and a natural shot of joi de vivre? Get moving in the fresh air. It's true that increasing your heart rate several times a week will give you more get-up-and-go. Start off with just a few minutes of exercise a day, then after a while, you'll have the energy to add a few more minutes to your routine.

With so many life-changing benefits, why does exercise often feel like such a chore, something that's simply unrealistic in your busy life—something for the young or the athletic, not for you? There are a lot of commonly-held myths about exercise that make it seem more arduous and painful than it has to be. Are any of the following myths holding you back? Let's separate facts from fiction to overcome your barriers to getting active.

Exercise Myths and Facts

Myth: Working out once a week won't help. Fact: Some exercise is always better than none. A small amount of exercise can often help you maintain or get into more of an active routine. Try to continue the minimal amount of exercise until you can gradually add more days.

Myth: No pain, no gain. If working out doesn't hurt, it isn't working. Fact: Strenuous exercise may make you breathe heavily and your muscles ache temporarily but exercise should not be painful. In fact, if it does, it may indicate an injury or muscle strain. Many great forms of exercise—like walking, swimming, or gentle stretching—get results without the discomfort.

Myth: Exercise tires you out. I'm already exhausted, and working out will just make it worse. Fact: Physical activity actually makes you more alert. Exercise releases endorphins that relax and energize your body and mind. If you are really feeling tired, promise yourself a five-minute walk. Chances are you'll be able to go five more minutes.

Myth: Exercise is not going to stop me from getting older. Why bother? Fact: While exercise cannot turn back the clock, it can make your body healthier and stronger. What's more, feeling good about yourself and your body is a huge confidence booster—it can make you feel and move as if you were younger.

Myth: You have to be in shape to work out. Fact: Even if you're starting at "ground zero," you can still work out. Exercise helps you get in shape. If you have no experience exercising, start slow with low-impact movement a few minutes each day.

Reaping the Benefits of Exercise Is Easier than You Think

Wondering just how active you should be? Current recommendations for physical activity suggest 30-minutes of moderate exercise five times a week. If that seems intimidating, don't despair. Take heart knowing that you don't have to train at the gym, sweat buckets, or run a single step to reap the benefits of physical activity.

Moderate exercise means two things:

- That you breathe a little heavier than normal, but are not out of breath (for example, you should be able to chat with your walking partner, but not easily sing a song)

- That your body feels warmer as you move, but not overheated or very sweaty

You might not have time for 30 minutes of exercise. Or maybe your body is telling you to take a break after 10 minutes. That's okay. Start with 10-minute sessions and slowly increase your time. Since exercising gives us more energy, eventually you'll feel ready for a little more. Remember, a few minutes of activity are better than none at all.

Do I Need Different Types of Exercise?

Different types of exercise benefits your health in different ways:

- **Aerobic activities** like running, biking, and swimming strengthen your heart and increase your endurance.

- **Strength training** like weight lifting or resistance training builds muscle and bone mass, improves balance, and prevents falls. It's one of the best counters to frailty in old age.

- **Flexibility** exercises like stretching and yoga help prevent injury, enhance range of motion, reduce stiffness, and limit aches and pains.

At first, just focus on getting any kind of exercise, whatever it may be. As exercising becomes your habit, try adding variety. If you keep at it, the benefits of exercise will begin to pay off.

Reaping the Benefits of Exercise: Easy Ways to Move More

Don't have 30 minutes to dedicate to yoga or a bike ride? Don't worry. Think about physical activity as a lifestyle rather than just a single task to check off. Look at your daily routine and consider ways to sneak in activity here, there, and everywhere. Need ideas? We've got them.

- **In and around your home.** Clean the house, wash the car, tend to the yard and garden, mow the lawn with a push mower, sweep up the sidewalk or patio with a broom.

- **At work and on the go.** Bike or walk to an appointment rather than drive, banish all elevators and get to know every staircase possible, briskly walk to the bus stop then get off one stop early, park at the back of the lot and walk into the store or office, take a vigorous walk during your coffee break.

- **With the family.** Jog around the soccer field during your kid's practice, make a neighborhood bike ride part of weekend routine, play tag with your children in the yard, go canoeing at a lake, walk the dog in a new place.

- **Just for fun.** Pick fruit at an orchard, boogie to music, go to the beach or take a hike, gently stretch while watching television, organize an office bowling team, take a class in martial arts, dance, or yoga.

Reaping the Benefits of Exercise: Tips for Getting Started

Exercise makes us feel great, but taking that first step towards getting active is easier said than done. If you're having trouble beginning, or just in a rut, you're not alone. Exercise obstacles are very real and we all face them.

Overcoming Obstacles to Exercise

- **Feeling uncoordinated.** Do you hide your head when the tennis ball approaches? Are you stumped at the difference between a foul ball and a free throw? Join the ranks. Don't worry if you're not sporty. Instead, find an activity like rowing, walking, or yoga that makes you feel good to be in your body.

- **Feeling bad about your body.** Are you your own worst critic? It's time to try a new way of thinking about your body. No matter what your weight, age, or fitness level, there are others like you with the goals of getting fit. Try surrounding yourself with people in your shoes. Take a class with people at a variety of fitness levels. Accomplishing even the smallest fitness goals will help you gain body confidence.

- **Feeling pressed for time.** If you work long hours, the thought of working out might seem overwhelming. If you have children, managing child care while you exercise can be a big hurdle. Just remember that physical activity helps us do everything else better. If you begin thinking of physical activity as a priority, you will soon find ways to fit small amounts in a busy schedule.

Tips for Getting Started in an Exercise Program

- **Take it slow.** The best thing you can do to ease yourself into a fitness plan is to take a moderate approach. Asking too much too soon leads to frustration and injuries. Start with what you feel comfortable, go at your own pace, and keep your expectations realistic. For example, training for a marathon when you've never run before may be a bit daunting, but you could give yourself the goal of participating in an upcoming 5k walk for charity.

- **Schedule it.** You don't go to important meetings and appointments spontaneously, you schedule them. If you have trouble fitting exercise into your schedule, consider it an important appointment with yourself and mark it on your daily agenda. Even the busiest amongst us can find a 10-minute slot to pace up and down an office staircase.

- **Expect ups and downs.** Don't be discouraged if you skip a few days or even a few weeks. It happens. Just get started again and slowly build up to your old momentum.

Safety Tips for Beginning Exercisers

If you've never exercised before, or it's been a significant amount of time since you've attempted any strenuous physical activity, keep in mind the following general health precautions:

- **Get medical clearance.** If you have special health issues such as an existing heart condition or high blood pressure, talk with your doctor or health practitioner and let him or her know your plans.

- **Stretch.** No matter what form of exercise you choose, you'll benefit from adding stretching exercises to gain flexibility and range of motion. Stretching is the best form of injury prevention for new exercisers.

- **Drink plenty of water.** Your body performs best when it's properly hydrated. Failing to drink enough water when you are exerting yourself over a prolonged period of time, especially in hot conditions, can be dangerous.

If you feel pain or discomfort while working out, stop and gently stretch. If you feel better, slowly and gently resume your workout. If you are sweating, even lightly, your heart rate has increased. In the beginning, there's no need to pressure yourself to exercise for a specific amount of time. Try exercising for even five minutes once or twice a day and gradually build up. And remember, short spurts of activity are just fine.

Reaping the Benefits of Exercise: Tips for Making Fitness Fun

You are more likely to exercise if you find enjoyable, convenient activities. Give some thought to your likes and dislikes, and consider that preferences can change over time. Here are some ways to find the right exercise for you.

Pair an Activity You Enjoy with Your Exercise

There are numerous activities that qualify as exercise. The trick is to find something you enjoy that forces you to be active. Pairing exercise with another activity makes it easier and more fun. Simple examples include:

- taking a dance or yoga class;

- blasting some favorite music and dancing with your kids;

- making a deal with yourself to watch your favorite TV shows while on the treadmill or stationary bike;

- work out with a buddy, and afterwards enjoy coffee or a movie;

- enjoying outdoor activities such as golf, playing Frisbee, or even yard work or gardening.

Make Exercise a Social Activity

Exercise can be a fun time to socialize with friends. For those who enjoy company but dislike competition, a running club, water aerobics, or dance class may be the perfect thing. Others may find that a little healthy competition keeps the workout fun and exciting. If this is your case, you might seek out tennis partners or join an adult soccer league, regular pickup basketball game, or a volleyball team.

Getting the Whole Family Involved

If you have a family, there are many ways to exercise together. The best part is that kids learn by example, and if you exercise as a family you are setting a great example for their future. Also, since physical activity promotes mental health by reducing stress, boosting self-esteem, and relieving anxiety, an active family is a happy family! Family activities might include:

- family walks in the evening if weather permits (infants or young children can ride in a stroller);

- walking the dog together;

- seasonal activities, like skiing or ice-skating in the winter and hiking, swimming, or bicycling in the summer, which can both make fun family memories and provide healthy exercise.

Reaping the Benefits of Exercise: Tips for Staying Motivated

The miracle of exercise is that if you ask your body to do a little bit more work, your body will respond. And if you continue to ask more of your body over an extended period of time, you'll vastly increase your ability to perform physical activities. Walking around the block becomes walking half a mile, and then a mile, and perhaps even several miles.

Find a few activities that will keep you healthy and strong, and stay with them for as long as they are enjoyable. If they lose their interest, it's time to shake up your routine. Add other activities or alter the way you pursue the ones that have worked so far. Relying on workout buddies for encouragement and support can also keep you going.

Make Exercise a Team Effort

For many, a workout partner is a great motivator. For example, if you won't get out of bed to swim yourself, but you would never cancel on a friend, find a swim buddy. Even if you prefer more solitary activities, exercising with a friend, in a class, or in a group helps keep you motivated and can provide positive feedback if you are getting frustrated. You might also have an easier time getting started if you participate in a more structured activity.

Other Tips for Keeping Your Exercise Program Going

- **Set goals.** Set some achievable goals that have to do with participation and effort, not necessarily how much weight you can lift, miles you can bike, or pounds you've lost. If you stumble in your efforts, regroup and immediately begin again. Decide how you'll celebrate when you arrive at your goals.

- **Be consistent.** Make your workouts habitual by exercising at the same time every day, if possible. Eventually you will get to the point where you feel worse if you don't exercise. That dull, sluggish feeling fitness buffs get when they don't work out is a strong incentive to get up and go.

- **Record your progress.** Try keeping an exercise journal of your workouts. In a matter of months, it will be fun to look back at where you began. Keeping a log also holds you accountable to your routine.

- **Keep it interesting.** Think of your exercise session as time to yourself. Enjoy that time by listening to music, chatting with friends, and varying locations. Exercise around natural beauty, new neighborhoods, and special parks. Above all, avoid workout boredom by mixing it up and trying new routines.

- **Spread the word.** Talking to others about your fitness routines will help keep motivation strong and hold you accountable to your exercise program. You'll be delighted and inspired hearing ways

211

your friends and colleagues stay active and on track. Who knows, you might even convince someone else to try to be more active.

- **Get inspired.** Read a health and fitness magazine or visit an exercise website and get inspired with photos of people being active. Sometimes reading about and looking at images of people who are healthy and fit can motivate you to move your body.

Section 18.2

Goal Setting

This section from "Motivation," "Define Your Goals," "Stay Motivated," and "Celebrate Your Achievements," *Physical Activity: Strength Training for Older Adults,* Centers for Disease Control and Prevention (www.cdc .gov), December 3, 2008.

If you want to make positive, lasting change in your life, it helps to spend some time thinking about motivation. What are your reasons for wanting to exercise? What are your personal goals? What obstacles do you anticipate and how might you overcome them? It's also a good idea to visualize your success and consider how you might celebrate your achievements.

Visualizing Your Goals

Believing in yourself—believing that you can leap barriers and achieve your goals—is the ticket to success. One of the most powerful tools for building self-confidence is visualization. This easy technique involves imagining the accomplishment of the changes or goals you're working to achieve. It is a process of "training" purely within the mind. By visualizing in detail your successful execution of each step in a given activity, you create, modify, or strengthen brain pathways that are important in coordinating your muscles for the visualized activity. This prepares you to perform the activity itself. The technique is useful in many areas of life—from avoiding anxiety during a stressful situation to performing well during competition. You may find it a powerful tool in physical fitness.

1. Identify the goal you want to visualize—for example, walking a golf course.

2. Find a comfortable place to sit and relax.

3. Eliminate all distractions—turn off the phone, television, etc.

4. Close your eyes and focus on feeling relaxed. Free your mind of intruding thoughts.

5. Now, imagine yourself on the golf course. Create a picture in your mind of the place—the sights, sounds, and smells. Imagine a perfect day, warm and sunny, with a gentle breeze. Picture yourself with your favorite golfing friends, talking and laughing. Now visualize yourself starting on your way, passing the golf carts, and setting off to walk the whole course.

6. Take a moment to feel the pleasure and excitement of achieving this goal.

7. Then imagine yourself walking from hole to hole, enjoying the sunshine, the views, the fresh air, the good company and excellent play.

8. Finally, visualize yourself finishing the course and feeling great, both physically and emotionally.

Define Your Goals

When taking on any challenge, it's a good idea to define your goals. You should identify what you want to accomplish and how you will carry out your plan. This is important when making positive change and will help you succeed.

Before starting your exercise program, set short-term and long-term goals. These goals should be SMART: specific, measurable, attainable, relevant, and time based.

For example, a specific short-term goal may be to start strength training; the long-term goal may be easing the symptoms of arthritis, improving balance, or controlling your weight. This goal is easily measurable: Have you or have you not begun the program? Indeed, this is an attainable goal, as long as your doctor approves, and this goal is certainly relevant to living a long, healthy life. Your goal should be time based: you should buy the equipment you need and set your exercise schedule within the next five days. Start the program within the following two to three days.

The goals and time frame are entirely up to you. You may want to focus your long-term goals on improving a specific health condition, such as reducing pain from arthritis, controlling diabetes, increasing bone density to help combat osteoporosis, or increasing muscle mass to help with balance or weight control. Or your goal may be to bowl or play tennis. Your success depends on setting goals that are truly important to you—and possessing a strong desire to achieve them.

Identifying Your Short-Term Goals

Identify at least two or three of your own short-term goals and write them down. Remember that each goal should be S-M-A-R-T—specific, measurable, attainable, relevant, and time based. Setting these short-term goals will help motivate you to make the program a regular part of your life.

Examples

1. I will talk to my doctor about starting this program.

2. I will buy the equipment I need and get ready to exercise within two weeks.

3. I will look at my calendar and schedule two or three 45-minute blocks of time for exercise each week.

4. I will invite my spouse/friend/family member to join me in these exercises.

Identifying Your Long-Term Goals

Identify at least two or three long-term goals and write them down. Are there activities that you want to do more easily over the long-term? Are there things that you haven't done in some time that you want to try again? Listing these goals will help you stay with the program, see your progress, and enjoy your success. (Don't forget to use the S-M-A-R-T technique.)

Examples

1. I will do each exercise two or three times each week. Within three months, I will do each exercise with five-pound weights.

2. After 12 weeks of the program, I will take the stairs instead of the elevator.

3. I will play golf.

4. I will reduce some of the pain and stiffness from arthritis.

Stay Motivated

Consider these factors that motivate people to begin and stick with their exercise program. Then identify which ones motivate you.

- **Pleasure:** People often really enjoy strength-training exercises; they find them less taxing than aerobic workouts and love the results.

- **Health and fitness benefits:** Strength training increases muscle mass and bone density. It makes you feel strong and energized, alleviates stress and depression, and gives you a better night's sleep. And it can help prevent the onset of certain chronic diseases or ease their symptoms.

- **Improvements in appearance:** Lifting weights firms the body, trims fat, and can boost metabolism by as much as 15%, which helps with weight control.

- **Social opportunities:** Exercising with friends or family gives you a chance to visit and chat while you work out.

- **Thrills:** People who start strength training later in life often find that they are willing and able to try new, exciting activities, such as parasailing, windsurfing, or kayaking.

Celebrate Your Achievements

Making any major lifestyle change can be trying. A great way to motivate yourself to keep with the program is to properly celebrate your achievements. This may be as important as setting goals and visualizing success. When you accomplish one of your short-term or long-term goals, make sure that you reward yourself well!

1. Buy yourself new workout clothes or shoes.

2. Make plans with good friends to see a movie or go hiking.

3. Go on a weekend getaway.

4. Treat yourself to a new piece of exercise equipment.

5. Plan a dinner at your favorite restaurant.

6. Get tickets to your favorite theater production or athletic event.

7. Pamper yourself with a massage, manicure, or pedicure.

8. Enroll in a class, such as ballroom dancing, yoga, or pottery making.

Chapter 19

Overcoming Barriers to Exercise

You know that physical activity is good for you. So what is stopping you from getting out there and getting at it? Maybe you think that working out is boring, joining a gym is costly, or doing one more thing during your busy day is impossible. Physical activity can be part of your daily life, and this chapter offers ideas to beat your roadblocks to getting active.

Why Should I Be Physically Active?

You may know that regular physical activity can help you control your weight. But do you know why? Physical activity burns calories. When you burn more calories than you eat each day, you will take off pounds. You can also avoid gaining weight by balancing the number of calories you burn with the number of calories you eat.

Regular physical activity may also help prevent or delay the onset of chronic diseases like type 2 diabetes, heart disease, high blood pressure, and stroke. If you have one of these health problems, physical activity may improve your condition. Regular physical activity may also increase your energy and boost your mood.

If you are a man and over age 40 or a woman and over age 50, or have a chronic health problem, talk to your health care provider before starting a vigorous physical activity program. You do not need to talk to your provider before starting an activity like walking.

"Tips to Help You Get Active," Weight-Control Information Network, National Institute of Diabetes and Digestive and Kidney Diseases (win.niddk.nih.gov), January 2009.

What Is Standing in My Way?

Personal Barriers

Barrier: Between work, family, and other demands, I am too busy to exercise.

Solutions: Make physical activity a priority. Carve out some time each week to be active, and put it on your calendar. Try waking up a half hour earlier to walk, scheduling lunchtime workouts, or taking an evening fitness class.

Build physical activity into your routine chores. Rake the yard, wash the car, or do energetic housework. That way you do what you need to do around the house and move around too.

Make family time physically active. Plan a weekend hike through a park, a family softball game, or an evening walk around the block.

Barrier: By the end of a long day, I am just too tired to work out.

Solutions: Think about the other health benefits of physical activity. Regular physical activity may help lower cholesterol and blood pressure. It may also lower your odds of having heart disease, type 2 diabetes, or cancer. Research shows that people who are overweight, active, and fit live longer than people who are not overweight but are inactive and unfit. Also, physical activity may lift your mood and increase your energy level.

Do it just for fun. Play a team sport, work in a garden, or learn a new dance. Make getting fit something fun.

Train for a charity event. You can work to help others while you work out.

Barrier: Getting on a treadmill or stationary bike is boring.

Solutions: Meet a friend for workouts. If your buddy is on the next bike or treadmill, your workout will be less boring.

Watch TV or listen to music or an audio book while you walk or pedal indoors. Check out music or audio books from your local library.

Get outside. A change in scenery can relieve your boredom. If you are riding a bike outside, be sure to wear a helmet and learn safe rules of the road. For more information about bike safety, read "Bike Safety Tips" from the American Academy of Family Physicians, available online at familydoctor.org/692.xml.

Mac in Tucson, Arizona, says, "I would take walks in the morning and see a lot of birds. Now I bring my camera along and get some great shots of birds. Taking pictures makes walking more fun. I don't get bored. I mail my pictures to my grandson and he enjoys them."

Barrier: I am afraid I will hurt myself.

Solutions: Start slowly. If you are starting a new physical activity program, go slow at the start. Even if you are doing an activity that you once did well, start up again slowly to lower your risk of injury or burnout.

Choose moderate-intensity physical activities. You are not likely to hurt yourself by walking 30 minutes per day. Doing vigorous physical activities may increase your risk for injury, but moderate-intensity physical activity carries a lower risk.

Take a class. A knowledgeable group fitness instructor should be able to teach you how to move with proper form and lower risk for injury. The instructor can watch your actions during class and let you know if you are doing things right.

Choose water workouts. Whether you swim laps or try water aerobics, working out in the water is easy on your joints and helps reduce sore muscles and injury.

Work with a personal trainer. A certified personal trainer should be able to show you how to warm up, cool down, use fitness equipment like treadmills and dumbbells, and use proper form to help lower your risk for injury. Personal training sessions may be cheap or costly, so find out about fees before making an appointment.

Barrier: I have never been into sports.

Solutions: Find a physical activity that you enjoy. You do not have to be an athlete to benefit from physical activity. Try yoga, hiking, or planting a garden.

Choose an activity that you can stick with, like walking. Just put one foot in front of the other. Use the time you spend walking to relax, talk with a friend or family member, or just enjoy the scenery.

Barrier: I do not want to spend a lot of money to join a gym or buy workout gear.

Solutions: Choose free activities. Take your children to the park to play or take a walk.

Find out if your job offers any discounts on memberships. Some companies get lower membership rates at fitness or community centers. Other companies will even pay for part of an employee's membership fee.

Check out your local recreation or community center. These centers may cost less than other gyms, fitness centers, or health clubs.

Choose physical activities that do not require any special gear. Walking requires only a pair of sturdy shoes. To dance, just turn on some music.

Barrier: I do not have anyone to watch my kids while I work out.

Solutions: Do something physically active with your kids. Kids need physical activity too. No matter what age your kids are, you can find an activity you can do together. Dance to music, take a walk, run around the park, or play basketball or soccer together.

Take turns with another parent to watch the kids. One of you minds the kids while the other one works out.

Hire a babysitter.

Look for a fitness or community center that offers child care. Centers that offer child care are becoming more popular. Cost and quality vary, so get all the information up front.

Barrier: My family and friends are not physically active.

Solutions: Do not let that stop you. Do it for yourself. Enjoy the rewards you get from working out, such as better sleep, a happier mood, more energy, and a stronger body.

Join a class or sports league where people count on you to show up. If your basketball team or dance partner counts on you, you will not want to miss a workout, even if your family and friends are not involved.

John from Chicago says, "When I moved to Chicago, I joined a basketball team that some people in my office put together. It's been great for building relationships with co-workers and getting rid of stress. We are all of different ages and abilities, but we are competitive too. It is social and fun."

Barrier: I would be embarrassed if my neighbors or friends saw me exercising.

Solutions: Ask yourself if it really matters. You are doing something positive for your health and that is something to be proud of. You may even inspire others to get physically active too.

Invite a friend or neighbor to join you. You may feel less self-conscious if you are not alone.

Go to a park, nature trail, or fitness or community center to be physically active.

Place Barriers

Barrier: My neighborhood does not have sidewalks.

Solutions: Find a safe place to walk. Instead of walking in the street, walk in a friend or family member's neighborhood that has sidewalks. Walk during your lunch break at work. Find out if you can walk at a local school track.

Work out in the yard. Do yard work or wash the car. These count as physical activity too.

Barrier: The winter is too cold/summer is too hot to be active outdoors.

Solutions: Walk around the mall. Join a mall-walking group to walk indoors year-round.

Join a fitness or community center. Find one that lets you pay only for the months or classes you want, instead of the whole year.

Exercise at home. Work out to fitness videos or DVDs. Check a different one out from the library each week for variety.

Jennifer from Detroit says, "I needed to find something to do to keep off the extra five pounds I gain every winter. I didn't feel like doing anything after work, when it is already dark. So, I started working out at a fitness center near my office at lunchtime. I do the treadmill and lift weights three days a week. It makes me feel great. Also, I don't pay for my membership during the summer, when I'd rather be outside."

Barrier: I do not feel safe exercising by myself.

Solutions: Join or start a walking group. You can enjoy added safety and company as you walk.

Take an exercise class at a nearby fitness or community center.

Work out at home. You don't need a lot of space. Turn on the radio and dance or follow along with a fitness show on TV.

Health Barriers

Barrier: I have a health problem (diabetes, heart disease, asthma, arthritis) that I do not want to make worse.

Solutions: Talk with your health care professional. Most health problems are helped by physical activity. Find out what physical activities you can safely do and follow advice about length and intensity of workouts.

Start slowly. Take it easy at first and see how you feel before trying more challenging workouts. Stop if you feel out of breath, dizzy, faint, or nauseated, or if you have pain.

Barrier: I have an injury and do not know what physical activities, if any, I can do.

Solutions: Talk with your health care professional. Ask your doctor or physical therapist about what physical activities you can safely perform. Follow advice about length and intensity of workouts.

Start slowly. Take it easy at first and see how you feel before trying more challenging workouts. Stop if you feel pain.

Work with a personal trainer. A knowledgeable personal trainer should be able to help you design a fitness plan around your injury.

What Can I Do to Break through My Roadblocks?

What are the top two or three roadblocks to physical activity that you face? What can you do to break through these barriers? Write down a list of the barriers you face and solutions you can use to overcome them.

You have thought about ways to beat your roadblocks to physical activity. Now, create your roadmap for adding physical activity to your life by following these three steps:

1. **Know your goal.** Set up short-term goals, like walking 10 minutes a day, three days a week. Once you are comfortable, try to do more. Try 15 minutes instead of 10 minutes. Then walk on more days a week while adding more minutes to your walk. You can try different activities too. To add variety, you can do low-impact aerobics or water aerobics for 30 minutes, two days a week. Then walk on a treadmill or outdoors for 30 minutes, one day a week. Then do yoga or lift weights for two days.

   Track your progress by writing down your goals and what you have done each day, including the type of activity and how long you spent doing it. Seeing your progress in black and white can help keep you motivated.

2. **See your health care provider if necessary.** If you are a man and over age 40 or a woman and over age 50, or have a chronic health problem such as heart disease, high blood pressure, diabetes, osteoporosis, or obesity, talk to your health care provider before starting a vigorous physical activity program. You do not need to talk to your provider before starting an activity like walking.

3. **Answer questions about how physical activity will fit into your life.** Think about answers to the following four questions. You can write your answers on a sheet of paper. Your answers will be your roadmap to your physical activity program.

   - **What physical activities will you do?** List the activities you would like to do, such as walking, energetic yard work or housework, joining a sports league, exercising with a video, dancing, swimming, bicycling, or taking a class at a fitness or community center. Think about sports or other activities that you enjoyed doing when you were younger. Could you enjoy one of these activities again?

- **When will you be physically active?** List the days and times you could do each activity on your list, such as first thing in the morning, during lunch break from work, after dinner, or on Saturday afternoon. Look at your calendar or planner to find the days and times that work best.

- **Who will remind you to get off the couch?** List the people—your spouse, sibling, parent, or friends—who can support your efforts to become physically active. Give them ideas about how they could be supportive, like offering encouraging words, watching your kids, or working out with you.

- **When will you start your physical activity program?** Set a date when you will start getting active. The date might be the first meeting of an exercise class you have signed up for, or a date you will meet a friend for a walk. Write the date on your calendar. Then stick to it. Before you know it, physical activity will become a regular part of your life.

Chapter 20

Measuring Physical Activity Intensity and Physical Fitness

Chapter Contents

Section 20.1

Measuring Physical Activity Intensity

"Measuring Physical Activity Intensity" and "Perceived Exertion," Centers For Disease Control and Prevention (www.cdc.gov), February 19, 2009.

Measuring Physical Activity Intensity

Here are some ways to understand and measure the intensity of aerobic activity: relative intensity and absolute intensity.

Relative Intensity

The level of effort required by a person to do an activity. When using relative intensity, people pay attention to how physical activity affects their heart rate and breathing.

The talk test is a simple way to measure relative intensity. As a rule of thumb, if you're doing moderate-intensity activity you can talk, but not sing, during the activity. If you're doing vigorous-intensity activity, you will not be able to say more than a few words without pausing for a breath.

Absolute Intensity

The amount of energy used by the body per minute of activity. The following list provides examples of activities classified as moderate intensity or vigorous intensity based upon the amount of energy used by the body while doing the activity.

Moderate Intensity

- Walking briskly (3 miles per hour or faster, but not race walking)
- Water aerobics
- Bicycling slower than 10 miles per hour
- Tennis (doubles)

- Ballroom dancing

- General gardening

Vigorous Intensity

- Race walking, jogging, or running

- Swimming laps

- Tennis (singles)

- Aerobic dancing

- Bicycling 10 miles per hour or faster

- Jumping rope

- Heavy gardening (continuous digging or hoeing)

- Hiking uphill or with a heavy backpack

Perceived Exertion (Borg Rating of Perceived Exertion Scale)

The Borg Rating of Perceived Exertion (RPE) is a way of measuring physical activity intensity level. Perceived exertion is how hard you feel like your body is working. It is based on the physical sensations a person experiences during physical activity, including increased heart rate, increased respiration or breathing rate, increased sweating, and muscle fatigue. Although this is a subjective measure, a person's exertion rating may provide a fairly good estimate of the actual heart rate during physical activity.*

Practitioners generally agree that perceived exertion ratings between 12 to 14 on the Borg Scale suggest that physical activity is being performed at a moderate level of intensity. During activity, use the Borg Scale to assign numbers to how you feel (see the following instructions). Self-monitoring how hard your body is working can help you adjust the intensity of the activity by speeding up or slowing down your movements.

Through experience of monitoring how your body feels, it will become easier to know when to adjust your intensity. For example, a walker who wants to engage in moderate-intensity activity would aim for a Borg Scale level of "somewhat hard" (12–14). If he describes his muscle fatigue and breathing as "very light" (9 on the Borg Scale), he would want to increase his intensity. On the other hand, if he felt his exertion was "extremely hard" (19 on the Borg Scale), he would need to slow down his movements to achieve the moderate-intensity range.

Instructions for Borg Rating of Perceived Exertion (RPE) Scale

While doing physical activity, we want you to rate your perception of exertion. This feeling should reflect how heavy and strenuous the exercise feels to you, combining all sensations and feelings of physical stress, effort, and fatigue. Do not concern yourself with any one factor such as leg pain or shortness of breath, but try to focus on your total feeling of exertion.

Look at the following rating scale while you are engaging in an activity; it ranges from 6 to 20, where 6 means "no exertion at all" and 20 means "maximal exertion." Choose the number that best describes your level of exertion. This will give you a good idea of the intensity level of your activity, and you can use this information to speed up or slow down your movements to reach your desired range.

Try to appraise your feeling of exertion as honestly as possible, without thinking about what the actual physical load is. Your own feeling of effort and exertion is important, not how it compares to other people's. Look at the scales and the expressions and then give a number.

6	No exertion at all
7	
	Extremely light (7.5)
8	
9	Very light
10	
11	Light
12	
13	Somewhat hard
14	
15	Hard (heavy)
16	
17	Very hard
18	
19	Extremely hard
20	Maximal exertion

9 corresponds to "very light" exercise. For a healthy person, it is like walking slowly at his or her own pace for some minutes.

13 on the scale is "somewhat hard" exercise, but it still feels okay to continue.

17, "very hard," is very strenuous. A healthy person can still go on, but he or she really has to push him- or herself. It feels very heavy, and the person is very tired.

19 on the scale is an extremely strenuous exercise level. For most people this is the most strenuous exercise they have ever experienced.

Borg RPE scale © Gunnar Borg, 1970, 1985, 1994, 1998.

*A high correlation exists between a person's perceived exertion rating times 10 and the actual heart rate during physical activity, so a person's exertion rating may provide a fairly good estimate of the actual heart rate during activity. For example, if a person's RPE is 12, then 12 x 10 = 120, so the heart rate should be approximately 120 beats per minute. Note that this calculation is only an approximation of heart rate, and the actual heart rate can vary quite a bit depending on age and physical condition. The Borg Rating of Perceived Exertion is also the preferred method to assess intensity among those individuals who take medications that affect heart rate or pulse.

Section 20.2

Resting and Target Heart Rates

"Resting Heart Rate" and "Target Heart Rates," reprinted with permission from www.americanheart.org. © 2010 American Heart Association, Inc.

Resting Heart Rate

What is resting heart rate?

This is a person's heart rate at rest. The best time to find out your resting heart rate is in the morning, after a good night's sleep, and before you get out of bed.

The heart beats about 60 to 80 times a minute when we're at rest. Resting heart rate usually rises with age, and it's generally lower in physically fit people. Resting heart rate is used to determine one's training target heart rate. Athletes sometimes measure their resting heart rate as one way to find out if they're overtrained. The heart rate adapts to changes in the body's need for oxygen, such as during exercise or sleep.

Target Heart Rates

AHA recommendation: Health professionals know the importance of proper pacing during exercise. To receive the benefits of physical activity, it's important not to tire too quickly. Pacing yourself is especially important if you've been inactive.

Target heart rates let you measure your initial fitness level and monitor your progress in a fitness program. This approach requires measuring your pulse periodically as you exercise and staying within 50 to 85% of your maximum heart rate. This range is called your target heart rate.

What is an alternative to target heart rates?

Some people can't measure their pulse or don't want to take their pulse when exercising. If this is true for you, try using a "conversational pace" to monitor your efforts during moderate activities like walking. If you can talk and walk at the same time, you aren't working too hard. If you can sing and maintain your level of effort, you're probably not working hard enough. If you get out of breath quickly, you're probably working too hard—especially if you have to stop and catch your breath.

When should I use the target heart rate?

If you participate in more-vigorous activities like brisk walking and jogging, the "conversational pace" approach may not work. Then try using the target heart rate. It works for many people, and it's a good way for health professionals to monitor your progress.

The Table 20.1 shows estimated target heart rates for different ages. Look for the age category closest to yours, then read across to find your target heart rate.

How should I pace myself?

When starting an exercise program, aim at the lowest part of your target zone (50%) during the first few weeks. Gradually build up to the higher part of your target zone (75%). After six months or more of regular exercise, you may be able to exercise comfortably at up to 85% of your maximum heart rate. However, you don't have to exercise that hard to stay in shape.

Table 20.1. Estimated Target Heart Rates

Age	Target HR Zone 50–85%	Average Maximum Heart Rate 100%
20 years	100–170 beats per minute	200 beats per minute
25 years	98–166 beats per minute	195 beats per minute
30 years	95–162 beats per minute	190 beats per minute
35 years	93–157 beats per minute	185 beats per minute
40 years	90–153 beats per minute	180 beats per minute
45 years	88–149 beats per minute	175 beats per minute
50 years	85–145 beats per minute	170 beats per minute
55 years	83–140 beats per minute	165 beats per minute
60 years	80–136 beats per minute	160 beats per minute
65 years	78–132 beats per minute	155 beats per minute
70 years	75–128 beats per minute	150 beats per minute

Your maximum heart rate is about 220 minus your age. The figures in the table are averages, so use them as general guidelines.
Note: A few high blood pressure medications lower the maximum heart rate and thus the target zone rate. If you're taking such medicine, call your physician to find out if you need to use a lower target heart rate.

Section 20.3

Calories Burned per Hour

"Calories Burned per Hour," reprinted with permission from the Wisconsin Department of Health and Family Services (www.dhfs.wisconsin.gov), 2005. Reviewed by David A. Cooke, MD, FACP, May 2010.

Find the activity you participate in and use the column closest to your body weight (130, 155, or 190 pounds) to estimate calories burned per hour.

Activity	Calories burned based on body weight		
	130 lbs	155 lbs	190 lbs
Aerobics, general	354	422	518
Aerobics, high impact	413	493	604
Aerobics, low impact	295	352	431
Archery (nonhunting)	207	246	302
Automobile repair	177	211	259
Backpacking, general	413	493	604
Badminton, competitive	413	493	604
Badminton, social, general	266	317	388
Basketball, game	472	563	690
Basketball, nongame, general	354	422	518
Basketball, officiating	413	493	604
Basketball, shooting baskets	266	317	388
Basketball, wheelchair	384	457	561
Bicycling, <10 mph, leisure	236	281	345
Bicycling, >20 mph, racing	944	1,126	1,380
Bicycling, 10–11.9 mph, light effort	354	422	518
Bicycling, 12–13.9 mph, moderate effort	472	563	690

Activity	Calories burned based on body weight		
Bicycling, 14–15.9 mph, vigorous effort	590	704	863
Bicycling, 16–19 mph, very fast, racing	708	844	1,035
Bicycling, BMX or mountain	502	598	733
Bicycling, stationary, general	295	352	431
Bicycling, stationary, light effort	325	387	474
Bicycling, stationary, moderate effort	413	493	604
Bicycling, stationary, very light effort	177	211	259
Bicycling, stationary, very vigorous effort	738	880	1,078
Bicycling, stationary, vigorous effort	620	739	906
Billiards	148	176	216
Bowling	177	211	259
Boxing, in ring, general	708	844	1,035
Boxing, punching bag	354	422	518
Boxing, sparring	531	633	776
Broomball	413	493	604
Calisthenics (push-ups, sit-ups), vigorous effort	472	563	690
Calisthenics, home, light/moderate effort	266	317	388
Canoeing, on camping trip	236	281	345
Canoeing, rowing, >6 mph, vigorous effort	708	844	1,035
Canoeing, rowing, crewing, competition	708	844	1,035
Canoeing, rowing, light effort	177	211	259
Canoeing, rowing, moderate effort	413	493	604
Carpentry, general	207	246	302
Carrying heavy loads, such as bricks	472	563	690
Child care: sitting/kneeling—dressing, feeding	177	211	259
Child care: standing—dressing, feeding	207	246	302
Circuit training, general	472	563	690
Cleaning, heavy, vigorous effort	266	317	388
Cleaning, house, general	207	246	302
Cleaning, light, moderate effort	148	176	216
Coaching: football, soccer, basketball, etc.	236	281	345
Construction, outside, remodeling	325	387	474

Activity	Calories burned based on body weight		
Cooking or food preparation	148	176	216
Cricket (batting, bowling)	295	352	431
Croquet	148	176	216
Curling	236	281	345
Dancing, aerobic, ballet or modern, twist	354	422	518
Dancing, ballroom, fast	325	387	474
Dancing, ballroom, slow	177	211	259
Dancing, general	266	317	388
Darts, wall or lawn	148	176	216
Diving, springboard or platform	177	211	259
Electrical work, plumbing	207	246	302
Farming, baling hay, cleaning barn	472	563	690
Farming, milking by hand	177	211	259
Farming, shoveling grain	325	387	474
Fencing	354	422	518
Fishing from boat, sitting	148	176	216
Fishing from river bank, standing	207	246	302
Fishing in stream, in waders	354	422	518
Fishing, general	236	281	345
Fishing, ice, sitting	118	141	173
Football or baseball, playing catch	148	176	216
Football, competitive	531	633	776
Football, touch, flag, general	472	563	690
Frisbee playing, general	177	211	259
Frisbee, ultimate	207	246	302
Gardening, general	295	352	431
Golf, carrying clubs	325	387	474
Golf, general	236	281	345
Golf, miniature or driving range	177	211	259
Golf, pulling clubs	295	352	431
Golf, using power cart	207	246	302
Gymnastics, general	236	281	345
Hacky sack	236	281	345

Activity	Calories burned based on body weight		
Handball, general	708	844	1,035
Handball, team	472	563	690
Health club exercise, general	325	387	474
Hiking, cross country	354	422	518
Hockey, field	472	563	690
Hockey, ice	472	563	690
Horse grooming	354	422	518
Horse racing, galloping	472	563	690
Horseback riding, general	236	281	345
Horseback riding, trotting	384	457	561
Horseback riding, walking	148	176	216
Hunting, general	295	352	431
Jai alai	708	844	1,035
Jogging, general	413	493	604
Judo, karate, kick boxing, tae kwon do	590	704	863
Kayaking	295	352	431
Kickball	413	493	604
Lacrosse	472	563	690
Marching band, playing instrument (walking)	236	281	345
Marching, rapidly, military	384	457	561
Motocross	236	281	345
Moving furniture, household	354	422	518
Moving household items, boxes, upstairs	531	633	776
Moving household items, carrying boxes	413	493	604
Mowing lawn, general	325	387	474
Mowing lawn, riding mower	148	176	216
Music playing, cello, flute, horn, woodwind	118	141	173
Music playing, drums	236	281	345
Music playing, guitar, classical, folk (sitting)	118	141	173
Music playing, guitar, rock 'n' roll band (standing)	177	211	259
Music playing, piano, organ, violin, trumpet	148	176	216
Paddleboat	236	281	345

Activity	Calories burned based on body weight		
Painting, papering, plastering, scraping	266	317	388
Polo	472	563	690
Pushing or pulling stroller with child	148	176	216
Race walking	384	457	561
Racquetball, casual, general	413	493	604
Racquetball, competitive	590	704	863
Raking lawn	236	281	345
Rock climbing, ascending rock	649	774	949
Rock climbing, rappelling	472	563	690
Rope jumping, fast	708	844	1,035
Rope jumping, moderate, general	590	704	863
Rope jumping, slow	472	563	690
Rowing, stationary, light effort	561	669	819
Rowing, stationary, moderate effort	413	493	604
Rowing, stationary, very vigorous effort	708	844	1,035
Rowing, stationary, vigorous effort	502	598	733
Rugby	590	704	863
Running, 10 mph (6 min mile)	944	1,126	1,380
Running, 10.9 mph (5.5 min mile)	1,062	1,267	1,553
Running, 5 mph (12 min mile)	472	563	690
Running, 5.2 mph (11.5 min mile)	531	633	776
Running, 6 mph (10 min mile)	590	704	863
Running, 6.7 mph (9 min mile)	649	774	949
Running, 7 mph (8.5 min mile)	679	809	992
Running, 7.5 mph (8 min mile)	738	880	1,078
Running, 8 mph (7.5 min mile)	797	950	1,165
Running, 8.6 mph (7 min mile)	826	985	1,208
Running, 9 mph (6.5 min mile)	885	1,056	1,294
Running, cross country	531	633	776
Running, general	472	563	690
Running, in place	472	563	690
Running, on a track, team practice	590	704	863
Running, stairs, up	885	1,056	1,294

Activity	Calories burned based on body weight		
Running, training, pushing wheelchair	472	563	690
Running, wheeling, general	177	211	259
Sailing, boat/board, windsurfing, general	177	211	259
Sailing, in competition	295	352	431
Scrubbing floors, on hands and knees	325	387	474
Shoveling snow, by hand	354	422	518
Shuffleboard, lawn bowling	177	211	259
Sitting—playing with children—light	148	176	216
Skateboarding	295	352	431
Skating, ice, 9 mph or less	325	387	474
Skating, ice, general	413	493	604
Skating, ice, rapidly, >9 mph	531	633	776
Skating, ice, speed, competitive	885	1,056	1,294
Skating, roller	413	493	604
Ski jumping (climb up carrying skis)	413	493	604
Ski machine, general	561	669	819
Skiing, cross-country, >8.0 mph, racing	826	985	1,208
Skiing, cross-country, moderate effort	472	563	690
Skiing, cross-country, slow or light effort	413	493	604
Skiing, cross-country, uphill, maximum effort	974	1,161	1,423
Skiing, cross-country, vigorous effort	531	633	776
Skiing, downhill, light effort	295	352	431
Skiing, downhill, moderate effort	354	422	518
Skiing, downhill, vigorous effort, racing	472	563	690
Skiing, snow, general	413	493	604
Skiing, water	354	422	518
Skimobiling, water	413	493	604
Skin diving, scuba diving, general	413	493	604
Sledding, tobogganing, bobsledding, luge	413	493	604
Snorkeling	295	352	431
Snow shoeing	472	563	690
Snowmobiling	207	246	302
Soccer, casual, general	413	493	604

Activity	Calories burned based on body weight		
Soccer, competitive	590	704	863
Softball or baseball, fast or slow pitch	295	352	431
Softball, officiating	354	422	518
Squash	708	844	1,035
Stair-treadmill ergometer, general	354	422	518
Standing—packing/unpacking boxes	207	246	302
Stretching, Hatha yoga	236	281	345
Surfing, body or board	177	211	259
Sweeping garage, sidewalk	236	281	345
Swimming laps, freestyle, fast, vigorous effort	590	704	863
Swimming laps, freestyle, light/moderate effort	472	563	690
Swimming, backstroke, general	472	563	690
Swimming, breaststroke, general	590	704	863
Swimming, butterfly, general	649	774	949
Swimming, leisurely, general	354	422	518
Swimming, sidestroke, general	472	563	690
Swimming, synchronized	472	563	690
Swimming, treading water, fast/vigorous	590	704	863
Swimming, treading water, moderate effort	236	281	345
Table tennis, ping pong	236	281	345
Tai chi	236	281	345
Teaching aerobics class	354	422	518
Tennis, doubles	354	422	518
Tennis, general	413	493	604
Tennis, singles	472	563	690
Unicycling	295	352	431
Volleyball, beach	472	563	690
Volleyball, competitive, in gymnasium	236	281	345
Volleyball, noncompetitive, 6–9 member team	177	211	259
Walk/run—playing with children—moderate	236	281	345
Walk/run—playing with children—vigorous	295	352	431
Walking, 2.0 mph, slow pace	148	176	216

Activity	Calories burned based on body weight		
Walking, 3.0 mph, moderate pace, walking dog	207	246	302
Walking, 3.5 mph, uphill	354	422	518
Walking, 4.0 mph, very brisk pace	236	281	345
Walking, carrying infant or 15-lb load	207	246	302
Walking, grass track	295	352	431
Walking, up stairs	472	563	690
Walking, using crutches	236	281	345
Wallyball, general	413	493	604
Water aerobics, water calisthenics	236	281	345
Water polo	590	704	863
Water volleyball	177	211	259
Weight lifting or body building, vigorous effort	354	422	518
Weight lifting, light or moderate effort	177	211	259
Whitewater rafting, kayaking, or canoeing	295	352	431

Section 20.4

Physical Activity Chart

"Monthly Physical Activity Sheet," reprinted with permission from the Wisconsin Department of Health and Family Services (www.dhfs.wisconsin.gov), December 2005.

To track your physical activity for a month, copy the chart shown in Figure 20.1 and track the points for activities you participate in during that month. Use the points-to-calories conversion based on your body weight to determine your monthly calorie expenditure related to your physical activities.

Name _____

Date	Activity	Length of Time	Points	Sub-total
1				
2				
3				
4				
5				
6				
7				
8				
9				
10				
11				
12				
13				
14				
15				
16				
17				
18				
19				
20				
21				
22				
23				
24				
25				
26				
27				
28				
29				
30				
31				

Total Points [   ]

Multiply by calories/point (see weight chart) x _____

Total calories burned this month [   ]

Figure 20.1. *Monthly physical activity sheet.*

1 point/4 minutes

Bicycling >16 mph
Handball, Squash, Racquetball
Rowing—vigorous
Running >7 mph
Cross-country skiing—racing

1 point/5 minutes

Boxing/sparring
Football
Martial arts
Rope jumping
Running, 6 mph
Soccer—vigorous
Swimming—vigorous
Cross-country skiing—vigorous

1 point/6 minutes

Basketball—game
Bicycling, 12–15 mph
Bicycling, stationary
Calisthenics—vigorous
Carrying heavy loads
Circuit training
Hockey
Rock climbing
Running, 5 mph
Cross-country skiing—moderate
Snow shoeing
Swimming—moderate
Tennis, singles
Volleyball, beach
Walking up stairs

1 point/10 minutes

Aerobic—general
Backpacking/hiking
Bicycling, 10–12 mph
Canoeing—moderate
Dancing—aerobic, fast
Jet-skiing, water
Jogging <5 mph
Moving boxes
Rowing—moderate
Shoveling snow
Skating—vigorous
Skiing—moderate
Sledding
Soccer—moderate
Swimming—leisure
Tennis—doubles
Weight lifting—vigorous
Walking—brisk, 4 mph

1 point/12 minutes

Badminton
Basketball—shooting
Construction/remodel
Dancing
Golf—without cart
Health club—general
Housework—vigorous
Hunting
Kayaking
Mowing lawn—walking
Play with kids—vigorous
Skate/roller blade
Softball or baseball
Volleyball—vigorous
Yard work, raking, etc.

Approximate calories burned during activity

1 point = 40 calories for a 105-pound person
1 point = 50 calories for a 130-pound person
1 point = 60 calories for a 155-pound person
1 point = 70 calories for a 180-pound person
1 point = 80 calories for a 210-pound person
1 point = 90 calories for a 235-pound person
1 point = 100 calories for a 260-pound person
Resting metabolic rate = about 1 to 2 points/hour

1 point/15 minutes

Archery
Auto repair
Bicycling <10 mph
Bowling
Canoeing—light
Golf—using motor cart
Home repair—carpentry, plumbing, etc.
Horseback riding
Housework—cleaning
Music—vigorous, drums
Play with kids—moderate
Sailing/sail board
Snowmobiling
Stretching, yoga
Table tennis
Walking—moderate, 3 mph
Water aerobics
Weight lift—moderate

1 point/20 minutes

Billiards/pool
Cooking
Fishing
Mowing lawn—riding
Music playing—general
Playing catch
Play with kids—light
Walking—slow, 2 mph
Yard games—croquet, Frisbee, darts, etc.

Section 20.5

Body Mass Index (BMI)

"About BMI for Adults," Centers for Disease Control and Prevention
(www.cdc.gov), July 27, 2009.

What is BMI?

Body Mass Index (BMI) is a number calculated from a person's weight and height. BMI is a fairly reliable indicator of body fatness for most people. BMI does not measure body fat directly, but research has shown that BMI correlates to direct measures of body fat, such as underwater weighing and dual energy x-ray absorptiometry (DXA).[1,2] BMI can be considered an alternative for direct measures of body fat. Additionally, BMI is an inexpensive and easy-to-perform method of screening for weight categories that may lead to health problems.

How is BMI used?

BMI is used as a screening tool to identify possible weight problems for adults. However, BMI is not a diagnostic tool. For example, a person may have a high BMI. However, to determine if excess weight is a health risk, a health care provider would need to perform further assessments. These assessments might include skinfold thickness measurements, evaluations of diet, physical activity, family history, and other appropriate health screenings.

Why does CDC [Centers for Disease Control and Prevention] use BMI to measure overweight and obesity?

Calculating BMI is one of the best methods for population assessment of overweight and obesity. Because calculation requires only height and weight, it is inexpensive and easy to use for clinicians and for the general public. The use of BMI allows people to compare their own weight status to that of the general population.

What are some of the other ways to measure obesity? Why doesn't CDC use those to determine overweight and obesity among the general public?

Other methods to measure body fatness include skinfold thickness measurements (with calipers), underwater weighing, bioelectrical impedance, dual-energy x-ray absorptiometry (DXA), and isotope dilution. However, these methods are not always readily available, and they are either expensive or need highly trained personnel. Furthermore, many of these methods can be difficult to standardize across observers or machines, complicating comparisons across studies and time periods.

How is BMI calculated and interpreted?

BMI is calculated the same way for both adults and children. The calculation is based on the following formulas:

Measurement Units	Formula and Calculation
Kilograms and meters (or centimeters)	**Formula: weight (kg) / [height (m)]^2**

With the metric system, the formula for BMI is weight in kilograms (kg) divided by height in meters (m) squared. Since height is commonly measured in centimeters (cm), divide height in centimeters by 100 to obtain height in meters.

Example:

Weight = 68 kg, Height = 165 cm (1.65 m)

Calculation: $68 \div (1.65)^2 = 24.98$

Pounds and inches   Formula: weight (lb) / [height (in)]² x 703

Calculate BMI by dividing weight in pounds (lbs) by height in inches (in) squared and multiplying by a conversion factor of 703.

Example:

Weight = 150 lbs, Height = 5'5" (65")

Calculation: [150 ÷ (65)²] x 703 = 24.96

For adults 20 years old and older, BMI is interpreted using standard weight status categories that are the same for all ages and for both men and women. For children and teens, on the other hand, the interpretation of BMI is both age and sex specific. For more information about interpretation for children and teens, visit the Child and Teen BMI Calculator (at apps.nccd.cdc.gov/dnpabmi).

The standard weight status categories associated with BMI ranges for adults are shown here:

BMI:	Weight Status
Below 18.5:	Underweight
18.5–24.9:	Normal
25.0–29.9:	Overweight
30.0 and Above:	Obese

For example, here are the weight ranges, the corresponding BMI ranges, and the weight status categories for a sample height:

Height	Weight Range	BMI	Weight Status
5' 9"	124 lbs or less	Below 18.5	Underweight
	125 lbs to 168 lbs	18.5 to 24.9	Normal
	169 lbs to 202 lbs	25.0 to 29.9	Overweight
	203 lbs or more	30 or higher	Obese

How reliable is BMI as an indicator of body fatness?

The correlation between the BMI number and body fatness is fairly strong; however the correlation varies by sex, race, and age. These variations include the following examples: [3, 4]

- At the same BMI, women tend to have more body fat than men.

- At the same BMI, older people, on average, tend to have more body fat than younger adults.

- Highly trained athletes may have a high BMI because of increased muscularity rather than increased body fatness.

It is also important to remember that BMI is only one factor related to risk for disease. For assessing someone's likelihood of developing overweight- or obesity-related diseases, the National Heart, Lung, and Blood Institute guidelines recommend looking at two other predictors:

- The individual's waist circumference (because abdominal fat is a predictor of risk for obesity-related diseases)

- Other risk factors the individual has for diseases and conditions associated with obesity (for example, high blood pressure or physical inactivity)

If an athlete or other person with a lot of muscle has a BMI over 25, is that person still considered to be overweight?

According to the BMI weight status categories, anyone with a BMI over 25 would be classified as overweight and anyone with a BMI over 30 would be classified as obese.

It is important to remember, however, that BMI is not a direct measure of body fatness and that BMI is calculated from an individual's weight, which includes both muscle and fat. As a result, some individuals may have a high BMI but not have a high percentage of body fat. For example, highly trained athletes may have a high BMI because of increased muscularity rather than increased body fatness. Although some people with a BMI in the overweight range (from 25.0 to 29.9) may not have excess body fatness, most people with a BMI in the obese range (equal to or greater than 30) will have increased levels of body fatness.

It is also important to remember that weight is only one factor related to risk for disease. If you have questions or concerns about the appropriateness of your weight, you should discuss them with your health care provider.

What are the health consequences of overweight and obesity for adults?

The BMI ranges are based on the relationship between body weight and disease and death.[5] Overweight and obese individuals are at increased risk for many diseases and health conditions, including the following:[6]

- Hypertension
- Dyslipidemia (for example, high LDL cholesterol, low HDL cholesterol, or high levels of triglycerides)
- Type 2 diabetes
- Coronary heart disease
- Stroke
- Gallbladder disease
- Osteoarthritis
- Sleep apnea and respiratory problems
- Some cancers (endometrial, breast, and colon)

For more information about these and other health problems associated with overweight and obesity, visit "Clinical Guidelines on the Identification, Evaluation, and Treatment of Overweight and Obesity in Adults" (at www.nhlbi.nih.gov/guidelines/obesity/ob_home.htm).

Is BMI interpreted the same way for children and teens as it is for adults?

Although the BMI number is calculated the same way for children and adults, the criteria used to interpret the meaning of the BMI number for children and teens are different from those used for adults. For children and teens, BMI age- and sex-specific percentiles are used for two reasons:

- The amount of body fat changes with age.
- The amount of body fat differs between girls and boys.

Because of these factors, the interpretation of BMI is both age and sex specific for children and teens. The CDC BMI-for-age growth charts take into account these differences and allow translation of a BMI number into a percentile for a child's sex and age.

For adults, on the other hand, BMI is interpreted through categories that are not dependent on sex or age.

References

1. Mei Z, Grummer-Strawn LM, Pietrobelli A, Goulding A, Goran MI, Dietz WH. Validity of body mass index compared with

other body-composition screening indexes for the assessment of body fatness in children and adolescents. *American Journal of Clinical Nutrition* 2002;7597–985.

2. Garrow JS and Webster J. Quetelet's index (W/H2) as a measure of fatness. *International Journal of Obesity* 1985;9:147–153.

3. Prentice AM and Jebb SA. Beyond Body Mass Index. *Obesity Reviews.* 2001 August; 2(3):141–147.

4. Gallagher D, et al. How useful is BMI for comparison of body fatness across age, sex, and ethnic groups? *American Journal of Epidemiology* 1996;143:228–239.

5. World Health Organization. *Physical status: The use and interpretation of anthropometry.* Geneva, Switzerland: World Health Organization 1995. WHO Technical Report Series.

6. National Heart, Lung, and Blood Institute. *Clinical guidelines on the identification, evaluation, and treatment of overweight and obesity in adults.* http://www.nhlbi.nih.gov/guidelines/obesity/ob_home.htm.

Chapter 21

Choosing Physical Fitness Partners

Chapter Contents

Section 21.1

Choosing a Health Club

What makes a fitness facility a place in which you have a safe, effective, fun exercise experience and also feel cared for?

A combination of the staff, the programs, the members, and physical environment work together to compose your ideal facility.

Most facilities will have people to give you a tour. Ask to see the entire facility. Observe the facility closely, ask questions, and use this section to compare two facilities that interest you.

Twenty-Two Points to Help You Choose a Quality Fitness Facility

1. Before you are allowed to work out, does someone at the facility give you a health screening form to fill out, ask you questions about your health (past or present injuries or illnesses), or find out if you are under a doctor's care?

A health screening will inform the instructors, trainers, and management of any injuries, illnesses, or limitations that you may have. It will help staff members evaluate your capabilities.

2. Does the facility have adequate room for the number of members who want to work out?

This is especially a concern if you plan to exercise during peak times (usually before work, during lunch, and after work).

3. Does the aerobics room have a floor that provides shock absorption?

Ask if the facility has installed a floor that was designed to reduce shock. The greater the shock absorption, the more protective the floor is, because shock absorption reduces impact forces. This can help prevent injuries.

4. Does the facility have the type of weight training and cardiovascular equipment you want to use?

Do you want to use weight machines or free weights? Do you like cycles or treadmills? Look for the types of equipment that interest you.

5. Is all equipment properly cleaned and maintained so that it is in working order?

You want to make sure that the equipment is maintained so that it will work when you want to use it. Clean equipment promotes good hygiene.

6. Are there signs or posters near the equipment that explain how to use it?

In the event that a staff member is not available to help you, signs near the equipment can help you figure out how to use it.

7. Is the facility kept at a comfortable temperature, and does it have good air circulation, either through the use of fans or through some kind of air circulation system?

You want to be comfortable when you exercise. Since you will probably sweat, you don't want to overheat.

8. Does the facility have established emergency procedures for the staff, and does it have first aid equipment and a trained person on-site to administer treatments?

In case of an injury, accident, or emergency, you want to make sure that someone can assist you immediately to forestall further problems.

9. Does the facility carry liability insurance?

If you get injured through negligence on the facility's part, it is important that the club have liability insurance.

10. Will you be allowed to try out the facility before committing to a membership?

Ask if you can obtain a free day pass to see if you like and feel comfortable in the facility.

11. Does the facility thoroughly explain payment methods, policies, and cancellation procedures?

You should find out how you will pay for membership and what will happen if you move or need to cancel your membership for some reason.

12. Does the facility belong to a professional association?

An association such as IDEA or IHRSA [International Health, Racquet & Sportsclub Association] keeps owners and instructors informed about current safety standards and enjoyable programs and provides a code of ethics that members adhere to.

13. Is the facility close to your home or work?

Research has shown that the number-one reason people leave a facility is because it is not conveniently located.

14. Does the facility hire qualified, certified fitness instructors?

To prepare a class that gives you a safe, effective workout, an instructor needs a good grounding in exercise technique. An exercise certification from an organization such as ACE [American Council on Exercise] or ACSM [American College of Sports Medicine] indicates that the instructor has basic knowledge or better in the areas necessary to teach a quality class. Instructors should be knowledgeable in anatomy, kinesiology, exercise physiology, injury prevention, monitoring of exercise intensity, and cardiopulmonary resuscitation (CPR). They should also be able to apply this knowledge for specific populations.

15. Is the facility service oriented, not sales oriented?

The staff should encourage you to *use* the facility, not just belong. Staff members should be happy to answer any questions you have about the facility's programs.

16. Are people available to help you if you have questions about the equipment? Will someone show you how to work the equipment?

You can't get much use out of the equipment if you don't know how to use it!

17. Do the instructors treat each member individually and offer exercise alternatives for different people, depending on their fitness level and goals?

Instructors should be able to show moves that are suitable for beginner, intermediate, and advanced participants and those with a variety of health concerns. They should encourage you to go at your own pace and stop and rest if you feel extreme discomfort or fatigue.

18. Do the employees seem to care about you as a person and not just as a revenue source?

Ask other members how happy they are with the customer service the facility provides. Ask if the employees build a personal relationship with the members. You want to know if employees are easily accessible, knowledgeable, and friendly.

19. Are you comfortable with the members at the facility?

Ask what type of people frequent the facility. What age range works out at the facility? Are you comfortable with the people you see there? Can you imagine yourself spending time there?

20. Will an employee be available to help you set up an exercise program?

If you are new to exercise or haven't exercised for years, it might be helpful to have someone advise you on what type of exercise would be best for you. The person can suggest classes you could take that you would enjoy and are at the appropriate level for you. He or she can also advise you on weight training and using the cardiovascular equipment.

21. Are the classes or programs you are interested in scheduled at times that are convenient for you?

You want to make sure the classes that appeal to you are convenient to your busy schedule. If you don't like those that are scheduled for your free times, you won't go, and that means less value for your dollar.

22. Does the facility offer a variety of programs that interest you?

Variety can improve adherence to an exercise program in the long run. Make sure the facility offers programs that you are excited about.

Section 21.2

Choosing a Personal Trainer

So you are thinking about hiring a personal trainer. That is terrific, because more people are working out with their very own exercise consultant than ever before. Personal trainers are not just for Hollywood stars and the "rich and famous" anymore! For good reason, since personal trainers can make the difference between a great workout and a ho-hum one—or even no workout at all. Your personal trainer will motivate you, keep you on track, and make sure your workouts are safe, enjoyable, and effective.

Of course, you want your personal trainer to exhibit the same qualities you demand of any provider of professional services, say, your tax preparer or dentist—a high degree of knowledge in their field, demonstrated expertise, plus a personality that's compatible with yours.

As The Health & Fitness Source, IDEA has provided information, education, and training to personal trainers for more than 10 years.

A recent IDEA survey showed that personal trainers provide a wide variety of clients with an extensive list of services, including nutritional guidance, fitness assessment, lifestyle management advice, weight control programs, and many more.

To help you choose the personal trainer who's just right for you, we've developed this handy guide. It takes you through the steps of identifying potential candidates and provides specific questions to ask. We recommend that you interview at least three personal trainers carefully before making your decision.

How to Locate Personal Trainers in Your Area

Personal trainers can be found through a variety of sources. If you are a member of a health club, fitness center, YMCA/YWCA [Young

Men's/Women's Christian Association], or JCC [Jewish Community Center] in your community, ask if they have a personal trainer on staff. Ask friends, health professionals, or your family doctor for referrals. Also, check your local yellow pages, newspapers, and magazines for listings. To choose a personal trainer near you, visit IDEA's Personal Trainer Locator [www.ideafit.com/find-personal-trainer].

Determine Your Goals, Needs, and Budget

Frequency: Are you merely looking for a one-time consultation about your exercise program, or do you want to establish a long-term working relationship? For a modest fee, many personal trainers will perform a fitness assessment and design a workout regimen tailored to your needs.

Location: Where do you want to work out? Many personal trainers will come to your home. Or, if you prefer, you can meet your personal trainer at a studio or health club nearby.

Budget: Personal training rates range from $20 to $100 per hour-long session, with the majority charging between $25 and $50. If that sounds high, remember, you are making an investment in your most important possession—your health. In addition, discounts are often available for multi-session purchases, for higher frequency (three times a week instead of two), and for training multiple clients at the same time.

Questions to Ask during Your Interview

The following questions will help you evaluate a personal trainer's credentials and determine whether his or her expertise is appropriate to your needs.

What is your exercise and educational background? Are you certified by a nationally recognized organization?

To properly design a safe and effective workout, a personal trainer should have a good grounding in exercise technique, including exercise physiology, anatomy, and injury prevention. A four-year degree in a fitness-related field or certification—or, preferably, both—indicates the personal trainer knows at least the basics of conducting a quality session.

What is your level of personal training experience? How do you keep current on the latest personal training techniques, research, and trends?

Fitness is a fast-moving field, and you want to be able to rely on your personal trainer for current information on fitness, exercise, and healthy lifestyle activities. Membership in a professional association such as IDEA is one way to tell the personal trainer is staying abreast of the latest information on a variety of important topics.

Are you certified in CPR and first aid?

While emergencies during training are extremely rare, be sure your personal trainer knows precisely what to do in case one should arise during your session.

Do you require a health screening or release from my doctor?

Many medical conditions or past injuries can affect your participation in a training session and the program your personal trainer designs for you. A quality personal trainer needs to know relevant details of your past medical history, including any medications you may be taking, before he or she can provide you with an effective workout. If you are under a doctor's care for certain conditions, your personal trainer will discuss any exercise concerns with your physician.

Can you give me references from other clients and industry professionals familiar with your knowledge and abilities?

People choose to hire a personal trainer for many reasons, including weight loss, cardiovascular improvement, marathon or triathlon training, injury or illness rehabilitation, pre/postnatal fitness, and many more. It is important to hire someone who has experience in the type of training you seek. Calling references can help you gauge whether the personal trainer has the expertise to properly serve your needs.

Will you keep track of my workouts, chart my progress, and update my medical history periodically?

Your personal trainer will help you establish realistic short- and long-term goals and assess your progress towards them. He or she might chart areas such as weight, percent body fat, body measurements, cardiovascular improvements, strength, and endurance. By updating your medical history from time to time, your personal trainer will also be able to adjust your workouts as necessary to reflect your new abilities.

Do you carry personal trainer liability insurance?

It is important for your personal trainer to have liability insurance in case you are injured while working out with him or her.

Do you provide clear-cut policies on cancellations, billing, and so on in writing?

Having all policies clearly stated in writing helps avoid any misunderstandings or confusion and protects your rights as a consumer.

What is your rate per session? Do you offer any discounts or package deals?

The personal trainer you select will most likely be an experienced professional with a high degree of expertise, and expects to be compensated as such. Expect to pay anywhere from $20 to $100 per hour-long session, and be sure to ask about any discounts available for multi-session purchases, for higher frequency (three times a week instead of two), and training two or more clients at a time.

What hours are you available to train?

If you're a professional with a full-time job, you probably want to work out either in the morning, at lunch, or in the evenings—all popular times demanded by clients. If not, you probably have more flexibility regarding workout times. However, do not feel "locked into" a time; should you need to change appointment times at a later date, be sure to ask what hours your personal trainer has available.

Will you help me focus on reasonable goals, not unattainable results?

No reputable personal trainer will promise that you will lose 30 pounds in 30 days, for example. It is vital both for your health and your motivation to set realistic, achievable goals. This prevents disillusionment and disappointment, raises your chances of success, and is a proven technique to keep you moving toward your goals.

Do you have a network of professionals, such as physicians, dietitians, physical therapist, and other fitness/health professionals?

A quality personal trainer will have established sources for specialized questions and referrals to provide you with the best service possible.

What is your communication style with your clients?

A quality personal trainer will always motivate you through positive, not negative, reinforcement and should never make you feel incompetent or inadequate. Your personal trainer should listen to you carefully to determine your goals and needs, communicate an understanding of them, and tell you why the program that has been designed is appropriate. He or she should also ask for your input on your program, and be prepared to put in writing the principles and reasoning behind exercise program decisions.

Parting Thoughts

Keep in mind that while personal trainers are business people, most got into the profession because they care about the well-being of their clients and want to see them succeed. Your personal trainer should ask questions about your lifestyle, including your eating habits, whether you smoke or drink, and other activities that could affect your ultimate health. He or she should also take steps to tailor your program to your unique needs and make you feel comfortable in the relationship. You should feel free to bring up questions or concerns you have at any time.

Give careful consideration to personality. Make sure your personal trainer's approach—energetic versus relaxed, aggressive versus low-key—fits your personal style. Gender is also important, since some people like working with a trainer of the same sex, while others prefer one of the opposite sex.

The bottom line is, you will experience good results if you are comfortable with your personal trainer. We hope you will use this section to go out and find the right personal trainer for you. Good luck, and stay active!

Section 21.3

Exercising with Friends

"Team Athletes Have Higher Endorphin Release when They Train To-gether," September 16, 2009, http://www.ox.ac.uk/media/news_releases_ for_journalists/090916.html. © 2009 University of Oxford. Reprinted with permission.

A study of Oxford rowers shows that members of a team who ex-ercised together were able to tolerate twice as much pain (an index of endorphin release) than when they trained on their own. In the study, published in the Royal Society journal *Biology Letters* on September 16 [2009], researchers from the University of Oxford's Institute of Cognitive and Evolutionary Anthropology found the pain threshold of 12 rowers from the Oxford Boat Race squad was greater after group training than after individual training. They conclude that acting as a group and in close synchrony seems to ramp up pain thresholds. The underlying endorphin release may be the mechanism that underpins communal-bonding effects that emerge from activities like religious rituals and dancing.

Each of the 12 rowers participated in four separate tests. They were asked to row continuously for 45 minutes in a virtual boat in the gym (as in normal training), in an exercise carried out in two teams of six, and then in a separate session as individuals, unobserved by other team members. After each of the sessions, the researchers measured their pain threshold by how long they could stand an inflated blood pressure cuff on the arm. The study found there was a significant increase in the rowers' pain threshold following exercise in both condi-tions (a well-established response to exercise of any kind), but there was a significantly larger increase in the group condition as compared with the individual condition.

Since close synchrony is the key to successful competition-class racing, these results suggest that doing a synchronised activity as a group increases the endorphin rush that we get from physical ex-ertion. The study says since endorphins help to create a sense of bonhomie and positive affect, this effect may underlie the experi-ence of warmth and belonging that we have when we do activities like dancing, sports, religious rituals, and other forms of communal exercise together.

Professor Robin Dunbar, head of the Institute of Cognitive and Evolutionary Anthropology at Oxford University, said: "Previous research suggests that synchronised physical activity such as laughter, music, and many religious activities makes people happier and is part of the bonding process. We also know that physical exercise creates a natural high through the release of endorphins. What this study shows us is that synchrony alone seems to ramp up the production of endorphins so as to heighten the effect when we do these activities in groups."

Lead author Dr. Emma Cohen, from the Institute of Cognitive and Evolutionary Anthropology, said: "The results suggest that endorphin release is significantly greater in group training than in individual training even when power output, or physical exertion, remains constant. The exact features of group activity that generate this effect are unknown, but this study contributes to a growing body of evidence suggesting that synchronised, coordinated physical activity may be responsible. Top-flight rowing teams must achieve an exceptional degree of synchrony and coordination so the Oxford squad gave us a wonderful opportunity to conduct this investigation. Follow-up research is required to investigate whether the effect would be reduced among teams that are less experienced, or under conditions of similar but non-synchronised physical activity."

Also involved as a researcher in this study was Robin Ejsmond-Frey, a double Blue in rowing and former President of the Oxford University Boat Club.

Section 21.4

Making Exercise Fun for the Whole Family

"Making Exercise Fun for the Whole Family," © 2010 Boys Town Pediatrics www.boystownpediatrics.org). Reprinted with permission. Additional information from the Substance Abuse and Mental Health Services Administration, U.S. Department of Health and Human Services is cited separately within the section.

Making Exercise Fun for the Whole Family

It is true that our society has become more relaxed to the idea of exercise. That's because we think of exercise as running laps at the track, lifting weights, or other rigorous, heart-pounding workouts. But, by the time you get home, feed the kids, and do a few chores around the house, exercise may be the last thing on your mind.

Not only do parents have to think of themselves, according to the American Academy of Pediatrics, children should get at least one hour of physical activity every day.

Boys Town Pediatrics recommends making exercise fun for the whole family. By doing activities together, parents and children will benefit from the physical exercise and, as a bonus, get to spend quality time doing fun activities together. Here are a few ideas that can help your family become more fit:

Parenting Tips

- **Walk to the park.** Bring Fido, stroll with your small children in a wagon, or race to the slide. And. while you're at the park, be sure to push each other on a swing, play tag, or climb on the monkey bars together!

- **Dance, dance, dance.** Turn on your favorite song and make up a dance routine. Each family member can make up his/her own dance moves and other family members can judge each other on talent and difficulty.

- **Run or walk for charity.** Pick a walk/run geared toward families with kid entertainment and activities. You will be putting in actual miles on the course, and there will be additional playtime during the post-race festivities.

- **Shoot some hoops.** Whether it's in your backyard or at your local recreation center, a quick pick-up game can boost agility while burning calories.

- **Bike the trails.** Pick a few trails or explore them all. Your family will be building muscle while encouraging each other to reach the top of the hill. After the ride, enjoy a family picnic.

- **Rake the leaves.** Gardening is hard work! It uses almost every muscle in your body. Jump in a pile of leaves or have your children help plant flowers. It's never exercise when you can have fun getting messy.

The best advice to help kids and families exercise is to make it fun! Think of what your family likes to do together, and make up your own exercise routine. A family that exercises together, stays fit together!

Making Exercise Fun

"Making Exercise Fun," Substance Abuse and Mental Health Services Administration, U.S. Department of Health and Human Services (www.samhsa.gov), September 18, 2007.

Children may not want to "exercise," but everybody loves to play. And young kids want to play with you. Here are a few ways to make your family "workouts" fun.

Play Games Outside or In

- Simon Says is an excellent game for stretching and flexibility. Start simply and build up to longer or more repetitive commands. For example: "Simon says, stand on your toes"; then, "Simon says, stand on your toes and count to five." Or, "Simon says, jump up high"; then, "Simon says, jump up high five times."

- Follow the Leader can help you and your child get aerobic exercise, especially if you play outside. It really doesn't matter whether you get creative with your actions; it's more important to keep moving. For example: If it's too difficult to climb over or under a fence, run around it. Or, if space is limited, do jumping jacks or run in place.

- Mirror Dancing provides the benefits of exercise with the fun of music. Put on music, either slow or fast, depending on whether you want an aerobic workout or slow stretching. Have your child stand directly in front of you and mimic whatever you do. Keep the steps easy; remember, the object is to get moving in time to the music. For example: Point your right foot to the front, to the side, and to the back. Repeat with the left foot. Do several slide steps to the right, then to the left. Bend at the waist, then rise up on tiptoe, arms stretched high. Do the twist or the bunny hop. Just have fun.

Be a Moving Role Model

- Climb the stairs with your child instead of taking the elevator or escalator.

- Park farther from the store and walk, rather than looking for the closest space.

- When a commercial comes on while you're watching TV, get on the floor and stretch for 2 or 3 minutes. If you do this five times during an hour show, you'll have exercised 10 or 15 minutes.

- Plan a family hike in the park or participate in a "fun run."

- Play together with all types of sports equipment: balls, hula hoops, jump ropes, scooters, and bikes.

- Use "Power Positive" on page 20 of the *Building Blocks Activity Book* (bblocks.samhsa.gov/media/bblocks/ActivityBook.pdf) to test your child's physical skills and build confidence.

Chapter 22

Evaluating Exercise Equipment and Exercise Program Claims

Author Information

David P. Swain, PhD, FACSM, is a professor of Exercise Science at Old Dominion University. He has published numerous research articles on the heart rate and oxygen consumption responses to exercise and is the originator of the VO2 reserve concept for exercise prescription. Dr. Swain is the author of *Exercise Prescription: A Case Study Approach to the ACSM [American College of Sports Medicine] Guidelines, 2nd Edition*, and the editor of the exercise prescription section of ACSM's *Resource Manual for Guidelines for Exercise Testing and Prescription, 6th Edition*.

Abstract

Learning objective: This chapter explains to readers how to cope with the sometimes incredible claims made by manufacturers about exercise equipment.

Infomercials and other forms of advertisement continue to make bold claims for exercise equipment. "Burns twice as many calories as a treadmill!" "Lose four inches from your waist in two weeks!" "Get a complete workout in just four minutes a day!" In most cases, the equipment can be effectively used to train clients, although the claims may be exaggerated.

"Exercise Equipment: Assessing the Advertised Claims," by David Swain, PhD, FACSM, *ACSM's Health & Fitness Journal*, September/October 2009, pp 8–11. © 2009 American College of Sports Medicine. Reprinted with permission from Wolters Kluwer Health, Inc.

How do exercise professionals decipher the claims and optimize their clients' success? Begin by remembering the following rules:

- If the claim seems incredible, it probably is not credible.

- Rely on one's knowledge of exercise physiology, not claims made by manufacturers, to explain to clients the benefits of exercise.

- Consult the scientific literature to determine if a given piece of equipment has been rigorously evaluated.

- When reputable scientific literature is not available, use one's personal expertise and body awareness to assess the equipment's muscle recruitment and energy requirements.

- Use reputable national recommendations, such as those available in ACSM's *Guidelines for Exercise Testing and Prescription, 8th Edition,*" and ACSM's *Resource Manual for Guidelines for Exercise Testing and Prescription, 6th Edition*, as the bases for designing exercise programs while being aware of special needs of individual clients.

Consider the following claims and misinformation regarding exercise equipment, especially cardio machines. Working through this information will allow us to better understand how to prescribe exercise with these devices and give us insight on working with newer pieces of equipment as they come along.

"Burns Twice as Many Calories as a Treadmill"

This claim is not credible based on basic knowledge of exercise physiology. The amount of energy expended during exercise depends on the amount of muscle mass used and on the intensity of effort used with that muscle. Up to a certain point, the more muscle that can be simultaneously engaged during exercise, the higher will be the maximum oxygen consumption (VO2 max) that can be attained in an incremental test.[2] However, the central cardiopulmonary system has an absolute limit on the amount of oxygen that can be transferred from the atmosphere to the blood and then pumped to the muscles, and the use of increasing amounts of muscle mass with various modes of exercise produces incrementally smaller increases in the mode-specific VO2 max (or VO2 peak) as the absolute VO2 max is approached. Running uphill on a treadmill generally elicits the highest VO2 of any mode of exercise because a large amount of muscle mass is engaged (especially hips and legs, but also back and upper body to a lesser extent). When athletes are highly trained in certain sports—cross-country skiing, bicycling, rowing—they may be able to slightly exceed their treadmill value (by 3%–5%) when performing sport-specific exercise tests.[5] Because the body has a central limit to oxygen delivery and because even elite athletes can only slightly exceed treadmill VO2, it is not feasible to think that a new mode of exercise can exceed treadmill VO2 by a huge amount.

How is it, then, that some manufacturers claim that their devices allow clients to achieve substantially greater caloric expenditure than on a treadmill? The website for a machine that claims "twice as many calories as a treadmill" adds "at the same speed" without clearly indicating that a hard resistance setting was chosen for the new machine while an easy grade was used on the treadmill. A deceptive tactic, but advertisers are in business to promote products, not to promote the full story. The website even states that studies were done at a university laboratory, but no references for these "studies" were provided. To search for published articles on the topic, one's first choice should be PubMed (http://www.ncbi.nlm.nih.gov/pubmed), a search engine from the U.S. National Library of Medicine and the National Institutes of Health that only indexes reputable scientific journals. A secondary search engine is SportDiscus, which must be used with caution as it indexes lesser-quality journals, including lay fitness magazines. A search of PubMed and SportDiscus reveals no peer-reviewed scientific articles that support the claims of this manufacturer.

The machine in this case clearly provides a cardiorespiratory workout that uses the major muscles of the hips and legs. It should be a fine machine for training clients who want an optional mode of exercise from treadmills and bicycles, but the exercise professional needs to caution clients not to expect twice the results, unless they are willing and able to work twice as hard.

An important consideration regarding the choice of aerobic machines is the amount of weight bearing and impact that they provide. Many advertisers tout "low impact" as though this was an important attribute. However, weight-bearing exercise, especially when it involves impact as in walking and running, provides mechanical loading of bones that is important in preventing osteoporosis. A low-impact exercise is useful for clients with certain orthopedic concerns, but most clients should be encouraged to judiciously include impact-generating exercise.

"Get Fit in Four Minutes"

Several manufacturers have claimed that major gains in fitness can be obtained with very brief periods of exercise. One extreme claim is that four minutes per day on a certain machine provides complete cardio, resistance, and flexibility training. It is true that intense efforts result in great increases in the capacity of the system being stressed, such as aerobic power, anaerobic power, or muscular strength. For example, a recent study compared three ways to train aerobic power: 50% of heart rate reserve (HRR) for an extended duration, 75% of HRR for a moderate duration, and 95% of HRR for five intervals of five minutes each.[4] Each group performed the same volume of exercise per week and increased their VO2 max by 10%, 14%, and 21%, respectively. These increases were all significantly different from each other.

Although brief bouts at a high intensity are very effective at raising VO2 max, it is unrealistic to assume that a single four-minute bout of exercise each day could accomplish similar results and also produce impressive increases in strength and flexibility. The website of the manufacturer cites three studies, but two are only abstracts and the third is a personal communication. Note that abstracts are preliminary reports of research studies. Most abstracts do not make it through the peer-review process to become published research articles in reputable scientific journals. Abstracts are useful as suggestions of possible information available on a topic but should not be given the weight of full articles. A search of PubMed and SportDiscus finds no peer-reviewed scientific articles in support of these incredible claims. However, as with the "twice as many calories" claim, this exercise machine seems to recruit major muscle groups and should be a useful mode of training.

Although high-intensity workouts are the most effective means of increasing the maximal capacity of stressed systems, there are many benefits of exercise that likely require a significant total volume to achieve; certainly, endurance is one and weight loss is another, as may be a variety of other health benefits. A large volume of exercise is more easily attained by holding a moderate intensity for a long duration than by performing high-intensity intervals for a large number of repetitions.

"Fat-Burning Zone"

Most cardio machines display a heart rate guide with suggested target heart rates for a "fat-burning zone" versus a "cardio fitness zone." Lower target values are given for "fat burning" than for developing "cardio fitness." The implication that lower intensities are better for fat burning and, therefore, for weight loss is based on a common misapplication of exercise physiology. Lower intensities of exercise rely more on fat as an energy substrate than do higher intensities, as demonstrated by the measurement of the respiratory exchange ratio (RER) during exercise. The RER is 0.7 when burning only fats and is 1.0 when burning only carbohydrates. As carbohydrates are the more efficient fuel, metabolic pathways shift to more carbohydrate usage as intensity of exercise increases, thus, RER rises, and 100% carbohydrates are used at approximately 90% of VO2 max and higher.[1] Therefore, it is true that a higher percentage of calories come from fat at lower intensities. However, the percentage of calories derived from fat during the exercise is not relevant to weight loss. The total number of calories burned, from any source, is the key factor. The body will adjust fat and carbohydrate stores during the day, and fat weight loss will be based on any deficit between the total number of calories consumed versus the total number of calories burned during days or weeks. Several studies have been conducted that compared the effect of different intensities of exercise on weight loss and found that as long as the total number of calories expended is the same, there is no intensity effect.[7] One potential advantage of a lower-intensity "fat-burning zone" is if the client is willing to stay at this intensity for a prolonged period of time. It is the total volume of exercise, intensity × duration × frequency, that determines caloric expenditure.

The "cardio fitness zone" is another matter. As explained earlier, higher intensities of exercise are indeed better for improving VO2 max than lower intensities of exercise.

Caloric Expenditure Reported by Machines

To determine the amount of fat weight loss that can be expected from exercise, the net energy expenditure (EE) is needed, that is, the EE caused by the exercise that is in excess of resting energy needs. The ACSM metabolic equations[6] provide gross oxygen consumption of certain modes of exercise, and this value can be corrected to net VO2 by subtracting resting VO2 ($3.5 \text{ mL·min}^{-1}\text{·kg}^{-1}$ on average) and then converted to net EE based on 5 kcal/L of oxygen consumed. For example, the net EE of a 136-lb (62 kg) person walking 1 mile (1.6 km) is 50 kcal. Running a mile has twice the energy cost, that is, 100 kcal. Knowing that 1 lb (0.45 kg) of body fat stores 3,500 kcal of energy, the amount of fat weight loss expected from exercise (assuming no change in dietary intake) can be calculated. For example, it would take 35 miles of running or 70 miles of walking to expend the 3,500 kcal in 1 lb of fat.

Gross EE while running a mile is a little more than 100 kcal, and gross EE for walking a mile approaches 100 kcal for very slow walking. The similarity of the gross values is caused by the longer duration needed for walking and, therefore, the inclusion of a longer period of resting metabolism in addition to the 50 kcal needed for the exercise itself. But the gross values should not be used in weight loss calculations because the resting metabolism would have occurred whether the client walked, ran, or did no exercise during a given period. Only the additional EE caused by the exercise should be used in determining the amount of weight loss the exercise may induce.

Most cardio machines report gross EE, which overestimates the potential effect of the exercise on body weight. Importantly, the lower the exercise intensity is, the greater the error between net and gross EE. For example, a check of two different brands of treadmills found that reported EE was 60% to 70% greater than the ACSM value for net EE when walking at 2 mph (3.2 kph), but only 10% to 20% greater when jogging at 6 mph (9.6 kph). The reported values were very close to the ACSM values for gross EE. A third brand of treadmill gave values inconsistent with the ACSM formulas. Therefore, exercise professionals need to recognize that caloric expenditure values provided by cardio machines are not necessarily accurate and may overestimate net EE, especially at low intensities.

A further point regarding caloric readouts on cardio machines is that they report either "calories per minute" or "calories per hour." These values are off by 1,000-fold! The proper units are kilocalories per minute or per hour. Unfortunately, it is common practice to mislabel kilocalories as calories because the food industry has been doing so for decades, even on packaged food labels. As exercise professionals, we should refer to kilocalories as kilocalories. We do not refer to kilograms as grams, nor do we refer to miles as inches. We should not accept this incorrect usage of units of measure and should encourage manufacturers of exercise equipment to correct their display panels.

Finally, the use of handrails or other support reduces the energy requirement of treadmills and many other aerobic machines. It is common to observe individuals using a steep grade on a treadmill while leaning back with their arms on the console or front handrails. Individuals on stair-stepping machines often push down on support rails with their hands, locking their elbows. In such cases, considerably less work is performed, and the caloric readouts on the machines will greatly overstate the actual EE. Clients should be taught to put their full weight on their feet and to use supports only as needed for balance.

"Lose Four Inches from Your Waist in Two Weeks"

Many pieces of equipment designed for training the abdominal muscles make excessive claims about their benefits. Often they claim to produce significant loss of body fat from the abdominal region. Of course, exercise physiologists know that such "spot reducing" is a fantasy. Exercising a given body part does not result in a loss of fat specifically from that region. Rather, if the caloric expenditure from the exercise causes the total EE over time to be greater than dietary intake, the person will lose body fat from adipose stores throughout the body. Typically, advertisements making claims for large fat reduction, such as the claim quoted, also include fine print stating that the "results are not typical" or that the fat loss can be expected "when combined with an overall exercise and diet program."

Other claims from "ab" machine manufacturers may be that the exercise is better at targeting the abdominal muscles than standard calisthenics, such as crunches. One needs to check to see if peer-reviewed research articles have been published that support the claims. Barring that, an exercise professional can try the device and note what muscle groups appear to be recruited. However, a well-trained individual may find a particular movement to be easier than an untrained client does, which could affect decisions regarding exercise selection. For example, Escamilla et al.[3] studied two "ab" exercisers and used electromyography to compare their muscle recruitment patterns with more traditional abdominal exercises. Performing a rollout with an exercise wheel elicited significantly greater activation of the rectus abdominis than did performing a standard crunch. However, performing a crunch while using a special frame designed to control the motion elicited a slightly lower activation than the standard crunch. Do these findings mean that an exercise wheel is the superior method of training the abdominals? For clients who already have strong abdominals, possibly so. But, as pointed out by Escamilla et al.,[3] an exercise wheel may be too difficult for less-fit clients or those with lumbar problems. This is where the expertise of the exercise professional is needed in examining an exercise and deciding how best to use it with his or her individual clients.

Many other novel exercise devices have been advertised via infomercials and other media. Are special tools needed to better perform pull-ups or push-ups? Will vibrating a large vertically held blade back and forth provide a good workout? Claims of manufacturers cannot be taken at face value. The exercise professional needs to look for peer-reviewed published research articles or evaluate new devices through personal use to determine whether they may be useful in training clients.

Condensed Version and Bottom Line

Incredible claims are often made about new exercise products. Exercise professionals need to rely on their knowledge of exercise physiology and peer-reviewed scientific literature to assess the claims. When reputable research on a specific device is not available, exercise professionals should personally evaluate the equipment to assess its muscle recruitment and energy requirements to determine its potential value to clients.

References

1. Achten J, Gleeson M, Jeukendrup AE. Determination of the exercise intensity that elicits maximal fat oxidation. *Med Sci Sports Exerc.* 2002;34:92–7.

2. Bergh U, Kanstrup IL, Ekblom B. Maximal oxygen uptake during exercise with various combinations of arm and leg work. *J Appl Physiol.* 1976;41:191–6.

3. Escamilla RF, Babb E, DeWitt R, et al. Electromyographic analysis of traditional and nontraditional abdominal exercises: Implications for rehabilitation and training. *Phys Ther.* 2006;86:656–71.

4. Gormley SE, Swain DP, High R, et al. Effect of intensity of aerobic training on VO2 max. *Med Sci Sports Exerc.* 2008;40:1336–43.

5. Stromme SB, Ingjer F, Meen HD. Assessment of maximal aerobic power in specifically trained athletes. *J Appl Physiol.* 1977;42:833–7.

6. Swain DP. Exercise prescription. In: Ehrman J, deJong A, Sanderson B, Swain DP, Swank AM, Womack CJ, editors. *ACSM's Resource Manual for Guidelines for Exercise Testing and Prescription.* 6th ed. Philadelphia (PA): Lippicott Williams & Wilkins; 2008.

7. Swain DP, Franklin BA. Comparative cardioprotective benefits of vigorous vs. moderate intensity aerobic exercise. *Am J Cardiol.* 2006;97(1):141–7.

Part Four

Exercise Basics

Chapter 23

Aerobic Exercise Basics and Equipment

Chapter Contents

Section 23.1

Aerobic Exercise Basics

This section excerpted from "Physical Activity and Your Heart,"
National Heart Lung and Blood Institute (www.nhlbi.nih.gov), May 2009.

The four main types of physical activity are aerobic, muscle strengthening, bone strengthening, and stretching. Aerobic activity is the type that benefits your heart and lungs the most.

Aerobic Activity

Aerobic activity moves your large muscles, such as those in your arms and legs. Running, swimming, walking, bicycling, dancing, and doing jumping jacks are examples of aerobic activity. Aerobic activity also is called endurance activity.

Aerobic activity makes your heart beat faster than usual. You also breathe harder during this type of activity. Over time, regular aerobic activity makes your heart and lungs stronger and able to work better.

Other Types of Physical Activity

The other types of physical activity—muscle strengthening, bone strengthening, and stretching—benefit your body in other ways.

Muscle-strengthening activities improve the strength, power, and endurance of your muscles. Doing push-ups and sit-ups, lifting weights, climbing stairs, and digging in the garden are examples of muscle-strengthening activities.

With bone-strengthening activities, your feet, legs, or arms support your body's weight, and your muscles push against your bones. This helps make your bones strong. Running, walking, jumping rope, and lifting weights are examples of bone-strengthening activities.

Muscle-strengthening and bone-strengthening activities also can be aerobic, depending on whether they make your heart and lungs work harder than usual. For example, running is both an aerobic activity and a bone-strengthening activity.

Stretching helps improve your flexibility and your ability to fully move your joints. Touching your toes, doing side stretches, and doing yoga exercises are examples of stretching.

Levels of Intensity in Aerobic Activity

You can do aerobic activity with light, moderate, or vigorous intensity. Moderate- and vigorous-intensity aerobic activities are better for your heart than light-intensity activities. However, even light-intensity activities are better than no activity at all.

The level of intensity depends on how hard you have to work to do the activity. To do the same activity, people who are less fit usually have to work harder than people who are more fit. So, for example, what is light-intensity activity for one person may be moderate intensity for another.

Light- and moderate-intensity activities: Light-intensity activities are common daily activities that don't require much effort. Moderate-intensity activities make your heart, lungs, and muscles work harder than light-intensity activities do.

On a scale of 0 to 10, moderate-intensity activity is a 5 or 6 and produces noticeable increases in breathing and heart rate. A person doing moderate-intensity activity can talk but not sing.

Vigorous-intensity activities: Vigorous-intensity activities make your heart, lungs, and muscles work hard. On a scale of 0 to 10, vigorous-intensity activity is a 7 or 8. A person doing vigorous-intensity activity can't say more than a few words without stopping for a breath.

Examples of Aerobic Activities

Depending on your level of fitness, these examples of aerobic activity can be light, moderate, or vigorous in intensity:

- Pushing a grocery cart around a store
- Gardening, such as digging or hoeing, that causes your heart rate to go up
- Walking, hiking, jogging, running
- Water aerobics or swimming laps
- Bicycling, skateboarding, rollerblading, and jumping rope
- Ballroom dancing and aerobic dancing
- Tennis, soccer, hockey, and basketball

Section 23.2

Elliptical Trainers

"Selecting and Effectively Using an Elliptical Trainer." Reprinted with permission of the American College of Sports Medicine. Copyright © 2005 American College of Sports Medicine. All rights reserved. Reviewed by David A. Cooke, MD, FACP, March 2010.

A Complete Physical Activity Program

A well-rounded program of physical activity includes aerobic exercise and strength training exercise, but not necessarily in the same session. This blend helps to maintain or improve cardiorespiratory and muscular fitness and overall health and function. Regular physical activity will provide more health benefits than sporadic, high-intensity workouts, so choose exercises you are likely to enjoy and that you can incorporate into your schedule.

ACSM [American College of Sports Medicine]'s physical activity recommendations for healthy adults, updated in 2007, recommend at least 30 minutes of moderate-intensity physical activity (working hard enough to break a sweat, but still able to carry on a conversation) five days per week, or 20 minutes of more vigorous activity three days per week. Combinations of moderate- and vigorous-intensity activity can be performed to meet this recommendation. Typical aerobic exercises include walking and running, stair climbing, cycling on a stationary or moving bike, rowing, cross-country skiing, and swimming.

In addition, strength training should be performed a minimum of two days each week, with 8–12 repetitions of 8–10 different exercises that target all major muscle groups. This type of training can be accomplished using body weight, resistance bands, free weights, medicine balls, or weight machines.

Staying Active Pays Off!

Those who are physically active tend to live longer, healthier lives. Research shows that even moderate physical activity—such as 30 minutes a day of brisk walking—significantly contributes to longevity. A physically active person with such risk factors as high blood pressure, diabetes, or even a smoking habit can get real benefits from regular physical activity as part of daily life.

As many dieters have found, exercise can help you stay on a diet and lose weight. What's more, regular exercise can help lower blood pressure, control blood sugar, improve cholesterol levels, and build stronger, denser bones.

The First Step

Before you begin an exercise program, take a fitness test, or substantially increase your level of activity, make sure to answer the following questions. This physical activity readiness questionnaire (PAR-Q) will help determine your suitability for beginning an exercise routine or program.

- Has your doctor ever said that you have a heart condition or that you should participate in physical activity only as recommended by a doctor?

- Do you feel pain in your chest during physical activity?

- In the past month, have you had chest pain when you were not doing physical activity?

- Do you lose your balance because of dizziness?

- Do you ever lose consciousness?

- Do you have a bone or joint problem that could be made worse by a change in your physical activity?

- Is your doctor currently prescribing drugs for your blood pressure or a heart condition?

- Do you know of any reason you should not participate in physical activity?

If you answered yes to one or more questions, if you are over 40 years of age and have been inactive, or if you are concerned about your health, consult a physician before taking a fitness test or substantially increasing your physical activity. If you answered no to each question, then it's likely that you can safely begin fitness testing and training.

Selecting a Home Elliptical Trainer

Elliptical trainers have become one of the most popular machines for cardiovascular exercise. These trainers engage the legs in a movement pattern that combines the motion of stair stepping with cross-country skiing, providing a low-impact workout. Some elliptical devices also include poles that can be maneuvered with the arms while the legs are in motion, similar to cross-country machines. This option increases the amount of muscle mass used to perform the exercise.

Following are guidelines that should be considered when purchasing an elliptical trainer. These recommendations will help you select a trainer that suits your specific needs. Before making any purchases, always be sure to try out the machine so that you can familiarize yourself with its options.

Safety

Make sure the equipment is properly fitted to your size and movement range. If the machine is motorized, there should be a safety turn-off control.

When in use, the machine should be very sturdy and should neither move nor have the tendency to tip over. The side rails should also be sturdy and provide for adequate balance.

Check the area around the machine for adequate headroom and space for leg and arm motion.

Maintenance and Durability

- Is the machine manufacturer reputable and reliable?
- Does the trainer come with a warranty?
- What does the warranty cover and how long is the warranty period?
- Is the machine durable, easily assembled, and easily maintained?
- Elliptical machines tend to be rather large—is the space in which it is to be used large enough?
- If it is to be stored between use, is there adequate space for storage?
- Are local technicians available for service?

Power, Performance, and Operation

- Is the trainer motorized or non-motorized?
- Does your home have the proper power supply? (Motorized machines may require 120 to 220 volts.)

- Does the trainer require calibration?

- How often does the trainer have to be serviced?

- Is the noise level acceptable?

- Is the trainer sturdy and stable?

- Is there a control panel/readout? Is it easy to read? Is it accurate?

- Does the control panel offer the information that is important for your needs (time, distance, resistance level, calories expended, etc.)?

- Is the instruction manual easy to read and follow?

Other Considerations

Make certain the pedals will comfortably accommodate the size of your feet. Pedals with a textured "non-slip" surface and high curved ridges will also prevent your feet from sliding around or even off the pedal when exercising.

The stride length permitted by the trainer is also an important factor. Avoid purchasing a trainer if the stride length is too limited for your leg movement range. Some machines allow you to adjust the stride length.

Overall fit is very important. A good fit should allow you to move comfortably and smoothly, with a good upright posture and without the chance of your knees bumping into the console. The fixed hand-support rails should also allow you to maintain a comfortable upright posture versus a tendency to lean too far forward (which can be stressful to the back).

If the machine provides upper-body handles or poles, make sure that the handles are sturdy, easy to reach, and that the handgrips are comfortable. Avoid trainers with upper-body poles that infringe on your range of motion or cause contact with your knees.

Familiarize yourself with the options that increase the intensity of the workout. Some machines have elevating ramps under each pedal. Others increase the intensity through faster movement or by changing the resistance of the pedals with a tension control.

Using an Elliptical Trainer

Follow the manual regarding directions for proper setup and use of the machine. Make certain the trainer operates properly and be sure that adequate space is available and that the power supply is nearby. Adjust the machine to suit your size and range of movement. Get comfortable with any programming features such as exercise time, distance goal, resistance level, speed level, and caloric expenditure.

When exercising, maintain the correct posture by keeping your shoulder back, head up, chin straight, abdominals tight, and arms relaxed. Do not lean forward or grab and grip the balance bars tightly. The participant's weight should be supported by the lower body.

Important Points to Remember:

Before you start exercising on the elliptical trainer, make sure that you are familiar with the controls that increase speed and/or resistance. Make sure that the emergency shut-off switch or button works.

Maintain a good posture: Shoulders should be back, head up and slightly forward, chin up, and abdominals tight. Look forward, not down at your feet. Do not grip the handrails too tightly. Make sure that your weight is evenly distributed and that your lower body supports the majority of your weight.

Stride: Relax and maintain a good stride going through your normal range of motion.

Make it a habit: An elliptical trainer is only as good for your health as the frequency with which you use it. Set a specific time of day, set a specific number of minutes, and make it routine. Start out slowly and make sure that you have checked with your doctor before beginning any exercise program.

Section 23.3

Treadmills

Selecting a Home Treadmill

Treadmills are a popular choice of equipment for those who want to engage in physical activity. This section contains useful guidelines for you to consider before making a purchase. Be sure to try it out before you buy. Doing so will allow you to find a treadmill that meets your specific needs. A treadmill may be either motorized or human powered. Manual treadmills are less expensive and safer because the running belt stops moving when you do. However, manual treadmills usually have smaller running belts, making it difficult to jog or run, let alone maintain a brisk walk. Often, the difficulty in getting the belt to move smoothly on a non-motorized treadmill increases the likelihood of holding on to the handrail in an effort to generate power, causing an inconsistent pace. This inconsistent pace may cause muscle strain or difficulty in elevating your heart rate. Additionally, the holding on may elevate blood pressure from breath holding. Exercise at home should be easy and something to look forward to. If it is difficult to get the machine to work, you are less likely to exercise. For these reasons, you may want to consider a motorized treadmill.

Safety

- Stability of platform when level and with elevation: feels solid, not wobbly.

- Doesn't have parts that hit you or cramp your movements in an unnatural fashion.

- Automatic emergency shut-off key, clip, or tether.

- Side rails or safety bars for balance: They should be reachable and sturdy, but out of the way of swinging arms.

Maintenance and Durability

- Is the company reliable and reputable?
- Can the treadmill be easily assembled and maintained?
- Cost of maintenance?
- Does the treadmill come with a warranty? What does the warranty cover and for how long?
- Are local technicians available for service?

Power and Performance

- Treadmill motor: should have a minimum continuous duty rating of 1.5 hp motor (2.5 to 3.0 hp is preferred). To test the motor, plant your feet firmly on the belt while the machine is running at its lowest speed, checking for any hesitation, groaning, or grinding.

- Power supply: Does the treadmill require 110 or 220 volts? 220 volts will probably require circuit alterations in the room where it will be used.

- Belt size: Should be at least 18 to 20 inches wide and 48 inches long. Narrow, short running belts make it more difficult and less enjoyable because the chances of tripping or falling off of the belt increase with a narrow belt. The platform should be low to the floor and have ample space to straddle the treadmill belt.

- Speed range should be 0.1 to a minimum of 8 mph. This speed range should satisfy most walkers as well as runners. Low starting speed is an important issue. We recommend a safe starting speed of 0.1 mph with slow incremental increase in belt speed. The stop should be smooth stop (not sudden). The motor should be able to maintain speed regardless of treadmill elevation and weight of user.

- Incline should range from 0% to at least 10%. Incline mechanisms can be either electric or manual. Manual cranks are found generally on lower end treadmills to keep the price down. The treadmill should not wobble at high elevations.

Operation

- Is the control panel accessible and easy to read?
- Does the control panel have the capacity for manual use separate from software used for automated programming?

- Is the noise level acceptable?

- Is the belt heavy duty as to not stretch with extended use?

Other Considerations

- Weight of treadmill.

- Space available and height of ceiling.

- Aesthetics.

- Storage potential.

- How accurate is the calibration?

Using a Home Treadmill

Treadmills should be positioned away from walls to avoid injury due to falls. Be sure that the back of the treadmill has at least six to eight feet of clearance from a ledge, wall, or window. The power supply and wiring should be located away from walking paths or taped to prevent tripping when stepping on or off of the running belt.

Make sure the running belt is properly adjusted before use. Belts that are too loose or too tight will cause wear and tear on the treadmill, which result in expensive repair or replacement costs. The deck beneath the belt should be laminated to protect it from friction wear and tear. This deck absorbs the hundreds of pounds of force from each step.

Make sure that you follow the directions included with purchase for maintaining the belt deck connection. Increased friction and heat will cause "amp draw," which pulls power away from the electrical components of your machine. Discuss appropriate lubrication and maintenance with the sales people at the store where you purchased your treadmill.

Your treadmill should come equipped with arm grips, side rails, or safety bars. These are excellent for defining the running/walking area for your exercise bout. They allow you to catch yourself if you trip or fall. When stepping off a treadmill while the belt is moving it is advisable to use these rails for safety.

The treadmill should come equipped with an emergency shut-off key, clip, or tether. These are a safety must, especially with young children around. The tether feature is preferred, since an automatic stop button may not be in reach as you fall.

Many treadmills come with sophisticated electronic displays that allow you to design workouts to your needs. For some, this programming is basically a motivation and selling point. All you need is enough variety to keep your workouts motivating and interesting. The bare minimum display and programming features should include distance, speed, time, incline, and possibly calories expended. It is important that you be able to use the treadmill in the manual mode.

Important Points to Remember:

Before you get on: Before you get on the treadmill, experiment with the controls. Speed it up, slow it down, increase and decrease the incline, and test the emergency off button.

Posture when walking or running: Shoulders back, head up and slightly forward, chin up, and abdominals tight. Look forward, not down at your feet.

Stride length: Relax and maintain the normal stride you would use when walking on the ground. Don't chop your steps.

Where you are: It is important to pay attention to where you are on the treadmill. Don't drift sideways or allow yourself to go to the back of the belt.

Make it a habit: A treadmill is only as good for your health as the frequency with which you use it. Set a specific time of day, set a specific number of minutes, and make it routine.

Section 23.4

Rowing Machines

Selecting a Rowing Machine

Rowing is an efficient and effective low-impact exercise that utilizes the arms, abdomen, back, and legs, providing a total-body workout. This activity offers the opportunity for a wide range of training from fat burning and aerobic conditioning to high-intensity anaerobic and interval VO2 max [maximal oxygen consumption] training. The rowing stroke is a smooth continuous, non-impact movement. If you have a history of low back pain, special attention must be given to developing proper rowing technique to prevent injury.

The rowing machine should mimic the smooth motion of rowing on the water. The machine and platform must be of sturdy construction and able to easily support the weight of the person rowing. The seat should be comfortable, but not too soft. The seat must slide back and forth smoothly and allow for full extension and flexion of the knees. There should be plenty of room in front of the person rowing to allow for full extension of the shoulders and arms at the beginning of the rowing motion. The "oar" handle should be centered in front and enable a full range of motion in a straight horizontal plane. There should be a smooth, seamless uptake of the resistance throughout the rowing stroke. Avoid machines that feature a jerky sensation of resistance change or sudden change in resistance. The rowing machine should allow for the easy adjustment of the resistance, even from one stroke to another.

Many rowing machines are equipped with a monitor that will indicate pace, distance, power output (watts), calories burned, and heart rate. Some may also be programmed for a workout including distance or time rowed and the rest period between intervals. More sophisticated monitors provide a visual display of the force of a stroke and/or continuous tracking against an imaginary "pace" boat for each interval in a workout. They may also keep a personal electronic log of your workout and results. One manufacturer even has an annual worldwide ranking online for various ages, body weights, and distance rowed and sponsors a world indoor rowing championship. Some machines provide detailed instruction on rowing technique and have websites for training tips, maintaining a personal workout log, and motivational competitions.

Rowing machines are manufactured with four different types of resistance: air, water, magnetic, and piston. The industry standard utilizes air resistance, and the less expensive machines are piston driven. Magnetic machines are the quietest. Air and magnetic machines allow for the fastest change in resistance. Water and air machines claim to provide the closest replication to the feeling of rowing on water. Water machines are the heaviest. The air machines should have a cover made of narrow mesh over the flywheel to prevent injury to the fingers. Some piston and air resistance machines can be folded for easy storage.

The rowing machine should mimic the smooth motion of rowing on the water. The following may be effective in developing a smooth and effective stroke.

The Rowing Stroke

The rowing stroke is a continuous motion. The starting point is generally referred to as the catch. At this point, the knees are flexed or bent with the shins vertical and the shoulders and arms reaching forward. This is the position that mimics the oar being placed into the water prior to the drive phase of the stroke. The drive phase is initiated by the legs as they extend. The arms remain straight until the knees are mostly extended, and then the elbows flex bringing the oar handle into the upper stomach. The drive ends at the finish when the legs are fully extended, shoulders are back, elbows are flexed, and the oar handle is against the upper stomach. The recovery phase is the phase of the rowing stroke where the rower returns to the catch position to initiate another drive phase. The recovery begins with the hands and arms moving away from the body and the elbows extending. The upper body moves forward over the hips as the hands move past the knees, the knees begin to flex, and the seat moves up the slide to the catch position.

Proper Use of a Rowing Machine

The rowing machine must be placed on a solid level surface. There must be open space around the machine to allow for the full arc of the rowing motion. Before purchasing a rowing machine, measure the space in which you intend to use it and store it to make sure it will fit. Some models allow for storage in a vertical position. The machine must be stable in this vertical position and not placed in an area where it may be knocked over.

A common error when rowing on a machine is allowing the knees to flex prior to the hands passing over the knees during the recovery. This forces the rower to lift the oar handle over the knees before the catch and may lead to injury. Another common mistake is allowing the seat to slide out from under the rower prior to the handle moving back on the drive. This puts the back in a weaker position and may lead to a back injury if done with enough force.

The effort put into the rowing stroke is a combination of the stroke rate and resistance setting. Generally there is a greater stress put on the back with the slower stroke rate. The resistance setting should be lower for the long aerobic workouts. Aerobic training for the beginner can start at 15 minutes with a five-minute warm-up and five-minute cool-down. When a person rows regularly for several weeks or months, and their fitness level increases, the time of the workout can increase to 20 minutes, then 25 and 30 minutes. To increase the intensity of the workout, the resistance and stroke rate can be increased. However, any attempt to combine a slower stroke rate with high resistance may lead to back injury.

In addition the rower should not suddenly pull as hard as possible in an attempt to achieve maximal effort in a single stroke or two. This places a sudden large stress on the lower back and may result in injury. The pace of a workout should be reached over three to five strokes or more. A warm-up consisting of slow, easy rowing for four to five minutes will help reduce the risk of injury and improve the benefits of a workout.

Care of a Rowing Machine

All rowing machines should be kept clean, with regular wiping of the handle with a disinfectant. The handle should fit comfortably in the hand and be covered with a non-slip rubber surface. Should a rower develop blisters and/or bleeding, the handle must be appropriately cleaned.

Special care must be taken to avoid twisting the chain or cord attached to the handle to avoid damage to the chain. When the rowing machine is not being used, the handle should be placed against the flywheel to avoid unnecessary stretching of the pull cord.

Regular maintenance and cleaning of the machine will help ensure the proper operation and safety. The manufacturer should clearly detail a maintenance program in the owner's manual and should provide a warranty.

Care of a Rowing Machine

- Make sure the machine has been properly cleaning and maintained prior to use.

- Make sure that the proper rowing technique is always used.

- Avoid twisting or excessively stretching the cord.

- Always warm-up before a workout session and increase the length and intensity of training gradually over weeks and months.

- Never start a rowing interval with maximal effort in a single stroke.

Section 23.5

Stair Climbers

"Selecting and Effectively Using a Stair Stepper/Climber." Reprinted with permission of the American College of Sports Medicine. Copyright © 2005 American College of Sports Medicine. All rights reserved. Reviewed by David A. Cooke, MD, FACP, March 2010.

Selecting a Stair Stepper/Climber

Stair steppers, elliptical trainers, and climbers are often thought of as similar pieces of equipment, but they are very different. The stair stepper provides only lower body strength training and aerobic exercise. The elliptical trainer has an orbital motion that encompasses walking, running, climbing, and related cardiovascular workouts. Additionally, some elliptical trainer models incorporate upper-body workouts, providing a total-body workout. The climber allows for upper-body and lower-body strength training as well as aerobic training. These machines provide the ability to tone thigh and gluteal muscles equally well when compared to other exercise programs or machines.

Spend some time analyzing your needs and interests to decide on the type of stepper or climber you want. For example, is this to be used as a basic daily exercise program, or are you training for a specific event? Many of these machines feature a console with programs that can range from basic to sophisticated. Training for a specific event may indicate a need for a wider range of options and programs, including the ability to customize programs to meet your specific needs. The more features, options, and programs, the more costly the stepper/climber.

Basic consoles should display calories burned, distance climbed, rate of speed, and intensity level. Intensity may be controlled manually, and some basic models may have a few programs from which to choose. The best way to select the right stair stepper is to try out a number of different models.

Safety

It is essential that your machine have solid construction and a stable frame. In steppers, the stepping action should be smooth and independent (pushing one step down should not push the other step up). Self-leveling pedals will allow the user to keep the step flat throughout the workout. It is important that these machines be ergonomically sound and that you position yourself to maximize the safety and effectiveness of your workout. This means that the handrails should be positioned so that your workout posture is upright with the knees behind the toes. Bending forward places a great amount of stress on the back. Using the handrails to support part of the body weight reduces the total caloric expenditure and may result in a posture that is biomechanically unsound. Last, but not least, read all of the manufacturer's instructions to get the most out of your machine!

Using a Stair Stepper/Climber

Steppers should be positioned so that there is easy access onto and off of the steps. The path immediately behind the steps should be free of power cords and other tripping hazards. The area immediately above the stepper should be open and allow plenty of room to stand tall, even when the steps are at the top of the stepping range.

Make sure the stepper responds according to the manufacturers directions. Test all of the arrows or buttons that control the intensity, and make sure the display screen is working properly.

The stepper should have side rails, a rail in the front, and/or moving posts on the side. When using the stationary rails, your hands should rest lightly to assist with balance. Posture should be upright. Make the legs do the work! If using the moving posts, again, use a light grip to assist with balance and to add upper-body movement to the workout.

Unlike the treadmill, there is no emergency shut-off key. You simply need to stop the motion of the pedals by riding the pedals to the floor. Step off, one foot at a time, and release the pedals gently.

Make sure you understand all of the machine's characteristics before engaging in a workout. Thoroughly understanding the instructions will result in a safer and more effective workout for you!

Important Points to Remember

Before you get on: Read the instructions.

Understand how to increase and decrease the intensity of the workout. Have your water bottle, reading material, and other necessary items prepared and safely stowed in an accessible place.

Just because you are not running does not mean you should step with any old shoe. Wear athletic shoes that support the foot, heel, and ankle. Dress comfortably by avoiding restrictive clothing.

Be sure your posture is upright! Stand tall and look forward. If you're looking down to read, rest your neck every few minutes by changing the head position.

Stepping rate: Choose an initial stepping rate that slightly raises the pulse rate. Remember, the faster the pedals move, the faster you must move to keep up! More pedal resistance allows you to slow your stepping rate. The height of each step should approximate the stepping action for climbing a normal step. The stepping height should feel comfortable on the knees and ankles.

Maintenance and Durability

- Is the manufacturing company reliable and reputable?

- Does the stepper require assembly? Can this be completed by the consumer?

- What costs are associated with lubrication and replacement of parts? Which parts are most likely to wear and where can those parts be purchased?

- Does the stepper come with a warranty? What does it cover and for how long?

- Are local technicians available for service?

Power and Performance

- Check on the weight limit of the machine. Is it safe for all users?

- Most home models require 110–220 volts—however, read the manufacturer's guidelines to be sure.

- Are you able to increase the difficulty of your workout as you increase your level of fitness? Check the range of stepping difficulty available on manual mode as well as the range of programs available on the machine.

- Be certain the machine is placed on a level floor.

Operation

- Is the control panel accessible and easy to read?

- Does the control panel have the capacity for manual use separate from software used for automated programming?

- Can you customize programs for yourself?

Other Considerations

- Do you have appropriate floor support for the weight of the machine? Are there rollers that allow you to move the stepper with reasonable ease?

- Does the ceiling height allow all users to use the machine safely?

- Determine your space considerations. Will you need to store the stepper periodically?

Chapter 24

Step Aerobics

Step aerobics, which revolutionized the fitness industry when it was introduced in the late 1980s, is a versatile training modality that can be made more or less intense by simply changing the height of the step, performing movements through different ranges of motion, or adjusting the step cadence. The research-supported benefits of step training include cardiorespiratory fitness, weight management, and mood enhancement.

Platform height: Platform height is dependent on the exerciser's level of aerobic fitness, current skill with step training, and degree of knee flexion when the knee is fully loaded while stepping up. Deconditioned individuals should begin on 4-inch steps, while highly skilled and experienced steppers can use 10-inch steps. The most common height is 8 inches.

Regardless of fitness level or skill, participants should not exercise on a platform height that causes the knee joint to flex deeper than 90 degrees when the knee is fully loaded (when all the body weight is on the leg of the first upward step). Individuals with chronic knee problems should seek their physician's approval to perform step training.

Posture: The head should be up, shoulders down and back, chest up, abdominals lightly contracted, and buttocks gently tucked under the hips. Do not hyperextend the knees or back at any time. When stepping up, lean from the ankles and not the waist to avoid excessive stress on the lumbar spine.

Stepping up: Contact the platform with the entire sole of the foot. To avoid Achilles tendon injury, do not allow the heel to land over the edge of the platform. Step softly and quietly to avoid unnecessary high impacts. Look at the platform periodically to ensure proper foot placement.

Stepping down: Step close to the platform (no more than one shoe length away) and allow the heels to contact the floor to help absorb shock. Stepping too far back while pressing the heel into the floor could result in Achilles tendon injury. If a step platform requires stepping a significant distance from the platform, do not push the heel into the floor. Keep the weight on the forefoot.

Leading foot: Change the leading foot (the foot that begins the step pattern) after no more than one minute. The leading leg experiences greater musculoskeletal stress than the non-leading leg.

Propulsion steps: Do not perform propulsion steps (in which both feet are off the floor or platform at the same time) for more than one minute at a time. Propulsion steps result in higher vertical impact forces and are considered an advanced technique.

All propulsion steps should be performed up onto the platform and not down from the platform.

Repeaters: To avoid stress to the support leg, do not perform more than five consecutive repeaters (in which the non-weight-bearing leg repeats the movement, such as in a knee lift) on the same leg.

Arms: Master the footwork before adding the arm movements. Avoid using the arms at or above shoulder level for an extended period of time, because this places significant stress on the shoulder girdle. Be sure to frequently vary low-, mid-, and high-range arm movements.

Music: Music tempos above 128 beats per minute (bpm) are not recommended. Technique and safety are seriously compromised when music speeds are too fast.

Weights: The use of weights during the aerobic portion of step training produces little if any increases in energy expenditure or muscle hypertrophy. However, the risk of injuring the shoulder joint is significantly increased when weights are rapidly moved through a large range of motion, especially if the arms are fully extended. It is recommended that weights be reserved for the strength segment of a step training class.

Chapter 25

Kickboxing

Are you looking for a total body workout that totally kicks butt? How about a way to increase your stamina, flexibility, and strength while listening to your favorite dance mixes?

If this sounds good to you, keep reading to find out what you need to know before you take the kickboxing challenge.

What Is Kickboxing?

Although the true roots of kickboxing date back to Asia 2,000 years ago, modern competitive kickboxing actually started in the 1970s, when American karate experts arranged competitions that allowed full-contact kicks and punches that had been banned in karate.

Because of health and safety concerns, padding and protective clothing and safety rules were introduced into the sport over the years, which led to the various forms of competitive kickboxing practiced in the United States today. The forms differ in the techniques used and the amount of physical contact that is allowed between the competitors.

Currently, one popular form of kickboxing is known as aerobic or cardiovascular (cardio) kickboxing, which combines elements of boxing, martial arts, and aerobics to provide overall physical conditioning and toning. Unlike other types of kickboxing, cardio kickboxing does not involve physical contact between competitors—it's a cardiovascular workout that's done because of its many benefits to the body.

Cardio kickboxing classes usually start with 10–15 minutes of warm-ups, which may include stretching and traditional exercises such as jumping jacks and push-ups, followed by a 30-minute kickboxing session that includes movements such as knee strikes, kicks, and punches. Some instructors may use equipment like punching bags or jump ropes.

After this, at least 5 minutes should be devoted to cooling down, followed by about 10 minutes of stretching and muscle conditioning. Stretching is really important because beginners can strain ("pull") their muscles, and slow, proper stretching helps relax muscles and prevent injury.

Instructional videos and DVDs are also available if you're interested in trying a cardio kickboxing routine at home.

The Basics

Before you decide to jump in and sign up for a class, you should keep a few basic guidelines in mind:

- **Know your current fitness level.** Kickboxing is a high-intensity, high-impact form of exercise, so it's probably not a good idea to plunge in after a long stint as a couch potato. You might try preparing yourself by first taking a low-impact aerobics course or less physical form of exercise and working up to a higher level of endurance. When you do begin kickboxing, allow yourself to be a beginner by working at your own pace and not overexerting yourself to the point of exhaustion.

- **Check it out before you sign up.** If possible, observe or try a class beforehand to see whether it's right for you and to make sure the instructor is willing to modify the routine a bit to accommodate people's different skill levels. Try to avoid classes that seem to move too fast, are too complicated, or don't provide the chance for any individual instruction during or after the class.

- **Find a class act.** Look for an instructor who has both a high-level belt in martial arts and is certified as a fitness instructor by an organization such as the American Council on Exercise (ACE). Also, try to start at a level that suits you and slowly progress to a more intense, fast-paced kickboxing class. Many classes call for intermediate levels of fitness and meet two to three times a week.

- **Comfort is key.** Wear loose, comfortable clothing that allows your arms and legs to move easily in all directions. The best shoes are cross-trainers—not tennis shoes—because cross-trainers allow for side-to-side movements. Gloves or hand wraps are sometimes used during classes—you may be able to buy these where your class is held. Give your instructor a call beforehand so you can be fully prepared.

- **Start slowly and don't overdo it.** The key to a good kickboxing workout is controlled movement. Overextending yourself by kicking too high or locking your arms and legs during movements can cause pulled muscles and tendons and sprained knee or ankle joints. Start with low kicks as you slowly learn proper kickboxing technique. This is very important for beginners, who are more prone to developing injuries while attempting quick, complicated kickboxing moves.

- **Drink up.** Drink plenty of fluids before, during, and after your class to quench your thirst and keep yourself hydrated.

- **Talk to your doctor.** It's always a good idea to see your doctor and have a complete physical exam before you begin any type of exercise program—especially one with a lot of aerobic activity like kickboxing. This is extremely important if you have any chronic medical conditions such as asthma or diabetes or are very overweight.

Moves You Can Use

Here are a few moves that you can try at home:

- **Roundhouse kick:** Stand with the right side of your body facing an imaginary target with your knees bent and your feet shoulders' width apart. Lift your right knee, pointing it just to the right of the target and pivoting your body toward the same direction. Kick with your right leg, as though you are hitting the target. Repeat with your other leg.

- **Front kick:** Stand with feet shoulders' width apart. Bend your knees slightly, and pull your right knee up toward your chest. Point your knee in the direction of an imaginary target. Then, kick out with the ball of your foot. Repeat with your other leg.

- **Side kick:** Start with the right side of your body facing a target. Pull your right knee up toward your left shoulder, and bend your knees slightly as you kick in the direction of your target. The outside of your foot or heel should be the part that would hit the target. Repeat with your other leg.

Why Kickboxing?

Besides keeping your body fit, kickboxing has other benefits. According to a study by ACE, you can burn anywhere from 350 to 450 calories an hour with kickboxing!

Kickboxing also reduces and relieves stress. Its rigorous workout—controlled punching and kicking movements carried out with the discipline and skills required for martial arts—can do wonders for feelings of frustration and anger. Practicing kickboxing moves can also help to improve balance, flexibility, coordination, and endurance.

Kickboxing is also a great way to get a total body workout while learning simple self-defense moves. Kickboxing fans say the sport helps them to feel more empowered and confident.

So get out there and jab, punch, and kick your way to fitness.

Chapter 26

Dancing

If television mimicked the real world, Americans tuning into such popular television shows as *So You Think You Can Dance* and *Dancing with the Stars* wouldn't think twice about jumping onto Mary Murphy's Hot Tamale Train or heating it up Latin-style with ballroom dancer's bad boy Maksim Chmerkovskiy or the lovely Chelsie Hightower.

Dream no more: The popularity of these shows has already set an entire railroad system in motion at a local dance studio near you. Whether you want to pack ballroom heels, hip-hop sneakers, tap shoes, ballerina flats, a belly dance costume, or even the hula hoop, fun dance classes are just around the corner.

With so many dance techniques to choose from, it's only a matter of time before you too can reap the benefits of feeling more energized and looking fit and toned. Dancing could even help you shed some extra pounds before the upcoming holiday season.

To help you find your own dance style that doesn't break the bank, ACE [American Council on Exercise] has consulted four acclaimed dance instructors to talk about their varied professional and coaching careers, client profile, and the ubiquitous health benefits one can reap from dancing at any age.

"So You Think You Can Dance? Well, Now You Can" © American Council on Exercise. Reprinted with permission from the American Council on Exercise (www.acefitness.org).

Jennifer Curry, Principal Ballerina of the California Ballet Company/Certified Pilates Instructor

At age 40, Curry is still dancing strong.

The principal ballerina for the California Ballet Company attributes her longevity as a professional dancer to her secret weapon—Pilates.

Pilates teaches awareness of breath and alignment of the spine, and aims to strengthen the deep torso muscles.

"It's been a tough journey," said Curry about her 30-year career path at the San Diego–based ballet company.

"For the body, it becomes more challenging to keep up with performance and class routines, but Pilates helped me sustain my career," said Curry, and added "I have better technique and better performances, because it gave me so much more core strength."

Curry's day begins in the morning with about two to five hours of ballet practice and continues with up to five hours of Pilates training and instruction, sometimes until 9 p.m. She offers private lessons at the Body Alchemist Pilates studio in San Diego. Her clients range from middle-aged working professionals to professional dancers. Curry charges $70 for a 60-minute private lesson; $26 a person for group sessions; and $35 per person for semiprivate lessons.

By popular demand, the California Ballet School, part of the California Ballet Company, also recently expanded its classical ballet training to offer a wider and more diverse curriculum.

"Lately with the dance infusion in pop culture, more people are getting interested in hip hop, jazz, tap, and lyrical (fusing contemporary, modern, and ballet)," Curry said.

The finalists of *So You Think You Can Dance* have all trained extensively in these techniques.

See the California Ballet School [www.californiaballetschool.com] for a class schedule. Additionally, for dance education information at the local, state, and national levels, check out the National Dance Education Organization [ndeo.org].

Curry said she is also excited about the heightened interest by high school students.

"It's becoming more cool," she said, noting an upsurge in the numbers of high school dance departments and arts programs. Meanwhile, the *Dancing with the Stars* series has bolstered interest in ballroom dancing among adults.

But you don't have to be a rising TV star or a youngster to start formal dance training, including in classical ballet, Curry said.

"Anybody at any age can get started," Curry said.

"Dance keeps you looking young and feeling young at heart." Curry is living proof that this is true.

Tesha Marie Jacobson, U.S. Latin Dance Champion and Ballroom Dance Instructor

Tesha Marie Jacobson left behind a successful career as an internationally acclaimed ballroom dancer to coach professional and aspiring ballroom dancers and amateur dancers.

She agrees with Curry that dance shows have bolstered interest in ballroom dancing.

"People want to learn ballroom dancing for wedding parties and I also got a lot more younger people involved," noted Jacobson. She began dancing at the tender age of 11 after watching a friend in a dance class.

Certainly, the earlier one starts formal dance training, the better the chances for a professional career. Hence, it's nice to see more studios pop up with kids in mind, she said.

Compared to Europeans, who enroll children at a young age in ballroom dance classes to learn about etiquette and classical dance, American children prefer dancing ballet or tap. But as more TV shows feature 20-somethings or younger partnering up to dance a Viennese waltz or Quickstep, the greater the "hip factor."

"*So You Think You Can Dance* has brought to light that ballroom and Latin dancing is a real art form that they have to train in," Jacobson said.

Partner dancing isn't merely a full body workout; it trains the mind as well.

"Having taught at so many levels, you learn how to dance and control your muscles while using your mind to control muscle action and to create timing," Jacobson said.

During formal competitions, partners sometimes dance up to five hours at a time.

Ladies dance in heels and are so graceful on their feet that their heavy costumes appear weightless.

Jacobson used to soak and rub her feet for hours to find relief. She didn't recognize until late in her career that adding weight lifting for strength and yoga for stretching can help significantly with injury prevention and overall performance.

"Since getting my ACE certification (as a Group Fitness Instructor) I know how muscles function and how the body works as I'm getting people ready for competition," Jacobson said. "I can pinpoint which muscles are working and make that movement happen."

And men, if you think partner dancing isn't a good workout, consider Jacobson's boyfriend.

A non-trained dancer, Jacobson said her boyfriend swears he gets a better cardio workout Latin dancing than playing basketball.

For local chapters on ballroom dancing visit USA Dance [www .usadance.org].

Valentina Martin, Hoop Dance Instructor and Owner of "Unity Hoops"

Valentina "Unity" Martin started belly dancing at the age of 12 with her mother.

It wasn't until 2007, when she met San Diego's Jennifer Quest, aka "HoopCharmer," at the annual Burning Man event, an underground arts festival held in Nevada, that Martin became hooked on "hooping."

Hooping or hoop dance uses a hula hoop, but these are not to be confused with the primordial version of hula hoops from the 1950s.

These handmade rainbow-colored hoops are offered in a variety of sizes, weights, and can be accessorized with LED lights and even fire for more advanced performers. Dancers use the hoop on virtually every part of their body, starting with basic moves around the waist and progressing to movements around the arms, legs, and up and down the entire body. The single prevailing element is the dancer's happiness.

Still an underground dance, Martin would love nothing more than to make hooping mainstream.

Her dance troupe "Hoop Unit" books live performances at multiple venues and events. But Martin loves the idea of teaching hooping to students who she vows will get a great workout along the way.

Martin teaches 60-minute hoop dance classes at the Point Loma Dance Studio and at University of California, San Diego recreation. Drop-in fees are $12 per person or $40 for five classes at the studio. Most students are between 18-40 years old and female, but everyone is welcome to hoop.

Class starts with a warm-up or basic hooping around the waist, working the abdominal muscles, followed by walking and turning with the hoop and moving the hoop around the hands, feet, and legs.

"I also teach them how to hoop on shoulders and around the body in an expressive way," Martin said. Advanced students learn even more tricks. Every class is taught with fun, upbeat music.

Martin said many people don't realize that hooping is a solid aerobic workout.

"It increases flexibility in your back, is low impact, and you can definitely feel it in your stomach, arms, legs, and glutes," Martin added. It's a sure way to tone your body.

Martin sells her hoop creations online. Every hoop is handmade, collapsible, and colorful. Prices range from $30–$50. Visit unityhoops. com for more detailed information or YouTube for a video demonstration of these portable hoops.

To locate hooping instructors in your area, the best place to start is the international website hooping.org. Another valuable resource is hulahooping.meetup.com to find "meetup" groups all over the world focused on hooping.

Leilainia Penix, Belly Dancer and Instructor; "Shimmy Sisters"

Leilainia grew up belly dancing with her mother and sister.

"My mother was a belly dancer," said Penix. "It's part of my culture and I grew up with it."

It wasn't until 2002 that Penix started looking at belly dance as a business. She formed her own entertainment company dubbed Nomad Artz Co.

Penix performs solo and with her sister under the name "Shimmy Sisters."

She also teaches belly dance, crediting singers Beyonce and Shakira for bringing belly dance into the mainstream through their videos and stage performances.

"One thing that is great about belly dancing is that you can start at any point of your life," Penix said. "You can be out of shape or overweight (it doesn't matter). It is one of those dances that you can grow with and that grows with you."

Penix teaches belly dance at the California Ballet School, Pure Fitness, and at Bamboo Yoga in San Diego to a variety of students of all ages.

"People come to lose weight and to have fun," she said. Some students look at belly dance as a hobby, yet others strive to become performers and to join Penix on stage.

Penix describes belly dance as an internal dance that allows you to view your body as beautiful regardless of shape or size. She said belly dancers can achieve tranquility and meditative qualities that are similar to practicing tai chi and qigong.

"You will have a more peaceful relationship with your body and will feel more energized," she said. She defies the stereotype of belly dance as being sexual and reserved for entertaining men.

"Belly dancing isn't about that," she said. "It's about finding a connection from within yourself and women dancing together. As people learn more about it, it broadens their awareness of the art."

Among the many health benefits of belly dancing are improved core balance and coordination, increased flexibility and strength, and enhanced physical appearance and posture. It can help tone the arms, abs, obliques, legs, and the back. One hour of belly dance can burn up to 400 calories.

See Leilainia.com for classes and more information. For a list of various belly dance classes by city and state, check out us.bellydanceclasses.net.

Chapter 27

Racquet Sports

The reasons for playing tennis are many and are listed and explained in this chapter. As for who should play, the answer is anyone—at any age and at any skill level. The following describes several groups of people and how, based on their stage of life, they can enjoy both the physical and psychological benefits of playing what many people call "the sport for a lifetime." To see for yourself how science has proved that tennis contributes to health and fitness, keep reading!

Young children (or their parents, who are looking for healthy activities for their children): Tennis not only provides children with much-needed exercise but also has been shown to help psychological skill development and improve bone growth and general fitness. (These benefits are very important to stemming the problem of childhood obesity). Physical activity also strengthens the immune system of every child who plays the game.

Preteens and teens: People in this age group will have tons of fun, increase their social skills, and build friendships. Tennis will help preteens and teens increase their self-confidence and generally feel better about themselves. Also, tennis can enhance their cognitive abilities, thus helping this group improve their grades.

This chapter excerpted from "Tennis—For the Health of It!" © 2008. This copyright material is reprinted with permission of the United States Professional Tennis Association and was originally published on its website at www.uspta.com.

Adults (ages 18–55): Tennis is a great fitness activity and good social outlet that provides general wellness by improving the immune system. It also boosts cognitive skills and emotional well-being.

Seniors (ages 55–up): Tennis is a tremendous activity for strengthening the immune system, thus improving longevity. It also assists in the development of a healthier bone structure and the prevention of osteoporosis. Basically, tennis will improve a person's overall fitness and general wellness.

Tennis is the Ultimate Exercise—Both Mentally and Physically

Tennis-specific research has discovered:

- People who participate in tennis three hours per week at a moderately vigorous intensity cut in half their risk of death from any cause, according to the late Dr. Ralph Paffenbarger, who was an internationally recognized exercise authority and studied more than 10,000 people for 20 years.

- Tennis players scored higher in vigor, optimism, and self-esteem while scoring lower in depression, anger, confusion, anxiety, and tension than other athletes and nonathletes, according to Dr. Joan Finn and colleagues at Southern Connecticut State University.

- Since tennis requires alertness and tactical thinking, it may generate new connections between nerves in the brain and promote a lifetime of continuing brain development.

- Tennis, as a racquet sport, outperforms golf and most other sports in developing positive personality characteristics, according to Dr. Jim Gavin, author of *The Exercise Habit*.

- Competitive tennis burns more calories than most other activities, according to studies in caloric expenditures. A detailed analysis in the January 2005 issue of *Consumer Reports* compared various activities and the calories burned. The article showed that tennis ranks among the top five activities that one could participate in to burn the most calories and, in fact, burns more calories than swimming, rowing, weightlifting, jazzercise, hiking, or golf.

With these facts in mind, review the 34 specific reasons why you should consider playing regularly!

Physical Reasons to Play Tennis

1. Aerobic fitness: Playing tennis burns fat, improves cardiovascular fitness, and helps the body maintain higher energy levels.

The American College of Sports Medicine has cited that more calories may be burned in high-intensity intervals of exercise interspersed with low to moderate intensity levels. That's exactly what tennis provides. It is interval training, due to the nature of how points are played. Because the heart rate gets into a fat-burning zone and then can easily go higher, tennis has been recognized as one of the leading activities that help to burn fat. Also, because the intensity of tennis can get fairly high, depending on how hard a player works while playing, and because tennis is purely an interval sport, more fat is burned after working out than during the time on court. Thus, physical capacity gets stronger and players have more energy later on for what matters most in life.

2. Anaerobic fitness: Playing tennis builds muscle power and improves physical capacity.

Since the average point in tennis is between 4 and 12 seconds long, tennis allows players to fully engage their anaerobic (or power) system. During the short duration of a tennis point, the body relies on the energy provided by a starch called glycogen that is stored in the muscles. This form of metabolism works without the aid of oxygen and a player goes into what scientists call oxygen debt. Following this, the body recovers to replenish this "debt" through improved heart and lung function. The natural repetition provided by tennis allows the body to adapt by building muscle and improving heart-lung function. In fact, Legros and colleagues found that the rate of phosphocreatine concentrations (PC) (a measure of anaerobic capacity/fitness) recovery was much faster in tennis players or active people than in sedentary subjects.

3. Improved acceleration: Tennis improves a person's ability to accelerate.

One of the key measures to athletic success is the ability to accelerate from a still position to maximum velocity. Regardless of the sport activity, accelerating and positioning are foundational to high achievement. This occurs naturally in tennis! In every point while playing tennis, you must explode, sprint, and recover for the next shot. This constant and repetitive "explosive movement" trains your body for forceful movements that truly expand your capacity. As the muscles adapt to the need for improved strength and power, you become quicker and more agile.

4. Enhanced power for first step: In tennis, what matters is the first step, which requires anticipation, quick reaction time, and explosive action.

5. Improved speed: Speed is the distance you travel divided by time.

6. Leg strength: You can build leg muscles through the hundreds of starts and stops that tennis requires.

The constant lunging, pushing off, or leaping to hit an overhead develops your legs unlike many other activities. Laforest, S., and other researchers, even found that the muscles of tennis players demonstrated a greater resistance to fatigue than those of sedentary people across two sets of age groups (ages 27 to 30 and ages 64 to 66). In fact, people often say that tennis players have "great legs." Why? Because of the natural repetitions that occur when they play.

7. Coordination: Tennis develops incredible coordination.

8. Enhanced gross motor control: You must move and perform ball-striking skills in tennis that require control of your large muscle groups.

9. Better fine motor control: In the great game of tennis, you often must slow the ball down and hit a gentle, soft return. We call these maneuvers either a drop shot or drop volley.

10. Agility: Tennis improves agility because it forces you to change direction as many as five times in 10 seconds during a typical point.

When playing a point, you must constantly change direction. Imagine if you do this over and over for the duration of an entire match or tennis workout, which could be well over an hour. The overall agility gained from playing tennis is great for your body. Also, coaches in other sports are always looking for ways to vary their practices and workouts. Cross-training has become a huge part of what athletes do, both for the improvement and/or maintenance of all forms of fitness as well as the improvement of general skills that will benefit them in their specific activity. Tennis provides great cross-training for other sports that require rapid changes in direction, including football, basketball, soccer, baseball, and volleyball.

11. Good dynamic balance: Dynamic balance—balance while moving—is as important in everyday life as it is in sports.

12. Cross-training: Tennis is a physically demanding sport that's fun and challenging for athletes of other sports.

13. Bone strength: For years, scientists and physicians have recommended "impact" exercises for people who want to increase bone strength and density and prevent osteoporosis.

Experts usually recommend running, jogging, or even walking to build bones, but when it comes to an activity that will create impact with the ground, as well as impact when striking the ball, nothing beats tennis. Bone development for children is critical, and bone growth and maintenance for seniors is equally important.

14. Improved immune system: Tennis, through its conditioning effects, promotes overall health, fitness, and resistance to disease.

Studies have demonstrated that the more active you are the stronger and healthier your immune system will be. And, the intensity of exercise helps to strengthen the immune system even more. It makes sense, then, that tennis, with its inherent demands for heart rate, interval training, impact, agility, etc., is one of the most beneficial activities in which you could participate. Schneider and Greenburg cited tennis specifically as an activity in which participants were less likely to be obese, smoke, or be involved in other forms of threatening activities than those who participate in team sports and an aggregate of other sports. And, Laforest, with other scientists, discovered that recreational tennis players who participate twice a week had a lower body fat percentage than age-matched control groups.

Finally, Houston and colleagues published a longitudinal investigation of more than 1,000 male students examined after an average of 22 and 40 years. Sustained playing of activities such as tennis was associated with a lower risk of cardiovascular disease. They inferred that a primary factor for this beneficial health profile may be that tennis was the sport played most often through mid-life.

15. Better nutritional habits: Tennis players learn how to eat to enhance energy production during a match and recovery after a match.

16. Good hand-eye coordination: Tennis players develop good hand-eye coordination because they must constantly judge the timing between the oncoming ball and the proper contact point.

17. Flexibility: Because tennis players continually stretch and maneuver to return the ball to their opponent they become more flexible.

Psychological Reasons to Play Tennis

18. Strong work ethic: Tennis improvement through lessons and practice reinforces the value of hard work.

19. Self-discipline: Tennis requires you to work on improving your skills during practice and to control the pace of play during competition, which builds discipline.

20. Recognize and manage mistakes: A tennis match can become a game of emergencies! More matches are won by players capitalizing on their opponents' unforced errors than by the players hitting outright winners.

21. One-on-one competition: The ability to do battle on court trains you in the ups and downs of a competitive world. During the 2008 match between Andy Roddick and Roger Federer at the Sony Ericsson Tournament (where Roddick overcame an 11-match losing streak with Federer), Roddick won a big point at particularly stressful time in the match. The commentators said, "Fortune goes to the brave!"

You must react and respond to what your opponent has done with the ball, how he or she wants to play the point, think while you are moving, plan while you are hurrying to the shot, execute your shot, and recover to your next position, while the whole time determining how you can take control of the point. The question you must learn to quickly answer: Do you need to be defensive and patient or do you take the offensive and set up to finish the point? All of this is learned in the great game of tennis.

22. Build responsibility: Tennis requires you to practice and "show up" for competition on time and with all of your equipment.

23. Manage adversity: Tennis players must learn to adjust to changing conditions and still be able to compete tenaciously.

24. Manage stress: The physical, mental, and emotional stress of tennis forces you to increase your capacity for dealing with stress.

When you play singles, you are out there on your own. Not only are you alone on the court during a singles match, but you must continually battle your opponent. And, then there's the battle with yourself.

Stress is actually the stimulus for growth, and recovery is when you grow. With no recovery, there is no growth. The key to successful living is to build recovery naturally into your life so that you can increase your capacity for stressful situations. When a person lives a linear lifestyle by just go, go, go, that life is dysfunctional! And, complete linearity in life can cause high blood pressure, the development of poor lifestyle habits, and even death. However, tennis helps you to build recovery in a natural way by the very essence of how it is played. You literally get to practice thinking and acting under stress, which is huge preparation for life skills. It is a continual battle with your opponent, but also with yourself. Every point has the capacity to become an emotional slap in the face. Yet, the more you play, the more effectively you learn to manage all of the stresses that life and tennis competition create.

25. Recover and adapt: Because of the nature of tennis, a player must learn to recover quickly, adapting to the stress that each point presents.

26. Planning and implementation: In tennis, you naturally learn how to plan and implement a strategy based on your anticipation of your opponent's moves.

27. Develop problem-solving skills: Tennis forces you to learn to solve problems based on angles, geometry, and physics.

28. Develop performance rituals: Tennis is a game of rhythm and preparation. In between points you will learn how to prepare yourself physically, emotionally, and mentally for the next point.

29. Sportsmanship: Tennis teaches all of us about fairness, honesty, integrity, and overall sportsmanship.

30. Win with grace and lose with honor: Gloating after a win or making excuses after a loss doesn't work in tennis or in life.

31. Teamwork: Successful doubles play depends on you and your partner's ability to communicate well and play as a cohesive unit.

32. Develop social skills: Tennis encourages participants to be social, especially recreational players. There are many opportunities for players to interact and communicate during a match—before play begins, during changeovers, and after a match.

33. Fun: People who play tennis experience healthy feelings of enjoyment, competitiveness, and physical challenge.

And, reason No. 34: Tennis is the sport for a lifetime.

When all is said and done, it's hard to argue against these reasons for playing tennis!

Tennis, as sports science supports, is a great choice for many reasons. Not only does it contribute to physical fitness and health, it also enhances mental focus, self-esteem, and a host of other personality traits that positively affect a person's overall sense of well-being.

At the end of the day, we invite you to speak with anyone who has played a lot of tennis in their life. We know from all our experience that these people will say one or more of several things:

- "I met some of my best friends on a tennis court."

- "Tennis is the greatest game in the world because it keeps me physically fit."

- "Tennis helped me to be more competitive in my business life, understanding more fully how to compete."

- "I learned how to work with people by playing tennis doubles."

- "I learned to control my anger through tennis. Managing mistakes was key to this."

To get started playing tennis, or to return to the game if you played previously, contact your local USPTA professional. Visit www .usptafindapro.com and search for a certified professional using your city, state, ZIP code, or a pro's last name.

Chapter 28

Aquatic Exercise

Chapter Contents

Section 28.1

Water Fitness

"Health Benefits of Water-Based Exercise,"
Centers for Disease Control and Prevention
(www.cdc.gov), December 23, 2009.

Swimming is the third most popular sports activity in the United States and a good way to get regular aerobic physical activity.[1] Just two and a half hours per week of aerobic physical activity, such as swimming, bicycling, or running, can decrease the risk of chronic illnesses.[2-3] This can also lead to improved health for people with diabetes and heart disease.[2] Swimmers have about half the risk of death compared with inactive people.[3] People report enjoying water-based exercise more than exercising on land.[4] They can also exercise longer in water than on land without increased effort or joint or muscle pain.[5-6]

Water-Based Exercise and Chronic Illness

Water-based exercise can help people with chronic diseases. For people with arthritis, it improves use of affected joints without worsening symptoms.[7] People with rheumatoid arthritis have more health improvements after participating in hydrotherapy than with other activities.[8] Water-based exercise also improves the use of affected joints and decreases pain from osteoarthritis.[9]

Water-Based Exercise and Mental Health

Water-based exercise improves mental health. Swimming can improve mood in both men and women.[10] For people with fibromyalgia, it can decrease anxiety, and exercise therapy in warm water can decrease depression and improve mood.[11-12] Water-based exercise can improve the health of mothers and their unborn children and has a positive effect on the mothers' mental health.[13] Parents of children with developmental disabilities find that recreational activities, such as swimming, improve family connections.[14]

Water-Based Exercise and Older Adults

Water-based exercise can benefit older adults by improving the quality of life and decreasing disability.[15] It also improves or maintains the bone health of post-menopausal women.[16]

A Good Choice

Exercising in water offers many physical and mental health benefits and is a good choice for people who want to be more active. When in the water, remember to protect yourself and others from illness and injury by practicing healthy and safe swimming behaviors.

1. U.S. Census Bureau. 2010 Statistical Abstract of the United States. Recreation Table 1212. Participation in Selected Sports Activities: 2007. Available at www.census.gov/compendia/statab/2010/tables/10s1212.pdf.

2. U.S. Department of Health and Human Services. 2008 Physical Activity Guidelines for Americans: Be active, healthy, and happy! In Chapter 2: Physical Activity Has Many Health Benefits. Available at www.health.gov/paguidelines.

3. Chase, N.L., Sui, X., Blair, S.N. 2008. Swimming and all-cause mortality risk compared with running, walking, and sedentary habits in men. *Int J of Aquatic Res and Educ.* 2(3): 213–23.

4. Lotshaw, A.M., Thompson, M., Sadowsky, S., Hart, M.K., and Millard, M.W. 2007. Quality of life and physical performance in land- and water-based pulmonary rehabilitation. *Journal of Cardiopulmonary Rehab and Prev.* 27: 247–51.

5. Broman, G., Quintana, M., Engardt, M., Gullstrand, L., Jansson, E., and Kaijser, L. 2006. Older women's cardiovascular responses to deep-water running. *Journal of Aging and Phys Activ.* 14: 29–40.

6. Cider, A., Svealv, B.G., Tang, M.S., Schaufelberger, M., and Andersson, B. 2006. Immersion in warm water induces improvement in cardiac function in patients with chronic heart failure. *Eur J Heart Fail.* 8(3): 308–13.

7. Westby, M.D. 2001. A health professional's guide to exercise prescription for people with arthritis: a review of aerobic fitness activities. *Arthritis Care and Res.* 45(6): 501–11.

8. Hall, J., Skevington, S.M., Maddison, P.J., and Chapman, K. 1996. A randomized and controlled trial of hydrotherapy in rheumatoid arthritis. *Arthritis Care Res.* 9(3): 206–15.

9. Bartels E.M., Lund H., Hagen K.B., Dagfinrud H., Christensen R., and Danneskiold-Samsøe B. 2007. Aquatic exercise for the treatment of knee and hip osteoarthritis. *Cochrane Database of Systematic Reviews.* 4: 1–9.

10. Berger, B.G., and Owen, D.R. 1992. Mood alteration with yoga and swimming: aerobic exercise may not be necessary. *Percept Mot Skills.* 75(3 Pt 2): 1331–43.

11. Tomas-Carus, P., Gusi, N., Hakkinen, A., Hakkinen, K., Leal, A., and Ortega-Alonso, A. 2008. Eight months of physical training in warm water improves physical and mental health in women with fibromyalgia: a randomized controlled trial. *J Rehabil Med.* 40(4): 248–52.

12. Gowans, S.E., and deHueck, A. 2007. Pool exercise for individuals with fibromyalgia. *Curr Opin Rheumatol.* 19(2): 168–73.

13. Hartmann, S., and Bung, P. 1999. Physical exercise during pregnancy—physiological considerations and recommendations. *J Perinat Med.* 27(3): 204–15.

14. Mactavish, J.B., and Schleien, S.J. 2004. Re-injecting spontaneity and balance in family life: parents' perspectives on recreation in families that include children with developmental disability. *J Intellect Disabil Res.* 48(Pt 2): 123–41.

15. Sato, D., Kaneda, K., Wakabayashi, H., and Nomura, T. 2007. The water exercise improves health-related quality of life of frail elderly people at day service facility. *Qual Life Res.* 16: 1577–85.

16. Rotstein, A., Harush, M., and Vaisman, N. 2008. The effect of water exercise program on bone density of postmenopausal women. *J Sports Med Phys Fitness.* 48(3): 352–9.

Section 28.2

Top 10 Reasons You Should Exercise in Water

"Top 10 Reasons Why You Should Exercise in Water," by Mark Grevelding. © 2008 Aquatic Exercise Association (www.aeawave.com). Reprinted with permission. Mark Grevelding is the owner of Fit Motivation, a fitness education and resource company based in Rochester, NY. He is a training specialist and continuing education provider with Aquatic Exercise Association.

Aquatic fitness has come out of the shadows and is drawing fans of all shapes, sizes, and ages. Men, women, and children are diving in and discovering fluid fun and cool challenges as they splash their way to a fitter body. Check out your local pool schedule and you may find aquatic kickboxing, cycling, boot camp, jogging, walking, Pilates, yoga, and much more!

Here are ten reasons to get wet!

#10: Follow the trend. The boomers are aging and so are their hips and knees. Watch out because new pool construction is going gang busters and will continue to do so over the next 15 years. Due to the fact that aquatic fitness is soaring in popularity, most locations are building more than one pool. A cooler pool is built for lap swimming and aggressive aquatic fitness programs, while a warmer pool meets the needs of senior programming, rehabilitation, and mind/body classes. New and exciting programming will continue to crop up as innovative aquatic equipment and technology develops due to increased demand!

#9: Provides excellent cross training. If you always do what you always did you will always get what you always got! Eventually your body will plateau on an exercise program if you do not introduce variation, or worse you could make yourself vulnerable to overuse injuries. Water offers the perfect solution to cross training. Do you like to jog? Try deep water jogging or lap swimming. Do you like to strength train with weights? Try an aquatic class that uses equipment or webbed gloves. Your body will thank you for introducing aquatic fitness into your exercise routine and that frustrating plateau will surely wash away!

#8: Sleep better. One of the first things a new aqua fitness participant notices is the incredible night of sleep that awaits them after a vigorous training session in water. Exercise in general has been proven to improve sleep patterns. However, aquatic exercise does even better due to the specific properties of the aquatic environment and their impact on the systems of the human body. Improved blood flow, changes in body temperature, and enhanced muscle conditioning all contribute to an absolutely delightful slumber under the sheets!

#7: You can't do that on land! The unique properties of water allow for creative and aggressive fitness programming. Kickboxing in the water lends itself to exciting kick adventures because *both* feet can come off the floor thanks to buoyancy in the water. Re-discover boot camp with an H_2O twist. The viscosity of water allows you to push, pull, run, jump, jack, and jog much harder! Get wet and discover moves you never would have thought possible. A jumping jack with a tuck and half turn, followed by ski moguls and two more jacks before letting your feet even touch the pool bottom? You can't do that in your living room or an aerobic studio!

#6: You get more in one workout. What happened to leisure activities and spare time? Most people would agree that there simply aren't enough hours in the day. Finding time to exercise is the biggest hindrance to people who want to get in shape. Aquatic fitness provides the perfect blend of cardio and muscle conditioning for people who are pressed for time. Exercising in the pool is like exercising in a liquid gym. Submerged in water you spend the entire exercise session working your muscles in pairs. On land, an arm curl would only work the bicep; in water the same arm curl works both the bicep and triceps thanks to submerged resistance. Furthermore, increased muscle demand creates increased oxygen consumption. Water fitness is an excellent choice for improving both cardiovascular health and muscle tone, especially when lack of time is an issue.

#5: You'll get more out of your core. Core training is all the rage now. In prehistoric times we simply referred to it as an ab workout. Fitness equipment manufacturers keep supplying the market with expensive core training devices and consumers can't get enough. Save yourself some money and get in the water! If you seriously want more out of your core take a deep water fitness class or simply put on a flotation belt and jog/walk in deep water. Maintaining vertical alignment in deep water keeps core musculature in a constant state of work. If you are skittish about deep water, consider putting the same flotation belt on in the shallow end and experiment with some suspended movement. Better yet, float onto your back and treat yourself to some killer crunches in the water.

#4: Exercising in water is fun. Let's face it—there are people who just don't like to exercise. Common psychology dictates that if you dislike an exercise activity you will distract yourself with every excuse you can think of to avoid it. On the other hand, if you enjoy a fitness activity you will move heaven and earth to participate in that planned exercise session. Exercising in water is *fun*! There is something about romping around in a pool that makes you feel young and vibrant. If you enjoy a fitness activity you will commit to an exercise plan. If you commit to planned exercise sessions over a period of time you will change your body, your mind, and your life!

#3: Exercising in water is a good workout. Everyone wants to work hard, including seniors! Water provides an excellent opportunity for allowing variations in the intensity of a workout. Unlike land fitness, working out in a pool you are surrounded by a source of resistance and each individual can decide how hard to push, pull, and move that resistance during the workout. Water exercise allows people of *all* fitness levels to work at a pace that is appropriate for their exercise goals. The more forceful you push the harder the workout. The secret must be getting out because aquatic fitness formats like kickboxing, boot camp, and cycling are bringing younger exercise enthusiasts into the pool along with more men!

#2: Reduced joint impact. Unlike today's children, the baby boomers participated in lots of sports and spent their childhoods playing outdoors. As they got older they kept in shape with running, aerobics, biking, and more. Unfortunately, joint impact issues have sidelined many boomers from the land fitness activities they once enjoyed. Doctors are encouraging water fitness for good reason. The buoyant property of water unloads joints and allows for vigorous physical activity with minimal or zero joint impact. For example, if you are in water that is at chest level you will be bearing only about 25–35% of your body weight. If you simply flex at your hips and knees and lower into the water at shoulder level you will virtually eliminate impact during fitness activity. It gets better! Deep water training is vigorous exercise with zero impact—100% of the time!

#1: Burn calories and lose weight. Whether you need to slim down or work hard at maintaining your weight, exercising in water is a safe and efficient method of burning calories. When you work out in

321

a pool you don't have to sweat or suffer through the aches and pains of joint impact. Submerged in water you don't have to endure numbing boredom on an exercise machine or the shame of stumbling through a complicated class—in full view of mirrors and windows in the aerobic studio. The obesity epidemic is a serious problem and aquatic fitness is a serious solution. The problem only gets worse when you look at the obesity issues facing children. Pools provide a great fitness playground for kids.

Countless people worldwide have transformed their bodies thanks to water exercise. The most un-athletic people suddenly discover their inner athlete unleashed in the pool as they learn how to work the water with power and force. People who have never exercised a day in their life suddenly get hooked with the fitness bug after just a few aquatic fitness classes. Water truly is the essence of life.

Get wet and get fit!

Chapter 29

Walking and Hiking

Chapter Contents

Section 29.1

Beginning a Walking Program

This section excerpted from "Walking: A Step in the Right Direction,"
National Institute of Diabetes and Digestive and Kidney Diseases
(www.niddk.nih.gov), March 2007.

Walking is one of the easiest ways to be physically active. You can
do it almost anywhere and at any time. Walking is also inexpensive—
all you need is a pair of shoes with sturdy heel support. Walking may
accomplish the following:

- Give you more energy and make you feel good
- Reduce stress and help you relax
- Tone your muscles
- Increase the number of calories your body uses
- Strengthen your bones and muscles
- Improve your stamina and your fitness
- Lower your risk of chronic diseases, such as heart disease and
  type 2 diabetes
- Give you an opportunity to socialize actively with friends and
  family

For all of these reasons, people have started walking programs. If
you would like to start your own program, read and follow the information in this section.

Is It Okay for Me to Walk?

Answer the following questions before you begin a walking program.

- Has your health care provider told you that you have heart trouble, diabetes, or asthma?
- When you are physically active, do you have pains in your chest,
  neck, shoulder, or arm?

- Do you often feel faint or have dizzy spells?

- Do you feel extremely breathless after you have been physically active?

- Has your health care provider told you that you have high blood pressure?

- Has your health care provider told you that you have bone or joint problems, such as arthritis?

- Are you over 50 years old and not used to doing any moderate physical activity?

- Are you pregnant?

- Do you smoke?

- Do you have a health problem or physical reason not mentioned here that might keep you from starting a walking program?

If you answered yes to any of these questions, please check with your health care provider before starting a walking program or other form of physical activity.

How Do I Start a Walking Program?

Leave time in your busy schedule to follow a walking program that will work for you. Keep the following points in mind as you plan your program:

- Choose a safe place to walk. Find a partner or group of people to walk with you. Your walking partner(s) should be able to walk with you on the same schedule and at the same speed.

- Wear shoes with proper arch support, a firm heel, and thick flexible soles that will cushion your feet and absorb shock. Before you buy a new pair, be sure to walk in them in the store.

- Wear clothes that will keep you dry and comfortable. Look for synthetic fabrics that absorb sweat and remove it from your skin.

- For extra warmth in winter, wear a knit cap. To stay cool in summer, wear a baseball cap or visor.

- Think of your walk in three parts. Warm up by walking slowly for five minutes. Then, increase your speed and do a fast walk. Finally, cool down by walking slowly again for five minutes.

- Do light stretching after your warm-up and cool-down.

- Try to walk at least three times per week. Each week, add two or three minutes to your walk. If you walk less than three times per week, you may need more time to adjust before you increase the pace or frequency of your walk.

- To avoid stiff or sore muscles and joints, start gradually. Over several weeks, begin walking faster, going further, and walking for longer periods of time.

- Set goals and rewards. Examples of goals are participating in a fun walk or walking continuously for 30 minutes.

- Keep track of your progress with a walking journal or log.

- The more you walk, the better you may feel and the more calories you may burn.

Experts recommend 30 minutes of moderate-intensity physical activity on most, if not all, days of the week. If you cannot do 30 minutes at a time, try walking for shorter amounts and gradually working up to it.

Safety Tips

Keep safety in mind when you plan your route and the time of your walk.

- If you walk at dawn, dusk, or night, wear a reflective vest or brightly colored clothing.

- Walk in a group when possible.

- Notify your local police station of your group's walking time and route.

- Do not wear jewelry.

- Do not wear headphones.

- Be aware of your surroundings.

How Do I Stretch?

Stretch gently after you warm up your muscles with an easy five-minute walk, and again after you cool down. Try doing the stretches listed here. Do not bounce or hold your breath when you stretch. Perform slow movements and stretch only as far as you feel comfortable.

Side Reach: Reach one arm over your head and to the side. Keep your hips steady and your shoulders straight to the side. Hold for 10 seconds and repeat on the other side.

Wall Push: Lean your hands on a wall with your feet about three to four feet away from the wall. Bend one knee and point it toward the wall. Keep your back leg straight with your foot flat and your toes pointed straight ahead. Hold for 10 seconds and repeat with the other leg.

Knee Pull: Lean your back against a wall. Keep your head, hips, and feet in a straight line. Pull one knee to your chest, hold for 10 seconds, then repeat with the other leg.

Leg Curl: Pull your right foot to your buttocks with your right hand. Stand straight and keep your knee pointing straight to the ground. Hold for 10 seconds and repeat with your left foot and hand.

Table 29.1. A Sample Walking Program

	Warm-Up Time	Fast-Walk Time	Cool-Down Time	Total Time
Week 1	Walk slowly 5 minutes	Walk briskly 5 minutes	Walk slowly 5 minutes	15 minutes
Week 2	Walk slowly 5 minutes	Walk briskly 8 minutes	Walk slowly 5 minutes	18 minutes
Week 3	Walk slowly 5 minutes	Walk briskly 11 minutes	Walk slowly 5 minutes	21 minutes
Week 4	Walk slowly 5 minutes	Walk briskly 14 minutes	Walk slowly 5 minutes	24 minutes
Week 5	Walk slowly 5 minutes	Walk briskly 7 minutes	Walk slowly 5 minutes	27 minutes
Week 6	Walk slowly 5 minutes	Walk briskly 20 minutes	Walk slowly 5 minutes	30 minutes
Week 7	Walk slowly 5 minutes	Walk briskly 23 minutes	Walk slowly 5 minutes	33 minutes
Week 8	Walk slowly 5 minutes	Walk briskly 26 minutes	Walk slowly 5 minutes	36 minutes
Week 9 and Beyond	Walk slowly 5 minutes	Walk briskly 30 minutes	Walk slowly 5 minutes	40 minutes

If you walk less than three times per week, give yourself more than a week before increasing your pace and frequency.

Hamstring: Sit on a sturdy bench or hard surface so that your left leg is stretched out on the bench with your toes pointing up. Keep your right foot flat on the floor. Straighten your back, and if you feel a stretch in the back of your thigh, hold for 10 seconds and repeat with your right leg. (If you do not yet feel a stretch, lean forward from your hips until you do feel a stretch.)

Taking the First Step

Walking correctly is very important.

- Walk with your chin up and your shoulders held slightly back.

- Walk so that the heel of your foot touches the ground first. Roll your weight forward.

- Walk with your toes pointed forward.

- Swing your arms as you walk.

Section 29.2

Selecting and Using a Pedometer

"Selecting and Effectively Using a Pedometer." Reprinted with permission of the American College of Sports Medicine. Copyright © 2005 American College of Sports Medicine. All rights reserved. Reviewed by David A. Cooke, MD, FACP, May 2010.

About Pedometers

The pedometer is a device about the size of a pager that typically attaches to the belt or waistband and is designed primarily to count steps. More recently, some pedometers are also capable of counting steps while placed in a shirt pocket or in a bag if it's held snug to the body. Interestingly, Leonardo da Vinci is credited with the invention of the pedometer. Although the early mechanical pedometers were deemed unreliable, the electronic pedometer developed in the early 1990s is significantly more accurate and reliable.

Pedometers are capable of recording ambulatory activity such as walking, jogging, or running. They will not count steps during activities such as cycling, rowing, upper body exercise, etc.

How Do Pedometers Differ?

Pedometers can differ in cost, internal mechanism, and features.

Cost: Pedometers typically range in cost from $10-$50 depending on the features.

Internal mechanism: There are different mechanisms by which pedometers function.

- One common type consists of a spring-suspended lever arm that moves up and down in response to vertical acceleration of the hip. This movement opens and closes an electrical circuit and a step is counted.

- Others use an accelerometer-type mechanism. Pedometers with this mechanism can distinguish between ambulatory activities of differing intensities. (If you shake the pedometer up and down and it does not produce a clicking sound, it probably has an accelerometer-type mechanism.)

Features: While steps are the fundamental unit of the pedometer, some devices also calculate distance walked and estimate calories burned. In general, pedometers are most accurate in counting steps, less accurate in calculating distance walked, and even less accurate at estimating caloric expenditure.

The calculation of distance walked requires the input of the user's stride length while the caloric expenditure feature requires the input of the user's body weight. Steps are the fundamental unit of the pedometer and all other features are dependent upon the device's step-counting accuracy. Some of the newer devices also estimate the total time spent walking at a moderate intensity.

Choosing a Pedometer

The following questions should be considered when selecting a pedometer:

What feature(s) am I most interested in? Step counting is what most pedometers do best. Therefore, purchasing an accurate step-counting pedometer should be a primary objective.

How can I test a pedometer's accuracy? One way to test a pedometer's accuracy is to perform a 20-step test. To do this, position the device on your belt or waistband in line with your knee on either side of the body and reset your pedometer to zero. Take 20 steps at your typical walking pace. Check to see if the pedometer reads between 18 and 22 steps. If it does, it is likely a reasonably accurate step counter. If not, try repositioning it on your belt or waistband and try the test again. If your pedometer repeatedly fails this test, look into purchasing a different type.

What factors can affect pedometer accuracy? Studies have shown that a variety of factors can potentially affect a pedometer's step counting accuracy, i.e. walking speed, waistband type, and abdominal size. In general, most pedometers are fairly accurate step counters at speeds of 2.5 mph and above. Even some of the more accurate pedometers miscount steps at slower speeds. With regard to waistband type, pedometers are generally more accurate step counters when attached to a firm waistband in an upright position. (Loose waistbands typically result in a significant underestimation of steps.) Abdominal size can also affect step-counting accuracy. Those with the horizontal lever arm mechanism appear to be more vulnerable to miscounting steps based on the tilt or angle at which the pedometer sits when fastened to the belt or waistband.

How Do I Use a Pedometer to Supplement My Walking Program?

First, determine your baseline physical activity level. To do this, wear the pedometer for one full week without altering your typical routine. If you are routinely active, continue being so but, if you are not habitually active, do not start during this one-week period.

Table 29.2. Step Index

Steps per Day	Activity Level
<5,000	Sedentary
5,000–7,499	Low Active
7,500–9,999	Somewhat Active
10,000–12,500	Active
>12,500	Highly Active

*Developed by C Tudor-Locke and DR Bassett Jr (2004).

You can use the step index in Table 29.2 to classify your activity level based on steps per day. (Keep in mind that if you regularly participate in non-ambulatory activity, your steps per day value will not accurately represent your activity level.)

For most healthy adults, 10,000 steps per day is a reasonable goal. If your baseline steps fall short of this value, try to increase your activity level by 1,000 steps per day every two weeks until you reach your goal. To put your step count into perspective, there are about 2,000 steps in a mile.

Children can also benefit from the use of pedometers. Typically active children should accumulate between 12,000 and 16,000 steps per day. Pedometers can be used to motivate children or youth to become more physically active.

To increase your daily step counts, look for opportunities to be more active. For example, take the stairs rather than the elevator, park at the far end of the parking lot (if it is safe to do so), go for walking breaks at work, etc. The instant feedback that a pedometer provides can serve as a motivator to accumulate more steps. Every step counts so even small increases added into your daily routine can make a difference.

Section 29.3

10,000 Steps a Day Walking Program

This section excerpted from "Walking Works," President's Council
on Physical Fitness and Sports (www.fitness.gov), 2005. Reviewed
by David A. Cooke, MD, FACP, May 2010.

Walking works—in many ways. A brisk-paced walk can help you
and your family look and feel better, increase energy, and pick up your
spirits.

Walking can work to improve your health, too. A daily routine of 30
minutes or more of brisk walking can help you control your weight, lower
cholesterol, strengthen your heart, and reduce the likelihood of serious
health problems down the road. And since America is spending more than
ever on preventable health problems such as obesity, heart disease, and
type 2 diabetes, every step you take can help build a healthier nation.

The U.S. Surgeon General reports that a minimum of 30 minutes of
moderate physical activity, such as brisk walking, on most days of the
week can produce long-term health benefits. The President's Council
on Physical Fitness and Sports recommends at least 30 minutes a
day, on five or more days a week, or 10,000 steps daily measured by a
pedometer. Not everyone can achieve 10,000 steps a day, but almost
everyone can find ways to build walking into each day to accumulate
at least 30 minutes of physical activity.

If you can't walk for 30 minutes at one time, take 5-, 10-, or 15-min-
ute walks throughout the day. It all adds up to better health.

You're probably already walking more than you think. And by taking advantage of opportunities all around you to walk more every day,
you'll be surprised at how quickly the steps add up! Walk up the stairs
instead of riding the escalator at the mall; take an after-dinner walk
with your family; choose the farthest spot in the lot at work; eat lunch
outdoors instead of at your desk. By walking 30 minutes or more a day
at a brisk pace, you're on your way to better health!

In this section, you'll find everything you need to start a regular
walking routine—no matter what your fitness level. It's easy. All you
need is a comfortable pair of shoes and the determination to stick to
your program.

You can make walking a family activity—and reward family members who reach their daily walking goals! Walking is a great way for grandparents to spend time with grandchildren while improving their own health.

To help you stay motivated and focused on your goal, use a walking log to help track your progress. You may want to consider using a pedometer, a small device that senses your body motion and counts your footsteps.

If you don't use a pedometer, count the number of minutes walked. Start with no less than 30 minutes a day and add more minutes as you build up endurance.

On Your Mark

Walking has gained acceptance as an excellent way to improve health and maintain a healthy weight. The President's Council on Physical Fitness and Sports reports that walking one mile burns about 100 calories, depending on intensity, pace, and speed. According to the Mayo Foundation for Medical Education and Research, when done briskly on a regular basis, walking can accomplish the following:

- Decrease your risk of a heart attack
- Decrease your chance of developing type 2 diabetes
- Help control your weight
- Improve your muscle tone
- Promote your overall sense of well-being

Regular physical activity helps prevent many chronic diseases and conditions, such as heart disease, colon cancer, type 2 diabetes, osteoporosis, and conditions associated with obesity, such as stroke and arthritis. If most Americans adopted a daily routine of brisk walking, the result would be a savings of billions of dollars in health-care costs related to these conditions (U.S. Department of Health and Human Services).

Get Set

Walking is a simple and flexible way to improve your health, and it's free. You can walk alone or with friends, indoors or outdoors, on a city sidewalk or a country trail, any time of the year. But before you start your walking program, be sure to follow a few basic principles to keep you safe and comfortable:

- If you have a health condition or have not done any regular physical activity for a long time (men over 40, women over 50), talk with your doctor before starting any new exercise program.

- Choose comfortable, supportive shoes, such as running, walking, or cross training shoes, or light hiking boots.

- If you are going to do stretching exercises, be sure your muscles are warmed up first. Walk briskly for 10 minutes before stretching. Maintain a brisk pace. You should work hard to keep up your pace but still be able to talk while walking. Practice correct posture—head upright, arms bent at the elbow and swinging as you stride.

- Drink plenty of water before, during, and after walking to cool working muscles and keep your body hydrated.

- If you're going for a long walk, include a cool-down period to reduce stress on your heart and muscles.

Go

It's important to know your own starting point before you set your personal walking goals. This knowledge will help you create a personalized walking program that is right for you.

Baseline

If you are using a pedometer, count your steps for seven days; if you don't have a pedometer, follow the recommendations of the President's Council on Physical Fitness and Sports—begin with 30 minutes of brisk walking at least five days each week. Keep a log to track the amount of daily walking activity you are currently doing. This will establish your baseline. Include all of your normal walking activities, such as walking up the stairs at home, walking to work, etc. At the end of each day, write down your total number of steps in the log. If you are not using a pedometer, keep track of the minutes you spend walking.

Benchmark

Your benchmark is the highest number of steps you walked on any given day while establishing your baseline the first week. Use that number as your daily goal for the second and third weeks. Log your daily walks, and at the end of the third week, review your log. If you averaged your goal, add another 500 steps or several more minutes to your daily goal for the fourth and fifth weeks.

Build

At the end of each two-week period, try to add 500 steps or several more minutes to your walking goal. If you had difficulty reaching your goal, walk at the same level until you build enough endurance to increase your target. Continue to log your activity to prevent slipping back or dropping out. If you find yourself falling behind your average daily goal, try not to become discouraged. To maintain your motivation, keep logging your progress and stay with the same number of steps or minutes instead of increasing your target.

Keep in mind that 10,000 steps per day may not be a realistic goal for everyone. That's why we're offering a flexible program to help you set your own personal goals. If you are very overweight or have other health problems, ask your doctor to help you determine a walking goal appropriate for you.

Make Daily Walking a Habit

There are ways you can increase your physical activity to maintain a basic level of fitness—without setting aside a big part of your busy day. The challenge is to think creatively about ways you might add steps to your day and make walking a habit.

- Take stairs instead of elevators or get off below your destination and walk up a few stairs.

- Park a few blocks from your destination or at the far end of the parking lot.

- Walk the last few blocks instead of riding the bus all the way to work.

- Park at the opposite end of the mall from where you need to shop.

- Walk around the field at your children's ball games.

- Consider adding other routine walking to your day by organizing a lunchtime walking group at work, or a before- or after-work group with friends or neighbors.

- Make family time active time. After dinner, get the whole family outside for a game of tag and a walk around the block.

Try not to get stuck in the "all or nothing" rut. Even if you don't have time for a long walk, you might be able to take several brisk walks to add up to your daily goal.

335

Keep Going

A key part of your walking program is to log your progress every day. Reward yourself as you make progress toward your goals. As you record your steps, take a few minutes to sit down and relax. Think about the good feelings exercise gives you and reflect on what you've accomplished. This type of internal reward can help you make a long-term commitment to regular walking.

There are other ways to help keep you motivated. When you reach your personal goal, consider treating yourself to a new pair of walking shoes or a new walking outfit or T-shirt. If you are walking as a family, treat children and teens to a special activity excursion—to the park, the beach, the skating rink, or other outdoor fun—as a reward for reaching their daily goals for the week. Avoid using food, snacks, or candy as a reward. Children can earn a Presidential Active Lifestyle Award from the President's Council on Physical Fitness and Sports for any kind of physical activity done for 60 minutes a day, five days a week, for six weeks.

Your commitment to a "healthier you" can also mean a healthier America. You and your family are eligible to take the President's Challenge and receive a Presidential Active Lifestyle Award. This award is sponsored by the President's Council on Physical Fitness and Sports to recognize Americans of all ages for committing to a program of regular physical activity. Adults and children can achieve the award together—it's a great way for families to work together—everyone benefits! Log on to www .presidentschallenge.org to find out more about America's way to recognize your commitment and achievement of a healthy, active lifestyle.

You're On Your Way

Congratulations for choosing to walk! A few weeks after you start the program, you will feel better than when you began. And by committing yourself and your family to a daily walking program, you will be steps closer to improving your health.

By walking, you are contributing to the nation's health. With each step you take, you are lowering your risk of developing serious health conditions, such as heart disease, colon cancer, type 2 diabetes, osteoporosis, and conditions related to obesity, such as arthritis. And that's important to the nation's health, because America is spending hundreds of billions of dollars on preventable health conditions such as type 2 diabetes and overweight/obesity.

Walking also helps you maintain a positive mental outlook to avoid depression and anxiety.

Every day each of us has opportunities to choose a healthy lifestyle. The choices we each make can change our lives.

Section 29.4

Hiking for Health

"Hiking: Take Steps to Enjoy the Great Outdoors," by Jeffrey Kress. Reprinted with permission of the American College of Sports Medicine, ACSM Fit Society® Page, Summer 2005, pp 1–3. Reviewed by David A. Cooke, MD, FACP, May 2010.

Hiking is a great way to exercise and develop an appreciation for the great outdoors. However, before hitting the trail, all hikers should adhere to some basic guidelines to have a safe and enjoyable experience.

Planning

Prior to leaving for any hike, take the time to properly plan. The first step is to obtain trail maps or guidebooks which include distances as well as the estimated times required to hike the trails. Maps should be securely placed in a waterproof plastic bag since they may come into contact with moisture from streams, rain, or perspiration. Once you have decided where you are going, let someone know where you will be hiking and when you expect to return.

You should plan to start early so that you have plenty of time to enjoy your hike and the destination. More importantly, you should plan to head back early; allowing extra time for unforeseen activities, accidents, or misjudgments is paramount for ensuring that you arrive back prior to losing daylight. Check the weather, as this information is critical for planning your choice of clothing as well as how much water you should bring.

One item that you should always keep on your person is a whistle. Three short bursts on a whistle means you are in trouble and need assistance. If you are injured and perhaps off the trail due to unforeseen circumstances, a whistle will be heard from a long distance and will alert others to your location.

Clothing

You probably own some or most of the clothing necessary for hiking. Ideally, hiking wear should hold sufficient heat for warmth but release surplus heat and moisture. This is best accomplished by wearing layers of clothing; to adjust to temperature changes and varying activity levels, you simply add or remove clothing accordingly.

Choose clothing made from synthetic or polyester materials such as Polartec, Synchilla, and Capilene, but avoid cotton. Cotton retains moisture and does not breathe, while the previously mentioned fabrics wick moisture away from the skin which will keep you warm when the temperature is cool and cool when it is warm.

If you are hiking in an area prone to rain, always carry some sort of waterproof outer layer. A thin shell made from Gortex or some other wind and waterproof material is all that it will take to turn a wet miserable venture into an enjoyable hike in the rain.

Your feet arguably deserve the most attention because if they hurt, you will not enjoy yourself. Your footwear should provide stability, warmth, and comfort. As a general rule, wear a hiking boot that's one-half size larger than your street shoe size. The extra room will help with blister prevention by allowing you to wear two layers of socks, a thin polyester sock liner to wick away moisture and a thicker outer sock to reduce friction. Wearing one sock means the material rubs directly against your foot creating a blister; with two, the socks' friction point is against each other, sparing your feet from pain.

Food

Since hiking will burn many calories, this is not a day when you should restrict your diet. You will need all of the energy possible to traverse the terrain and complete the hike. Therefore, you should pack snacks that are high in calories and will not spoil. Do not pack empty calories, but instead, bring along high-quality fuel foods that are simple to pack and carry, such as dried fruits, nuts, trail mix, or any high-energy bar. Just remember to pack out whatever you pack in.

Water

Whether hiking in the cold or heat, your body will require a lot of water. A good rule is to bring along at least two to three quarts per person and always drink before you are thirsty. Avoid drinking soda or alcohol when hiking, as these beverages will dehydrate you. Also avoid drinking the untreated water found in streams, rivers, and creeks.

These water sources likely contain the organism *Giardia lamblia*, which if ingested may cause diarrhea within 48 hours. Normally this illness can last from one to two weeks, but chronic cases have been known to last from months to years. If you plan to drink from an un-treated source, use either a water purification system or water tablets to treat the water.

Insects

If you are hiking, chances are there will be insects around. Most are merely annoying and not harmful, while others such as mosquitoes and black flies swarm and bite.

Steps you can take to avoid being the target of most insects:

- Avoid applying scented products to your skin and hair.
- Keep cool, as insects are attracted to your sweat.
- Apply an insect repellant.
- Wear light-colored, long-sleeved clothing.

While most insects are only bothersome, ticks should not be taken lightly since they can transmit Lyme disease. This is the most common arthropod-borne illness in the United States and it is often difficult to diagnose. Avoid exposure to ticks by wearing a light-colored, long-sleeved shirt tucked into your pants. You should frequently check yourself and have someone else check you for ticks since finding and removing a tick within 36 hours is the key to the prevention of Lyme disease. If you find one, gently pull it from your skin while taking care to avoid pinching it.

Poison Oak, Ivy, and Sumac

Most hiking trails encounter potentially harmful plants such as poison oak, ivy, and sumac, which can lurk under shrubs or take the form of vines. One tiny drop (a billionth of a gram) of the urushiol oil present on these plants is all it takes to get a nasty rash. The oil is present during all times of the year, and thus should be avoided. If you are exposed to a harmful plant, you should wash the area immediately with soap and cold water. Urushiol oil can also remain on clothing for months at a time, so thoroughly wash all of your hiking clothes immediately. While the old saying, "leaves of three, let them be" holds true for both poison oak and ivy, poison sumac has leaf cluster of 7 to 13 per branch.

Following these guidelines will aid in your hiking enjoyment. But remember above all else, a little common sense goes a long way. If you feel uncertain, ask a park ranger. They are there to assist you and ensure that your hiking experience is both safe and enjoyable. So, get out there and enjoy what millions of other outdoor enthusiasts have found. For more information, contact outdoor agencies such as the American Hiking Society or the Sierra Club.

Chapter 30

Bicycling

Chapter Contents

Section 30.1

Biking and Walking for Transportation and Obesity Prevention

This section excerpted from "Active Transportation for Americans: The Case for Increased Federal Investment in Bicycling and Walking," by Thomas Gotschi, PhD, and Kevin Mills, JD. © 2008 Rails-to-Trails Conservancy (www.railstotrails.org). Reprinted with permission. The complete text of this report is available at http://www.railstotrails.org/resources/documents/whatwedo/atfa/ATFA_20081020.pdf.

Approximately 300,000 premature deaths per year in the United States are caused by being obese or overweight. In 2005, more preventable diseases and deaths occurred from excessive weight than from cigarette smoking. Our country has struggled for more than a decade to overcome the obesity epidemic, without notable success.

Simply put, obesity results from an imbalance between energy intake and energy output. We eat more calories than we burn through physical activity.

In 2007, less than half of all Americans met the Centers for Disease Control and Prevention's (CDC) recommendation of at least 30 minutes of modest physical activity on most days.

America's car-focused transportation system is a major contributor to our sedentary lifestyles. Not only are cars now used for almost all trips, including the shortest, but the large volumes of motorized traffic combined with the lack of adequate infrastructure have made bicycling and walking difficult and dangerous in many communities.

Investing in bicycling and walking offers a unique opportunity to reintegrate physical activity into our daily routines.

Obesity—An Epidemic of Unprecedented Dimensions

In recent decades we have consistently increased our calorie intake while decreasing our activity levels. In the 1990s the consequences became apparent in sharply increased obesity rates—the beginning of the obesity epidemic. Since then, we have seen the standardization of food labels to inform consumers about caloric and fat content; the rise of fat-free, low-calorie, and diet products; multitudes of fad diets promising weight loss; sporadic bans of unhealthy foods; the development of pharmaceutical weight-loss drugs; gastric bypass surgery; and even lawsuits against fast food companies. However, none of these efforts have reduced obesity rates.

Today, 32% of American adults are obese, and 67% are overweight or obese. America's weight problem doesn't spare our youth either: Nineteen percent of all teenagers and 17% of all children between ages 6 and 11 are overweight. The childhood obesity rate has almost tripled since 1980 and the adolescent rate has more than quadrupled.

The childhood obesity epidemic is "a national catastrophe," says acting U.S. Surgeon General Steven Galson. And "there's a huge burden of disease that we can anticipate from the growing obesity in kids," according to William H. Dietz, director of the Division of Nutrition, Physical Activity, and Obesity at the federal CDC.

The costs in medical expenses and loss of productive lives associated with the obesity epidemic place a heavy financial burden on our nation's future. The annual medical costs of physical inactivity have been estimated at $76 billion, or close to 10% of all medical expenses. The human burden is of no less relevance. Because obesity decreases life expectancy by several years, for the first time in history, the current generation of youth may not live as long as their parents.

Obesity is a major risk factor for many of our most deadly diseases. The number one cause of death is heart disease, and five of its six risk factors are associated with obesity: excessive weight, inactivity, high blood pressure, high cholesterol, and diabetes. Diabetes is the sixth leading cause of death in the United States. More than 21 million Americans (7% of the population) have Type 2 diabetes. Obesity is the number one risk factor for this dramatically expanding disease, which had 1.5 million new diagnoses in 2005.

Childhood Obesity Is "a National Catastrophe": How Obese Children Suffer

- Five years shorter life expectancy

- High cholesterol is two to three times more likely

- Fatty liver disease occurs in one third

- Twenty-five percent are at high risk to develop diabetes

- Asthma occurs two times more often

- Medical costs are three times higher

Physical Activity—The Challenge of Bringing Movement into Sedentary Lifestyles

CDC Recommendations for Physical Activity

- 30 minutes of moderate exercise on most days
  - Equivalent to: 1.5 miles of walking or
  - 5 miles of bicycling or
  - 1 less slice of pizza

In 2007, less than half of all Americans met the CDC's recommendations for physical activity from work, transportation, or leisure-time exercise, and 13.5% did not get any physical activity at all.

During the past century, the benefits of an increasing standard of living were accompanied by ever-decreasing amounts of physical activity in all aspects of life. This reduction in physical activity was due to a reduction in manual labor on the job and the adoption of labor-saving devices in the home. Many Americans have benefited from this trend in the form of better paying jobs, safer and healthier work conditions, and more leisure time.

Unfortunately, much of this newly found leisure time is spent in sedentary activities such as watching television and increasingly using computers or playing video games. Taken together, this trend away from physical activity at work, at home, and at play has contributed to an imbalance between our energy intake and energy output.

Our modern lifestyles have also been characterized by a reduction in physical activity in the transportation sector. Decades of car-centered transportation planning have left us with a transportation system that requires very little physical effort to get around. We now make almost 90% of our trips in cars and spend on average more than 30 miles driving every single day. Worse than that, many communities are designed in a way that renders bicycling and walking unfeasible, or even dangerous.

In 1996 the Surgeon General published an alarming report on physical activity and health. In it, medical professionals agreed that prevention of obesity requires not only healthier diets but, in addition, a substantial increase in physical activity.

Economic Effects of Obesity

- General Motors: $286 million in medical expenses per year due to obesity
- Medicare: 15% more expenses for obese beneficiaries

- Absenteeism: Obese employees miss 12 times more work days than their normal-weight colleagues

Do the Math: Exercise Gains from Bicycling and Walking for Transportation

The information in Tables 30.1 and 30.2 is based on average speed of 3 mph for walking and 10 mph for bicycling. Bicycle share among active transportation miles is assumed to increase from 20% (Status Quo) to 30% (Modest) and 50% (Substantial) across scenarios. Per person averages are based on U.S. population of 300 million. CDC recommendation is 30 minutes of moderate exercise on most days.

Table 30.1. Underlying Assumptions for Health Benefits Calculations

Factor	Status Quo	Modest Scenario	Substantial Scenario
Percent of those bicycling or walking who do now not meet activity recommendations	0%	20%	50%
Bicycle share of total miles walked and biked	20%	30%	50%

Table 30.2. Health Benefits from Bicycling and Walking (averaged over all Americans)

	Daily Exercise Gain (minutes)			Daily Energy Burned (calories)		
Factor	Status Quo	Modest Scenario	Substantial Scenario	Status Quo	Modest Scenario	Substantial Scenario
Trips <1 mile	2	3	4	10	17	25
Trips 1–3 miles	1	2	4	5	12	26
Totals	3	5	9	15	29	51

Physical activity provides additional health benefits independent of body weight, such as the prevention of cardiovascular disease, osteoporosis, arthritis, and mental disorders like anxiety and depression. In short, active people are likely to be healthier and happier people. Active workers are also more productive and have significantly lower health costs than their obese colleagues.

To date, attempts to increase physical activity have mostly focused on leisure-time activity for adults and physical education in school for children. Neither approach has succeeded with the majority of Americans.

When we reduce physical activity to "exercise" that is separate and apart from our daily routines, we encounter obstacles related to time, money, or motivation that make it difficult to maintain such activity over time. Reintroducing activity into daily routines is a practical way to overcome such obstacles.

Imagine a weight loss solution that requires little extra time, relatively small amounts of effort, no additional motivation, no major expenses, no specific skills, and no particular qualifications.

Bicycling and walking offer a compellingly simple remedy. Take a routine we all engage in every day—getting from Place A to Place B, also known as transportation. By leaving the motor at home, one can get to a destination while being active at the same time. Active transportation drives active living.

Burn calories: Most American adults gain weight gradually, typically about two pounds a year. This is equivalent to an excess of only about 100 calories a day. Bicycling or walking for less than 30 minutes daily would be sufficient to burn this amount of excess energy and keep body weight stable.

Safe Routes to School Program

Marin County, California, was a Safe Routes to School pioneer. There is broad community involvement in planning and executing a comprehensive set of measures including education, encouragement, safety, and infrastructure improvements. Seeded by a federal pilot project, Marin nearly doubled the percentage of children bicycling or walking to school in the first two years of their program and has extended the effort with state grants and local sales tax revenue.

Another Bay Area community, Alameda County, California, concluded from a survey among school children from three different grades that 68% were not physically fit. The county has responded with plans to expand its Safe Routes to School program, which currently targets 50 schools, to every school in the county, enabling more than 100,000 children at 226 schools to walk or bike to school.

Burlington, Vermont, C. P. Smith Elementary School's walking school bus has operated since March 2005. Before the walking school bus began, approximately six children walked this route to school. Now on Walking Wednesdays there are between 25 and 40 children and the traffic congestion along the route has all but disappeared.

How Much Activity Could Result from Bicycling and Walking for Transportation?

Transportation offers opportunities to routinely engage in physical activity because many trips are short and ideal for bicycling and walking. About half of all trips taken in the United States are three miles or less.

By replacing some of these short car trips with bicycling or walking, many Americans could significantly increase their activity levels. Using the CDC recommendation of 30 minutes of daily activity as a benchmark, it is a reasonable estimate that insufficiently active Americans would, on average, need to increase their daily level of activity by 15 minutes. Shifting some of these trips as outlined in our scenario calculations would result in an average of 5 (Modest Scenario) to 9 minutes (Substantial Scenario) of additional exercise for each American, every day, or the recommended 30 minutes of daily exercise for 50 (Modest) to 90 million (Substantial) Americans.

Commuting two or three miles by bicycle takes only 15 minutes, and the complete round-trip satisfies the recommendations for daily physical activity.

Similarly, a two-mile, round-trip walk to run errands, access transit, or take children to school provides the recommended 30 minutes of physical activity. Nearly two-thirds of all households say they have satisfactory shopping available within walking distance of their home. Fifty-seven percent of parents with children 13 years or younger live within one mile of a public elementary school.

Bicycling and walking for short trips require little additional time, if any at all, fitting into very tight schedules because the activity occurs during time already allocated for transportation. The additional time needed for walking trips of less than a mile, compared to using a car, is at most minimal due to the short distance and elimination of the need for parking. Currently, two-thirds of these short trips are taken by car.

Bicycling and walking are physical activities which require no training or preparation, and anyone can engage in them. Young children find great joy through bicycling and love this form of physical activity. For elderly people, bicycling and walking provide safe, low-impact exercise that helps maintain their health.

A crucial advantage of bicycling and walking as transportation, rather than solely for exercise, is the motivation factor. For utilitarian trips, much less motivation and discipline are required to participate in it regularly because the person must make the trip anyway. For example, once the decision is made to commute to work by bike, this exercise easily becomes a routine. Bicycling and walking therefore offer an ideal opportunity to increase activity levels among those individuals who are not responsive to calls to increase leisure-time activity.

Further, individuals who want to increase their leisure-time activity levels find an easy and low-cost opportunity to do so when appropriate bicycling and walking facilities are available to them. Children who live in safe places to bicycle and walk can transport themselves to outdoor activities without having to wait for someone who can drive them, making it more likely that they will engage in additional physical activities outdoors.

Billings, Montana: The Sneakers, Spokes, and Sparkplug Challenge pits bicyclists, pedestrians, and drivers against one another in completing a set of tasks around Billings, Mont. The bicyclists won, with pedestrians often finishing before the car drivers. This popular event is the lighter side of a set of serious local initiatives to improve public health by integrating physical activity into everyday activities. Connecting places where people live, work, shop, and play with bicycle and pedestrian infrastructure is a key component of such efforts. Billings is using Health Impact Assessments to infuse health as a criterion for decision-making into community projects and plans. And a general obligation bond was passed to provide local funds to match federal funds invested in trails.

Declining Activity Levels

- 1969: 50% of students walk to school.

- 2004: 14% of students walk to school.

- The average miles each American drives have more than doubled since 1960, to now almost 30 miles per day.

Bottom Line—Transportation: First a Driver of the Problem, Now a Step toward the Solution!

"Bicycling is a big part of the future. It has to be. There's something wrong with a society that drives a car to work out in a gym." —Bill Nye the Science Guy

In light of all the advantages of increasing physical activity in our daily routines, it is obvious that, from a public health perspective, current levels of bicycling and walking are much too low.

America is at a crucial crossroad in the battle against obesity. Only by providing Americans with routine opportunities to engage in physical activity are we likely to prevent this epidemic from putting an unfathomable burden on our society.

Therefore it is important to think of our transportation system as more than just a means to get around. Transportation infrastructure defines the built environment we live in, and as such has a tremendous influence on our levels of activity and our general well-being. For this reason, the impact of transportation projects on public health should be taken into consideration just as routinely as we evaluate the financial costs of a project or its effects on the environment.

For decades, car-focused transportation investment has contributed to a steady reduction in physical activity. To achieve an increase in physical activity through investments in transportation infrastructure, urban designers, city planners, medical professionals, and transportation engineers must realize the potential of routine bicycling and walking. Once bicycling and walking are widely accepted and treated as legitimate, viable, and healthy transportation modes, health professionals can recommend active transportation as an efficient and safe form of physical activity, allowing Americans to improve their health by bicycling and walking.

To assure the maximum health benefits for our society from bicycling and walking, transportation policy must be held accountable for its impact on public health and make investing in bicycling and walking a priority.

Section 30.2

Spinning/Indoor Cycling

Imagine taking your trusty old three-speed—or your rugged new mountain bike—onto the open road for an exhilarating 40-minute ride. It's a beautiful day . . . there's a gentle breeze . . . and before you know it, you're back home, tired but refreshed from a workout that seemed more like fun than work.

The simple pleasure of riding a bicycle is so appealing that this traditional pastime has been revived as a hot new way to exercise indoors—where weather, traffic, terrain, and plain old lack of motivation are less likely to foil your good intentions.

Indoor cycling classes are popping up in gyms and studios around the world. If you haven't witnessed the real thing, no doubt you've seen the advertisements: groups of exercisers huddled over stationary bikes, looking determined and even a little euphoric as they listen intently to an instructor and pedal their hearts out. Have you ever wondered about joining them?

Taking Your First Indoor Ride: Indoor Cycling Tips

Feel a little intimidated at the thought of trying a class? You're not alone. The most common misconception is that indoor cycling is an intense, overwhelming experience that only the very fit can handle, says San Diego–certified Spinning™ instructor Jill Flyckt. I tell newcomers to remember they're in charge of their own ride. They set the pace and they do it privately—unlike in other classes where everyone can see if they make a wrong step.

Ultra-endurance cyclist, motivational trainer, and internationally acclaimed fitness expert Johnny G, who created the original Spinning program that sparked the indoor cycling trend, says the beauty of indoor cycling is that you set your own level of intensity by adjusting the bike's resistance, so your age, size, or fitness level doesn't matter. The goal is to help you find the champion within.

Fitness experts agree that indoor cycling is an excellent cardiovascular workout, providing the same health and weight management benefits as other aerobic activities. It is particularly versatile because it's a nonimpact activity, ideal for postrehab patients, pre/postnatal women, and people with overuse injuries, back pain, or arthritis.

Perhaps the most unique aspect of indoor cycling is its special brand of motivation.

Indoor cycling consists of continuous coaching, music, and visualization (which transports you to some imaginary terrain, such as a mountain or wilderness) that help you achieve your personal best. It's about physical, mental, and emotional development, says Johnny G. You can learn how to challenge yourself, overcome obstacles, and build inner strength to reach your goals.

What to Expect From Indoor Cycling

Indoor cycling classes often last 40 to 45 minutes, but some beginner sessions are only 30 minutes. Your instructor may speak to you through a speaker system or through headphones you wear during class. Various types of indoor cycling programs and bikes are available.

Here are answers to two common indoor cycling questions:

Will I get big quads from indoor cycling? Your muscle size is a matter of genetics; it depends on your parents, not your indoor cycling class.

Will I get really sore from indoor cycling? Soreness and muscle ache in the quadriceps, lower legs, and pelvis are common after your first indoor cycling classes but will diminish if you keep cycling two or three times a week.

Indoor Cycling Tips for Getting Started

To help you ease into the indoor cycling experience, remember the following tips:

Take control of the ride. Don't come out of the gate too fast. This is the most common mistake beginners make. Pace yourself!

Come prepared. Wear comfortable clothes, including padded bike shorts and low-top shoes with stiff midsoles (cross trainers or cycling shoes). Bring plenty of water and a towel.

Talk to your indoor cycling instructor. Describe your fitness history, goals, and injuries. Ask about proper posture and learn how to adjust resistance and speed. Make sure your seat height and angle are correct.

Make a commitment. Don't let initial discomforts scare you off. Try this activity for several weeks, rather than giving up too soon. Indoor cycling may provide just the boost your fitness program needs—so get on your bike and ride!

Chapter 31

Running

Chapter Contents

Section 31.1

Running for Beginners

"Tips for Beginning Runners," U.S. Customs and Border Protection, Department of Homeland Security (www.cbp.gov), February 26, 2009.

- **Take stock of your current health and fitness level.** If you have been sedentary; have or suspect health problems such as heart disease, diabetes, high blood pressure, high cholesterol, joint problems, etc.; or are over 40, it is recommended that you have a physical with your doctor before starting a vigorous exercise program. If you know you have no major health problems, starting a light- to moderate-intensity exercise program such as brisk walking usually does not require a physical, but check with your doctor for his or her opinion in your specific case. Remember that the health risks of a sedentary lifestyle are much greater than the risks of exercise. A renowned exercise physiologist, Per Olaf Astrand, quipped that if one plans a sedentary lifestyle, one should have a physical to see if the heart can stand it!

- **Be safe.** Don't run/walk in "high crime" areas. When running after dark, be sure to wear reflective clothing, carry a small flashlight, and assume drivers don't see you. Well-lighted neighborhoods are a good choice. Women should run with a partner or a dog if possible and consider carrying pepper spray. Runners and walkers should never use headphones outdoors, as it makes it impossible to hear traffic or an approaching attacker. Always carry ID.

- **Start slowly and build up gradually.** Most people should start with a brisk walking program and progress to a mix of alternating walking and jogging. Eventually you should be able to run the entire distance you desire at a comfortable pace. At that point you can increase weekly mileage about 10% every third week, depending on your goals. For health and fitness there is generally no need to run more than about 15 miles per week, along with some strength and flexibility training. Those wishing to progress to competitive running should seek out experienced runners or coaches for advice. Check the Road Runners Club of America website for a running club in your area (www.rrca.org).

- **Using the right type of shoes helps prevent injuries.** Shin splints and runner's knee are preventable with proper conditioning *and* the right running shoe type. There are three basic types for different running mechanics:

  1. Motion control: Generally best choice for flat feet and "floppy ankles" (over pronation or rolling too far to the inside after foot touches down). Shoes should be straight lasted and often will have a full board last inside plus a harder rubber or plastic area on the inner (arch support) side of heel to control excess movement.

  2. Stability: Generally best for normal arches, will have a semi-curved last and a moderate amount of motion control.

  3. Cushioned: Generally best for high arches and "clunk foot"; these feet are usually very rigid and "under pronate," i.e., feet do not roll to the inside far enough after foot touches down and therefore make poor shock absorbers. Shoes should have a curved or semi-curved last, extra cushioning, a full slip last (no board inside), and be very flexible.

Another choice, for off-road running, are trail running shoes. These are made low to the ground and more stable to help prevent ankle sprains, have good traction, and help prevent foot bruises from roots, rocks, etc.

Don't use any type running shoes for other sports, as they are not made for lateral movements, making ankle sprains more likely. They also last longer and maintain cushioning better if only used for running. Use only good quality court shoes or cross-trainers for other conditioning activities. Wrestling shoes are recommended for defensive tactics training on matted floors.

- **Do the "wet test" to see what type of foot you have.** Wet feet and step onto some paper on a hard surface. (Even better is to run a short distance barefoot on sand.) A "blob" footprint with little arch indicates flat feet. Two "islands" with a lot of space between the heel and ball indicates high arches. A normal arch will look like the classic cartoon footprint.

- **Make sure the shoe fits!** The best shoe for you is one that fits your foot type and running mechanics and also is the right length and width. Try on running shoes with the socks you plan to run in, and toward the end of the day when feet are larger. You should have about one thumb's width of room between your longest toe and the end of the shoe. Shoes should be wide enough that foot does not feel pinched on the sides, but not a sloppy fit or one that slips at the heel. Jog a bit in the store to see how the shoes feel and fit. Most running specialty stores such as Fleet Feet in Savannah or 1st Place Sports in Jacksonville will have the expertise and take the time to fit you properly in several models and watch you run in them before you choose. Don't count on the employees of a general sporting goods or discount footwear store understanding any of the aforementioned running shoe information!

- **Dress for the weather.** In cold weather wear several light-weight layers, a hat, and gloves to trap body heat. You can unzip or remove layers if you get too warm. In hot weather wear as little as the law allows, and don't forget the sunscreen. Drink plenty of fluids throughout the day to avoid dehydration and plan ahead so you can get fluids during longer runs.

- **Run with good form.** Shoulders should be relaxed with elbows bent to about 90 degrees as arms swing smoothly forward and back with no twisting of the torso. Arms should not cross the center of body and hands should pass just above the "hip pocket" on each forward and backward motion. The upper body should be nearly upright, with a very slight forward lean. Don't run on the toes or hit hard with the heel, but rather land as softly as possible with foot nearly flat. The foot should be flexed upward slightly just before foot lands. Breathe naturally through both the nose and mouth. If you're gasping for air—slow down!

- **Most running injuries are avoidable!** Following the tips on proper footwear, form, and starting slowly will greatly reduce your chances of common beginners' complaints such as shin splints and knee pain. Basic strength and flexibility exercises can prevent and correct muscle imbalances responsible for most running injuries. If you do have a running injury, find the cause rather than just treating the symptoms.

- **Ignore the myths.** The bulk of scientific evidence shows that running, even in ultra-marathon runners, does not cause osteo-arthritis in the hips or knees if these joints were healthy to begin with. In fact, weight-bearing exercise such as running probably prevents arthritis, since the incidence in long-time runners is about half that of non-runners, including swimmers.

- **Further information sources:**

  - *Runner's World* (magazine): a great resource for advice on current running shoes on the market, injury prevention and treatment, training information, and other beginning to advanced runner advice (www.runnersworld.com).

  - *Running Times* (magazine): a great resource for intermediate to advanced runners, plus good shoe reviews and advice (www.runningtimes.com).

  - Road Runners Club of America: find a running club in your area suitable for beginners to advanced runners, plus loads of other running information (www.rrca.org).

  - *Lore of Running* by Tim Noakes, MD. The definitive book on running, recently revised.

  - *Bill Rodgers Lifetime Running Plan* by Bill Rodgers.

Section 31.2

Training to Run Your First 5K

So you've started a walking program and, after a few weeks of consistent improvement, you feel you're ready to pick up the pace and run your first 5K race.

A 5K—a 3.1-mile race—is the perfect length to aim for as a beginner. Begin by setting a realistic training schedule to keep you motivated and give yourself ample time to move to the next level. Beginning a running program may improve many facets of your life, as it builds your cardiovascular system, may boost your self-esteem, and may strengthen ties within your community while also allowing you to appreciate the outdoors.

From the novice to the expert runner, a local 5K race is a great way to get in shape and improve your sense of health and well-being.

Set Attainable Goals

While the length of a 5K may be a relatively easy goal to achieve as a novice runner, designing the training program can present quite a challenge. Start out with a simple program that allows you to succeed and move forward only when you feel comfortable with your current stage. To avoid burnout or injury, do not push your limits.

Remember that your main goal is to reach the finish line. For your first race, you should enjoy the run and feel good for having reached your goal, rather than going for a certain time.

Take Your Time

Depending on your training base, a five-week program should be just enough time to have you running for the full 3.1 miles. Your first step should be a complete medical exam to make sure it is safe for you to begin a running program.

Begin with a walk/run program four times per week for 20 to 25 minutes. Plan to add a little variety to your training by alternating every other day with 20 to 30 minutes of an aerobic cross-training activity to build your cardiovascular fitness.

Select a starting distance that you are comfortable with. Perhaps it is 1.0 to 1.5 miles. Increase the distance (and duration) by approximately 10 to 15% each week. For example, increase the duration of your walk/run from 25 minutes to 28 minutes in week two.

Vary your runs during the week to break the monotony. Choose one or two days a week to run your distance, and use the remaining days to focus on shorter, harder runs or interval-type sessions. Make sure to take one to two days off per week to let your body recover. Gradual training is the key to long-term success and rest time is just as important as the time you spend training.

Be Smart and Safe

Be sure to have proper running shoes that suit your individual needs, and be aware of the surface on which you are running. The best running surface is a rubber track. If you do not have access to a track, asphalt is better than concrete, and dirt or silt alongside the road is even better.

Nutrition and Hydration

Never run on an empty tank. Consume a light carbohydrate snack one to one-and-a-half hours before your runs and be sure to adequately hydrate. Drink plenty of fluids, but make sure you drink at least 16 ounces two to three hours before your run. Plan to drink 7 to 10 ounces of fluids every 15 minutes during your run and eat a light carbohydrate and protein snack soon after the run if possible. Monitor your hydration by weighing yourself before and after the run, making sure you drink enough fluids after your run to replace the weight lost.

Race Day

If you aren't familiar with the race course, check it out on one of your training runs or do a drive-by. It's easy to get mentally and physically fatigued when you don't know where your run ends and how much farther you have to go. Also, be sure to avoid running at a pace that is faster than your training pace.

For your first race, there is some running etiquette that you should be aware of:

- Don't cut someone off unless you're at least two paces in front of them.

- Make sure there is no one behind you if you're going to spit or throw away a cup from the water stations.

- When you cross the finish line, don't stop moving. Keep walking down the chute to prevent a traffic jam.

- If you're on a team, cheer on teammates that finish behind you. That extra encouragement may be the boost they need to finish hard.

Support Your Community

Since running is relatively inexpensive and a great way to stay in shape, the popularity of 5K races has dramatically increased over the past few years. By running a 5K and donating money through your entry fee or raising money through donations, you are supporting a larger cause and meeting new people who share similar interests and goals.

Chapter 32

Strength and Resistance Exercise

Chapter Contents

Section 32.1

Strength/Weight Training Basics

Why should I do strength training?

- Sedentary individuals (someone who does little or no regular exercise) can lose up to 30% of their muscle between ages of 20 and 70, averaging several pounds of muscle per decade.

- Muscle is an active tissue. A pound of muscle burns 30 to 50 calories per day just to maintain itself. Add three pounds of muscle and burn 630 to 1,050 extra calories per week. A pound of fat only burns 3 calories per day. So you can see by lifting weights and gaining muscle you will burn more calories every day.

- Strength training can increase your muscle mass, and this can happen at any age.

What are the benefits of strength training?

Strength training increases or improves:

- metabolism (your body will burn more calories);
- muscle mass and strength;
- stamina, energy, and endurance;
- functional mobility;
- balance and coordination;
- mental alertness;
- ability to perform challenges of daily life with less chance of injury;
- muscle strength, tone, and firmness;
- strength of tendons and ligaments;

- bone density and strength;
- personal appearance.

You will feel and look great!

How do I get started on a strength training program?

First you need to review and understand strength training guidelines:

- Warm up before you start. You need to warm up to increase blood flow to your muscles. Do this by walking briskly, biking, or stair climbing for three to five minutes.
- Work the largest muscle groups first (chest, back, legs), then proceed to smaller muscle groups (shoulders, biceps, triceps).
- Repetitions (reps) are the number of times you repeat an exercise. Usually you will do between 8 and 15 repetitions.
- Sets are groups of repetitions. Eight to 15 repetitions make up one set. Begin with one set of each exercise. As you progress in your program, you may want to increase to two to three sets.
- Frequency: To increase or maintain muscular strength, you need to lift a minimum of two to three times per week (every other day). Rest your muscles for 48 hours between workouts. This allows the muscle to rebuild.
- Intensity: Lift a weight that is just heavy enough to tire (where you cannot lift the weight again due to muscular fatigue) your muscle in 8–15 repetitions.
- Progression: Progressive resistance training is the most important principle of strength training. Gradually increase the amount of weight you are lifting to continue to develop muscular strength. When you can do 15 to 20 repetitions with ease it is time to increase your weight by the smallest unit available.
- Safety: Perform each exercise slowly and with proper form.

Form

- When you start losing your form or control of your muscles, *stop*. You have reached muscular fatigue for that set.
- Timing: Lift the weight on a "2 count" and lower on a "4 count."

363

- Lifting in a slow and controlled manner is essential for getting the most out of each set and to prevent injury.

- Breath: Do not hold your breath while lifting; exhale upon exertion (while pushing or pulling the weight).

- Intervals range between 0 seconds to 60 seconds between sets but may very depending on the type of workout you are performing.

Performing Your First Workout

- Begin with 8 to 10 exercises focusing on the major muscle groups (for example, chest or back if time permits).

- Begin with one set and after three to four weeks (6 to 12 workouts) add a second set.

- Begin with resistance which requires a "pretty good effort" to reach 15 repetitions but does not cause muscle fatigue.

- Keep a record or log of each workout session; this will allow you to properly and consistently progress in your strength program.

- Be sure to stretch after your workout.

Dumbbells can be purchased at sporting goods stores and/or discount stores. Consult your physician before starting any exercise program.

Section 32.2

Progression and Resistance Training

This section excerpted from "Progression and Resistance Training," President's Council on Physical Fitness and Sports (www.fitness.gov), September 2005. The full text of this document, including references, is available at www.fitness.gov/digest-september2005.pdf.

The popularity of resistance training has increased in recent times. Not only is resistance training used to increase muscular strength, power, endurance, and hypertrophy in athletes, but the adaptations to resistance training have been shown to benefit the general population as well as clinical (i.e., those individuals with cardiovascular ailments, neuromuscular disease, etc.) populations. Both scientific and anecdotal evidence points to the concept that progression is needed in order to create a more effective stimulus to promote higher levels of fitness. In fact, a threshold of activity/effort is necessary beyond the initial few months (which is characterized by enhanced motor coordination and technique) in order for the body to produce further substantial improvements in fitness. This threshold continually changes as one's conditioning level improves and is specific to the targeted goals of the exercise program. It is also bounded by each individual's genetic ceiling for improvement. Resistance training at or beyond this threshold level leads to progression.

In 1998, the American College of Sports Medicine published a position stand entitled "The Recommended Quantity and Quality of Exercise for Developing and Maintaining Cardiorespiratory and Muscular Fitness, and Flexibility in Healthy Adults." In this document, an initial starting point consisting of performance of one set per exercise (8–10 exercises) for 8–12 repetitions (10–15 for older adults) two to three days per week was recommended. This initial recommendation has been shown to be effective for progression during the first few months of training, but then benefits tended to plateau during subsequent months when variation in the program design was minimal. However, the question then arose, "what type of programs would be recommended for those individuals who desire a higher level of fitness?" Because it is important to make exercise a lifetime commitment, recommendations based on scientific research were needed to provide specific directives for those who desire to make further goal-specific improvements via resistance training. In response to this need, the American College of Sports Medicine later published a position stand providing basic recommendations for progression during resistance training. In this document, recommendations were given to novice, intermediate, and advanced individuals who sought to improve muscle strength, power, endurance, hypertrophy, and motor performance. The general conclusion was that there were numerous ways to progress as long as one adhered to basic tenets regarding the proper manipulation of the acute program variables. How much one can progress depends on the individual's genetic makeup, program design and implementation, and training status or level of fitness (i.e., slower rates of improvement are observed as one advances). In this section, we will discuss the critical elements to progression during resistance training and the current recommendations for manipulating the acute program variables. It is important to note that the amount of progression sought is individual-specific, as moderate improvements have been shown to elicit significant health benefits. Once the desired fitness level is achieved, programs can be used to maintain that current level of fitness.

Basic Components of Resistance Training Programs

Maximal benefits of resistance training may be gained via adherence to three basic principles: 1) progressive overload, 2) specificity, and 3) variation.

Progressive overload necessitates a gradual increase in the stress placed on the body during training. Without these additional demands, the human body has no reason to adapt any further than the current level of fitness.

Specificity refers to the body's adaptations to training. The physiological adaptations to resistance training are specific to the muscle actions involved, velocity of movement, exercise range of motion, muscle groups trained, energy systems involved, and the intensity and volume of training. The most effective resistance training programs are designed individually to bring about specific adaptations.

Variation is the systematic alteration of the resistance training program over time to allow for the training stimulus to remain optimal. It has been shown that systematic program variation is very effective for long-term progression.

Table 32.1. General Benefits of Resistance Training

Increased muscular strength

Increased muscular power

Increased muscular endurance

Increased muscle size

Reduced body fat

Increased balance, coordination, and flexibility

Enhanced speed and jumping ability

Enhanced motor performance and ability to perform activities of everyday living

Increased bone mineral density

Increased basal metabolic rate

Lower blood pressure

Reduced cardiovascular demands to exercise

Greater insulin sensitivity and glucose tolerance

Improved blood lipid profiles

Reduced risk for injury and disease (i.e., osteoporosis, sarcopenia, low back pain, etc.)

Enhanced well-being and self-esteem

Progression and Resistance Training Program Design

The resistance training program is a composite of acute variables. These variables include: 1) muscle actions used, 2) resistance used, 3) volume (total number of sets and repetitions), 4) exercises selected and workout structure (e.g., the number of muscle groups trained), 5) the sequence of exercise performance, 6) rest intervals between sets, 7) repetition velocity, and 8) training frequency. Altering one or several of these variables will affect the training stimuli, thus creating a favorable condition by which numerous ways exist to vary resistance training programs and maintain/increase participant motivation. Therefore, proper resistance exercise prescription involves manipulation of the variables to the specificity of the targeted goals.

Muscle Actions

The selection of muscle actions revolve around concentric (CON), eccentric (ECC), and isometric (ISOM) muscle actions. Most resistance training programs include mostly dynamic repetitions with both CON

367

and ECC muscle actions, whereas ISOM muscle actions play a secondary role. Eccentric muscle actions result in larger forces generated and less motor unit activation per tension level, require less energy per tension level, are very conducive to muscle hypertrophy, and elicit greater muscle damage compared to CON actions. Muscular strength is enhanced to a greater extent when ECC actions are included. It is recommended that both CON and ECC muscle actions be included in novice, intermediate, and advanced resistance training programs. The use of ISOM actions is beneficial but adaptations to ISOM are mostly specific to joint angles trained so ISOM actions need to be performed throughout the range of joint motion.

Resistance

The amount of weight lifted is highly dependent on other variables such as exercise order, volume, frequency, muscle action, repetition speed, and rest interval length, and has a significant effect on both the acute response and chronic adaptation to resistance training. Individual training status and goals are primary considerations when considering the level of resistance. Light loads of approximately 45–50% of one repetition maximum (1 RM) or less can increase muscular strength in novices who are mostly improving motor coordination at that level. As one becomes progressively stronger, greater loading is needed to increase maximal strength (i.e., 80–85% of 1 RM for advanced training). These findings have also been recently supported by a meta-analysis, which demonstrated that 85% of 1 RM yielded the highest effect size for strength gains in athletes.

There is an inverse relationship between the amount of weight lifted and the number of repetitions performed. Several studies have indicated that training with loads corresponding to 1–6 RM (i.e., the maximal amount of weight that can be lifted 1 to 6 times) were most conducive to increasing maximal dynamic strength. This loading range appears most specific to increasing dynamic 1 RM strength. Although significant strength increases have been reported using loads corresponding to 7–12 RM, it is believed that this range may not be as specific to increasing maximal strength in advanced resistance-trained individuals compared to 1–6 RM (although it is very effective for strength training in novice and intermediate trainees). Although heavy loading (1–6 RM) is effective for increasing muscle hypertrophy, it has been suggested that the 7–12 RM range may provide the best combination of load and volume in direct comparison. Loads lighter than this (13–15 RM and lighter) have only had small effects on maximal strength and hypertrophy but have been very effective for enhancing local muscular endurance.

Each "training zone" on this continuum has its advantages and, in order to avoid encountering training plateaus or overtraining, one should not devote 100% of the training time to one general RM zone. It appears that optimal strength, hypertrophy, and endurance training requires the systematic use of various loading strategies. Therefore, the American College of Sports Medicine recommends 60–70% of 1 RM loading for novice, 70–80% of 1 RM for intermediate, and 70–100% of 1 RM (periodized) for advanced strength training.

Training Volume

Training volume consists of the total number of sets and repetitions performed during a training session. Altering training volume can be accomplished by changing the number of exercises performed per session, the number of repetitions performed per set, or the number of sets per exercise. Volume and intensity are inversely related such that use of heavy loads results in lower volumes whereas use of light to moderate loads results in higher training volumes. Typically, high volume programs are synonymous with training for muscle hypertrophy and local muscular endurance whereas low volume programs are synonymous with strength and power training.

The vast majority of studies that examined volume and resistance training have investigated the number of sets performed per exercise. Most comparisons have been made between single- and multiple-set programs. In novice individuals, similar results have been reported from single- and multiple-set (mostly three sets) programs, whereas some studies have shown multiple sets superior. Thus, either may be used effectively during the initial phase of resistance training. However, periodized (i.e., varied), multiple-set programs have been shown to be superior as one progresses to intermediate and advanced stages of long-term training in all. Within multiple-set training programs, two, three, four-five, and six or more sets per exercise have all produced significant increases in muscular strength in both trained and untrained individuals. Therefore, it appears that similar improvements, at least in novice-trained individuals, may be gained within various multiple-set protocols. Less is known with intermediate and advanced training. Typically, three to six sets per exercise are common during resistance training, although more and less have been used successfully. Based on the aforementioned data, the American College of Sports Medicine has made the following strength training recommendations: 1) novice: 1–3 sets per exercise x 8–12 repetitions per set; 2) intermediate: multiple sets of 6–12 repetitions per set; and 3) advanced: multiple sets of 1–12 repetitions per set (periodized).

Exercise Selection

Two general types of free weight or machine exercises may be selected in resistance training: single- and multiple-joint. Single-joint exercises stress one joint or major muscle group whereas multiple-joint exercises stress more than one joint or major muscle group. Although both are effective for increasing muscular strength, multiple-joint exercises (e.g. bench press, squat) have generally been regarded as most effective for increasing muscular strength because they enable a greater magnitude of resistance to be used. Exercises stressing multiple or large muscle groups have shown the greatest acute metabolic and anabolic (e.g., testosterone, growth hormone family) hormonal responses, which may play a role in muscle size and strength increases. The American College of Sports Medicine (2002) recommends that novice, intermediate, and advanced resistance training programs incorporate single- and multiple-joint exercises with emphasis on multiple-joint exercises for advanced training.

Exercise Order and Structure

The sequencing of exercises significantly affects the acute expression of muscular strength. In addition, sequencing depends on program structure. There are three basic workout structures: 1) total body workouts (e.g., performance of multiple exercises stressing all major muscle groups per session), 2) upper/lower body split workouts (e.g., performance of upper body exercises only during one workout and lower body exercises only during the next workout), and 3) muscle group split routines (e.g., performance of exercises for specific muscle groups during a workout). All three structures are effective for improving muscular strength and it appears that individual goals, time/frequency, and personal preferences will determine which one(s) will be used. Once the structure has been developed, the sequencing of exercise will ensue. For strength training, minimizing fatigue and maximizing energy are critical for optimal acute performance—especially for the multiple-joint exercises. Studies have shown that placing an exercise early vs. later in the workout will affect acute lifting performance.

Rest Intervals

Rest interval length depends on training intensity, goals, fitness level, and targeted energy system and affects acute performance and training adaptations. Acute force production may be compromised with short (i.e., one minute) rest periods. We have recently developed a continuum for rest interval length for the bench press in which three-to-five-minute rest

Table 32.2. General Sequencing Strategies for Strength Training

Total Body Workout:

1. Large before small muscle group exercises
2. Multiple-joint before single-joint exercises
3. Rotation of upper and lower body exercises or opposing (agonist-antagonist relationship) exercises

Upper and Lower Body Split Workout:

1. Large before small muscle group exercises
2. Multiple-joint before single-joint exercises
3. Rotation of opposing exercises (agonist-antagonist relationship)

Muscle Group Split Routines:

1. Multiple-joint before single-joint exercises
2. Higher intensity before lower intensity exercises

intervals were most effective for maintaining acute lifting performance, but 30 seconds to two minutes of rest produced significant reductions in set performance. Rest intervals will vary based on the goals of that particular exercise, i.e., not every exercise will use the same rest interval. Muscle strength may be increased using short rest periods but at a slower rate, thus demonstrating the need to establish goals (i.e., the magnitude of strength improvement sought) prior to selecting a rest interval. The American College of Sports Medicine recommends one-to-two-minute rest intervals for novice training, two-to-three-minute rest intervals for core exercise, and one-to-two-minute rest intervals for others for intermediate training, and at least three-minute rest intervals for core exercises and one-to-two-minute rest intervals for others for advanced strength training.

Repetition Velocity

The velocity at which dynamic repetitions are performed affects the responses to resistance exercise. When discussing repetition velocity, it is important to note that velocity applies mostly to submaximal loading. Heavy loading requires maximal effort in order to lift weight. For dynamic constant external resistance (also called isotonic) training, significant reductions in force production are observed when the intent is to lift the weight slowly. There are two types of slow-velocity contractions, unintentional and intentional. Unintentional slow velocities are used during high-intensity repetitions in which either the loading and/or fatigue facilitate the velocity of movement (i.e., the resultant velocity is slow despite maximal effort). Intentional slow-velocity repetitions are used with submaximal loads where the individual has greater control of the velocity. The American College of Sports Medicine recommends slow to moderate velocities for novice training (i.e., with light loads while correct technique is learned), moderate velocities for intermediate training, and unintentionally slow (with heavy weights) and moderate to fast (with moderate to moderately heavy weights) for optimal strength training.

Frequency

Frequency refers to the number of training sessions performed during a specific period of time (e.g., one week) and/or the number of times certain exercises or muscle groups are trained per week. It is dependent upon several factors such as volume and intensity, exercise selection, level of conditioning and/or training status, recovery ability, nutritional intake, and training goals. Numerous studies have successfully used frequencies of two to three alternating days per week in novices. Progression does not necessitate a change in frequency for training each muscle group, but may be more dependent upon alterations in other acute variables such as exercise selection, volume, and intensity. Advanced training frequency varies considerably. It has been shown that football players training four to five days/week achieved better results than those who trained either three or six days/week. Other advanced athletes have used frequencies higher than this (i.e., 8–12 workouts per week or more). It is important to note that not all muscle groups are trained specifically per workout using a high frequency. Rather, each major muscle group may be trained two to three times per week despite the large number of workouts. The American College of Sports Medicine recommends two to three days per week for novice training, two to four days per week for intermediate training, and four to six days per week for advanced strength training.

Summary

Resistance training poses numerous health and fitness benefits to all individuals, providing that a threshold of activity/effort is reached. Progressive overload, specificity, and variation are critical elements to resistance training programs targeting progression. These elements may be attained by proper manipulation of the acute program variables in order to obtain specific, individualized goals.

The act of resistance training itself does not result in health-promoting benefits unless the training stimulus exceeds the individual's fitness threshold. Progression in program design entails gradual progressive overload, specificity, and variation in the training stimulus in order for the individual to improve his or her level of fitness.

Section 32.3

Best Ab-Strengthening Exercises

Strong abdominal muscles can protect you from low-back pain and help you perform your daily activities efficiently. Bill Bejeck, CSCS, CCS, owner of HealthSport Fitness and Sport Training Services in the Washington, DC, area, offers some guidance on training the abdominals.

The Muscles Involved

The "abdominals" include several muscle groups: the rectus abdominis, the obliques, and the transversus abdominis. Also important in any program designed to strengthen the abdominals are the erector spinae. Though not abdominal muscles themselves, these lower-back muscles add greatly to trunk strength and stability.

The rectus abdominis: The rectus abdominis muscles—sometimes called the "six-pack"—are the most superficial muscles in the core region. They stabilize the pelvis during walking and flex and rotate the lumbar spine. To work the rectus abdominis, perform a standard crunch or crunch over a stability ball. For a good combination exercise, crunch and rotate the elbows in an alternating fashion, right elbow to left knee and left elbow to right knee.

The obliques: The internal and external obliques lie at the sides of the core area. When activated on one side, they help perform moves that involve trunk rotation (twisting) or lateral flexion (bending to one side). When contracted on both sides simultaneously, these muscles aid in flexing the vertebral column and compressing the abdominal wall. To work the obliques, attach one end of a piece of rubber tubing to a secure object (i.e., a railing or heavy beam). Hold the other end in both hands. Turn 90 degrees, so one side of your body is toward the secure object, and extend your arms out in front of you. You should be far enough away from the attachment to feel tension on the tubing. From this starting position, rotate the trunk away from where the tubing is attached. Then return to the starting position. Perform 15 to 20 reps on each side.

The transversus abdominis: The transversus abdominis muscles contain the deepest fibers of the abdominal wall. These muscles increase trunk stability and help maintain proper posture and low-back stability. To activate the transversus abdominis, lie flat on your back with knees bent and feet flat on the floor. Draw the belly button toward the spine. Maintain this position for a slow count of five. Do not perform pelvic tilts. For more challenge, lift your feet off the ground and bring your thighs up until the kneecaps point toward the ceiling. Keeping the stomach drawn in, slowly extend one leg and bring it back to its previous position. Perform 10 to 15 repetitions per leg. If at any point the abdominal muscles push out, stop, put your feet down, and draw your stomach back in.

The erector spinae: These important low-back muscles add to trunk strength and stability and help maintain posture. To work the erector spinae, lie face down on the floor with arms extended. Simultaneously raise both arms and both legs off the floor. Keep the legs as straight as possible and squeeze the gluteus muscles. Hold briefly at the top and then lower the arms and legs to the floor. Perform 15 to 20 reps.

"Functional" Exercises

Functional abdominal exercises are valuable because they require all the muscles in the abdominal region to work together, as they often must do in real life. Here is one example: Kneel about 18 inches behind a stability ball. Lean forward and rest the forearms on the ball, clasping the hands together. Slowly push the ball away from the body until the arms are fully extended, then pull the ball back. To protect the lumbar spine, maintain a posterior tilt while performing this exercise. Perform 15 to 20 reps.

Section 32.4

Using Stability Balls and Resistance Bands

About Stability Balls

Stability balls provide an inexpensive, low-tech, lightweight, colorful, and fun means of improving core stability, muscular strength and endurance, balance, flexibility, and functional fitness. Stability balls were developed in Italy in the 1960s. They were first used in rehabilitative therapy by Dr. Susanne Klein-Vogelbach, founding director of a physical therapy school in Switzerland. The balls were introduced in the United States in 1989. Stability balls (aka Swiss balls or physioballs) can help anyone improve his or her fitness, they allow a variety of exercises with or without external resistance, and they can be used to overload the muscles. Stability balls also work the core muscles (abdominals, back muscles, hip flexors and extensors). Because the ball itself is unstable, these muscles are actively engaged throughout each exercise.

Selecting a Stability Ball

Stability balls range from small to extra-extra-large. Choose a ball size that allows you to sit on it with erect posture with your hips and knees at 90 degrees based on your height and leg length:

- 30–35 cm if <4'10" (<145 cm) tall
- 45 cm for 4'8"–5'5" (140–165 cm)
- 55 cm for 5'6"–6'0" (165–185 cm)
- 65 cm for 6'0"–6'5" (185–195 cm)
- 75 cm for those over 6'5" (>195 cm)
- 85 cm ball for heavier or long-legged exercisers

A smaller ball may be more useful as a handheld object for sitting or standing range of motion and balance exercises. A smaller ball can also be used to perform crunches with the ball between or behind the knees.

Maintenance and Durability

Stability balls are durable and will last a long time with proper care:

- Follow the manufacturer's directions for proper inflation and check inflation on a regular basis.

- Use stability balls on a clean, smooth surface (floor or carpet), free of debris and sharp objects that could produce wear on the balls' surfaces or puncture them.

- Clean stability balls regularly with water or mild soapy water for comfort and sanitary reasons. Avoid using chemical cleaners that may damage the covering.

- Stability balls can be stored on racks made specifically for that purpose, on stackers, or in a net suspended from the wall or ceiling to save space.

Safety

Using a stability ball safely starts with proper inflation and care (described earlier). To increase your safety while using a stability ball:

- Maintain the natural curves in your back while exercising.

- Increase your stability by placing your feet about shoulder-width apart (or wider for better balance). Put a mat in front of the ball to act as a cushion in case of a fall.

- Use a wall behind the ball to keep the ball from rolling out backwards from underneath you and to prevent you from falling directly to the floor should the ball slip forward.

- Place chairs on either side of the ball to provide lateral stability if needed while exercising in a seated position.

- Always use good movement technique and control.

- Remember to breathe throughout each exercise.

- Avoid ballistic movements (bouncing or fast movements of the joints) on the stability ball because they reduce your control of the movement and increase the risk of muscle strain and/or joint sprain.

In addition, it is important to follow a proper exercise progression to reduce your risk of injury and gain optimal training benefits. Begin by developing the ability to maintain your balance while sitting on the ball before adding movement of the limbs or trunk or adding external resistance with free weights, resistance bands, or a medicine ball.

Other Considerations

As your core stability, balance, and strength improve, you can achieve a progressive overload (i.e., challenging yourself further in different ways in order to achieve additional fitness benefits) in a number of ways:

- Practice transitions from one position to another.

- Make your base of support less stable by moving feet or hands closer and farther away from the ball.

- Vary your position on the ball so it supports less of your body weight (e.g., in crunches or push-ups) so you are lifting more weight against gravity.

- Add a dynamic balance challenge by adding movement on, over, or around the ball with one or both limbs (on the same or opposite sides of the body). Increase your volume of training (e.g., increase the resistance used, or repetitions or sets performed). Use a larger stability ball, rather than a smaller one, for added challenge.

Using Stability Balls

Stability balls can be used in a variety of ways to achieve different aspects of fitness.

- **Stretching:** lying over the ball on your back to stretch abdominal muscles, on your stomach to stretch back muscles, on your side to stretch abdominal oblique muscles. Sit on the ball with legs in front and reach forward to stretch the hamstrings.

- **Increase muscle strength/endurance without external weight:** lie on your back on ball and perform crunches; perform push-ups with knees, shins, or feet on ball; lie on your stomach on ball and perform back extensions; or perform squats by placing the ball between your back and a wall and move up and down.

- **Increase muscular strength and endurance by performing exercises with dumb bells or other external resistance:** lying supine (chest presses, triceps extensions) or prone on the ball (flies), or other exercises while sitting on the ball.

Important Points to Remember

Stability balls have multiple applications: improving core stability, static and dynamic balance, strength, flexibility, and can enhance functional performance of activities of daily living, or ADLs. Stability balls can be used to improve sports performance. They can also be incorporated as part of an injury rehabilitation program. You can do an entire workout with a stability ball or you can use one as part of a well-rounded exercise program for greater variety and effective development of core stability.

The following are additional sources of helpful information on stability ball exercises:

- American Council on Exercise (2002). *Stability Ball Training.* Monterey, CA: Healthy Learning.

- Flett, Maureen (2003). *Swiss Ball for Strength, Tone, and Posture.* London: PRC Publishing Ltd.

- Goldenberg, Lorne, and Twist, Peter (2002). *Strength Ball Training.* Champaign, IL: Human Kinetics.

- Lang, Annette (2003). *Foundations of Core Stability and Balance Training* (video). Monterey, CA: Healthy Learning.

- Prouty, Joy, and Gardiner, Josie (2000). *Fit over Fifty: Stability Ball Workout* (video). Monterey, CA: Healthy Learning.

- Verstegen, Mark, and Williams, Pete (2004). *Core Performance.* Rodale Press.

- Westlake, Lisa (2002). *Get on the Ball: Develop a Strong Core and a Lean, Toned Body.* New York: Marlowe & Company.

About Rubber Band Resistance Exercise

Originally used to train older adults in nursing homes, flexible bands now provide exercise options for beginning to advanced exercisers and athletes. The more you know about flexible bands, rubberized resistance cords, and the machines that use them, the better you can choose the method that's right for you. It's all about finding the resistance that matches the exercise you need.

Elastic bands offer no resistance at first, then more and more resistance as they are stretched to their limit. The resistance changes again as the bands return to resting position. This pattern—changing from extension to return—is known as hysteresis.

Rubber bands, by their nature, offer very little resistance when first stretched (for example, over the first 10–30 degrees of their range of motion). It is important to feel resistance early in the stretch—more easily accomplished with single rubber bands than with some resistance machines.

Strength Curves

Every exercise can be illustrated by a curve showing the force used over a range of motion. The three primary strength curves are:

- ascending (force increases over the range of motion);

- bell (force is greatest in the middle of the range of motion);

- descending (force decreases over the range of motion).

Variations among exercises and individuals can affect the shape of these curves as well as the timing and degree of force used in each exercise. Exercise loading should match the strength curve to ensure that appropriate force is applied to the muscle.

Take, for example, arm curl exercises using elastic bands. Too much resistance would prevent smooth motion through the entire range. Resistance that is below the starting strength of the arm curl movement allows normal repetition of the movement.

It is important to be able to choose resistance to suit the exercise. For example, chest presses need more resistance than arm curls.

The graph in Figure 32.1 shows the resistance of an elastic band (dotted line) compared with the strength curves of two different users. Greater strength gives User 1 force greater than the band's resistance, while User 2 has insufficient force throughout the entire range of motion. Neither user is well matched with this particular band.

Choosing Resistance Bands

When choosing from among the wide variety of rubberized resistance equipment available, ask:

- What exercises will I perform with the resistance bands? This tells you what range of resistance you'll need to adequately develop the muscle.

- What are the bands made of? Natural rubber latex, with its superior strength and elasticity, makes the best bands. Synthetic rubber is reinforced with additives that can cause the band to become harder and less elastic.

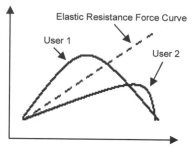

Figure 32.1. *The resistance of an elastic band compared with the strength curves of two different users.*

- How are the bands constructed? Understanding how bands are made can help you determine quality of construction and how they can be used in a variety of exercises. While any rubberized band provides resistance, heavier use requires a more durable product.

Some Features of Bands

- **Bonded ends:** A quarter-inch strip of rubber is bonded at the ends to make a continuous band. This joint is a weak spot that can break during exercise.

- **Extruded rubber:** Strands of rubber are wound together like spaghetti, making it very strong. The bonded ends, though, are a weak spot.

- **Over-layered:** A strip of rubber is overlapped and bonded into a continuous band. The center of the overlapped section is very strong, but both ends are weak.

- **Layered on mandrills:** Bands are built in layers, forming a continuous band. The first and last layers should finish on different planes, at least three inches apart. This forms a one-piece band with no weak spots.

Exercises

Rubber band exercises can be used for a variety of drills, such as:

- running and agility side-to-side drills;

- power exercises such as squat jumps and conventional resistance exercises;

- traditional exercise such as chest press, arm curl, and squats.

As always, safety is the primary consideration. Consider band strength.

Safety Questions

Before using a resistance band or rubber band machine, ask a number of questions, especially when there are multiple users. Rubber bands should be checked at rest and then when stretched to their usable length. Examine them carefully, asking:

- Is the resistance smooth and flexible in use?

- Are there signs of wear from repetitive use, including cracks or worn endings?

- Are there signs of weather exposure—such as sun, water or cold—making the rubber cracked or pale?

Chapter 33

Stretching and Flexibility for Healthy Aging

We all age a little each day, and with aging come some physiological changes to our musculoskeletal system and our flexibility. Losses in flexibility are as much the result of disuse as they are to aging. Reductions in joint range-of-motion affect mobility and balance, impacting routine physical functional status and the ability to perform basic and instrumental activities of daily living (ADLs/IADLs). Routinely performing flexibility and stretching exercises can limit the losses of flexibility over time. Although many of us exercise regularly, stretching before and after our exercise routines, we may not be doing enough to maintain flexibility and physical function.

Defining Flexibility

To appreciate the impact of aging, we must establish a common definition of flexibility and understand the physiological changes affecting flexibility during aging. Flexibility enables muscles and joints to move through their full range of motion. It has been defined as the absolute range of movement in a joint or series of joints that is attainable in a momentary effort with the help of a partner or a piece of equipment. Flexibility varies for each muscle and joint group. The condition of the muscles, joints, and connective tissues—including muscle fascia, ligaments, tendons, collagen, and elastin—affects flexibility.

"Flexibility in Aging: Stretching to Mend the Bend," by Diane Austrin Klein. Reprinted with permission of the American College of Sports Medicine, ACSM Fit Society® Page, Summer 2003, pp 5, 11. Reviewed by David A. Cooke, MD, FACP, May 2010.

Aging and physical inactivity contribute to the loss of flexibility over time. The notion of "use it or lose it" is highly applicable to flexibility and later affects ability to function in our daily routines. Several physiological changes affecting flexibility occur with aging:

- Increased calcification, fraying, or cracking in cartilage and ligaments

- Erosion of cartilage in heavily used joints—particularly of the knees and hands

- Decreased elasticity in joint capsules, tendons, and ligaments with the development of cross-linkages between adjacent fibrils of collagen

- Increased dehydration and loss of joint lubricants in connective tissue

- Changes in the chemical structure of the tissues

Older adults experience greater flexibility losses than younger adults, but activity can minimize losses. It has been suggested that performing flexibility and stretching exercises stimulates production and retention of connective tissue lubricants and can reduce flexibility losses.

Toward Healthier, Successful Aging

Experts say three components for "successful aging" include 1) avoiding disease and disability; 2) maintaining high cognitive and physical function; and 3) continuing to engage in life (and with others). These components focus on overall lifestyle behaviors—good dietary management, continuing education, socialization, and exercise. The exercise component, particularly for strength and flexibility, enables high physical function and avoidance of disability.

Physiological changes in aging muscles and joints affect mobility and limit locomotion, including reduced muscular work capacity and loss of muscle mass. Increases in connective tissues and cross-linkages add to muscle stiffness, soreness, and tension. For older adults, flexibility exercise is essential for aging muscles to retain their flexibility and protect them from injury. Older adults are more susceptible to muscle injury and it takes longer for their injuries to heal properly. In many cases, healed muscles may not perform as well as prior to the injury.

Recommendations from the Centers for Disease Control and Prevention and the American College of Sports Medicine have identified a need for older adults to perform flexibility exercises, preferably daily.

Flexibility and stretching exercises should be performed in a slow, sustained manner, holding stretches for 30 seconds. The stretch should be felt in the muscle, not the joint. If arthritis or muscle weakness is an issue, stretching and flexibility exercise can be performed in a warm pool to provide muscle warming and buoyancy.

Stretching and Flexibility Exercises

Flexibility training should be balanced with strength training to prevent connective tissues from becoming too loose and weak and being subject to damage through overstretching or sudden, powerful muscular contractions. The key is to strengthen what we stretch and stretch what we strengthen. When performing both a stretching program and a regular weight-lifting strength training program, stretching should occur after the weight-training program so that muscles are warmed before the stretching activity.

A variety of stretching and flexibility exercise techniques attract older adults because they are fun, easy to do, and highly effective. These include tai chi, yoga, Pilates, and water exercises, because of their ability to safely develop both strength and flexibility. This results in improved balance and mobility and the ability to perform ADLs and IADLs, maintaining functional independence.

Older adults beginning exercise programs should first obtain medical clearance and then work with a certified instructor. While exercise improves overall "fitness," their rate of adaptation will be slower. Long-term goals are achieved through slow progression, as they adapt. Older adults should begin at lower frequencies (two times/week), start with shorter time periods (15–20 minutes), and at lower intensities. As strength and endurance increase, frequency, duration, and intensity may be increased. Always begin the training session with a warm-up and end with a cool-down.

Chapter 34

Combined Exercise

Chapter Contents

Section 34.1

Cross Training

Are you tired of doing the same exercise day after day? Do you have trouble sticking to a fitness program? Or, do you get bored easily with the different exercise programs you have tried? If you answered yes to any of the questions, cross training may be the perfect fitness program for you.

According to the American Association of Orthopaedic Surgeons, cross training involves three components including: aerobic exercise, strength training, and flexibility.

Aerobic exercise, such as walking, stair climbing, and rollerblading, will improve your cardiovascular capabilities. Weight lifting, push-ups, which are forms of strength training, help develop muscle mass, while flexibility exercises keep you limber. By incorporating these three components and picking fun activities, you are more likely to stick to your program.

"For those individuals starting an exercise program, cross training is excellent," said Dr. Mark DiLella, orthopaedic surgeon at Ortho-Indy.

"Cross training uses different muscle groups, providing a total body workout. It also allows individuals to pick activities they are interested in, keeping them engaged in the workout, decreasing the chances of quitting," said Dr. DiLella. "Not only will you more than likely stick to the program, but you will decrease your chances of having an injury."

Like any fitness activity, there is a chance for injury. Individuals who only do one type of exercise are more prone to injury because they are focusing on a small group of muscles. Overuse injuries are decreased in a cross training program because you are working a number of muscles instead of a select few, more frequently.

"There are always risks associated with sports, however by cross training, you will increase your endurance, flexibility, and lessen the chances of injuries associated with your activities," said Dr. DiLella.

In most cases, if an injury occurs to an individual that only does one specific workout, he or she may be unable to perform their normal workout routine. However, if you are cross training, there is a high chance that you will not give up all the components of your program and will continue to work out.

Cross training isn't just for serious athletes. If you are looking for a program to get fit and not quit, starting a cross training program is perfect for you.

Starting a Cross Training Program

- Consult your physician to determine if it is safe to start the program.
- Select an activity that interests you, such as dancing or gardening.
- Do activities that you have prior experience in, such as a high school sport.
- Twice a week do 30 minutes of strength training, working each muscle group.
- Stretch every day to increase flexibility and decreases the chance of injuries.
- Like any exercise, your cross training program will increase your chances for a longer and healthier life.

For further information on cross training, please call OrthoIndy at 317-802-2000 or visit www.orthoindy.com.

Section 34.2

Interval Training

Do you want to increase your fitness level? Then interval training, also known as interval conditioning, may be for you. Douglass Brooks, MS, co-owner of Moves International and author of Program Design for Personal Trainers, describes how to use this method no matter how fit you are. If you have questions or would like a demonstration, ask your personal trainer.

1. **Understand the work-rest concept.** Interval conditioning utilized repeated cardiovascular work intervals performed at intensities above your typical exercise levels. To sustain and repeat these higher intensity work intervals, follow them with cardiovascular recovery (rest) intervals performed at a lower intensity. A work interval followed by a recovery interval is called a cycle.

2. **Learn the benefits of interval training.** Intervals help you build endurance, increase fat loss and calorie burning, and/or improve your performance in a sport or activity.

3. **Build your lactate threshold.** If you are not used to interval training, lactic acid in your muscles will most likely increase and accumulate quickly at 50 to 55% of your maximal aerobic capacity, also known as heart rate reserve (HRR). If you are highly conditioned, your threshold may not occur until 80 to 85%. When you accumulate too much lactic acid, you will have difficulty breathing and will be unable to continue exercise at the same intensity. You will need an active recovery period to accelerate lactic acid recovery and help prevent muscle cramps and stiffness.

4. **Start with spontaneous speed play.** If you are new to interval training, try this method during your workout: Speed up a little for 30 seconds, then continue the cardiovascular activity for 90 seconds at an easy effort. Do as many cycles as you desire.

5. **Monitor intensity.** For the following models, measure intensity by using the rating of perceived exertion (RPE) scale: 1 is your easiest effort, and 10 is the most difficult. As your fitness level improves, you can train harder at a given RPE.

6. **Use the fitness model.** More structured than speed play, this model has you exercising cardiovascularly for three to five minutes at an RPE of 4 to 6 (somewhat hard to very hard), then recovering for three to five minutes at a 2 to 3 RPE. Perform as many cycles as you can comfortably, increasing the number of cycles as you become more experienced.

7. **Work up to the challenging fitness model.** To use this model, you should be moderately to extremely fit. Exercise hard for 30 to 90 seconds, then recover for three times the length of the work interval. For example, recover for 180 seconds if you've exercised hard for 60 seconds. Perform work intervals at an RPE of 7 to 10 and rest intervals at a 2 to 3 RPE. Repeat a number of times.

8. **Train for sports with the performance model.** If you are a competitive athlete or highly conditioned, use the performance model to increase cardiovascular fitness. Utilize the fitness model explained earlier, but work at an 80 to 85% HRR for three to five minutes before recovering.

9. **Advance to the difficult performance model.** If you are an advanced athlete who is experienced at interval training, try this workout model. Exercise for 30 to 90 seconds, then recover for just twice the time. Work at an RPE of 8 to 10 (extremely intense!) and rest by exercising at a 2 to 3 RPE. Repeat for a number of cycles.

10. **Train safely.** Precede intervals with a warm-up of at least 5 to 10 minutes and follow it with a cool-down of at least 5 minutes. Interval training should be challenging, yet enjoyable. Use common sense. If you need more time to recover after a work interval, give yourself more time! Interval train no more than twice a week. These programs are for apparently healthy adults. If you are pregnant or have special medical concerns, plan a program in conjunction with a physician and personal trainer.

Section 34.3

Boot Camp Workouts

Fitness fads come and go, but boot-camp workouts are still among the most popular.

Back in the spring of 1998, the American Council on Exercise [ACE] first spotted the rapid growth of instructor-led workouts based loosely on the calisthenics used (like push-ups, squat thrusts, punches, kicks, etc.) to whip new recruits into shape in the U.S. Army's basic-training program. Ten years later, take a look at the class schedules of gyms and fitness centers across the country and you'll still find boot camp. According to recent stats from the International Health, Racquet & Sportsclub Association, a trade organization for health clubs, 955 of its 3,306 member clubs offer boot camp–style fitness classes. And it's not just hot in the gyms. A quick scan of the exercise videos offered on Amazon.com yields more than 30 different boot-camp videos.

"There's a certain element of getting back to the basics and a more functional-training approach," says ACE's chief science officer Cedric X. Bryant, PhD. "People are looking for different experiences. With boot camps, you're giving them something outside the traditional club environment."

Maybe the boot-camp trend is still going strong because it's not really trendy at all. The workout is simple and not tied to a single piece of equipment. Or maybe it's the motivating team-oriented atmosphere that's created as fellow exercisers "survive" the workouts together.

Whatever the reason, boot camp remains wildly popular, yet surprisingly its efficacy has never been formally studied. "Boot camp is becoming more and more popular in the health club setting so obviously people want to know if they're really going to get something out of it, and if it's going to be worth their time," says Kirsten Hendrickson, a graduate student in exercise and sports science at the University of Wisconsin. "So we decided to take a look at it."

The Study

To analyze the health and fitness benefits of boot camp–style workouts, a team of exercise scientists from the University of Wisconsin, La Crosse Exercise and Health Program, led by John Porcari, PhD, and Hendrickson, recruited six men and six women ages 19 to 29.

All volunteers were given an exercise test on a motorized treadmill to determine each subject's maximal heart rate (HR max) and maximal oxygen consumption (VO2 max) to establish a baseline of fitness. Ratings of perceived exertion using the 6–20 Borg Scale, a measure of how hard subjects feel they're exercising, were also recorded throughout the exercise testing.

Once that baseline was established, the subjects were invited back into the lab to view a 40-minute recorded boot-camp exercise video. Naturally there are many boot camp–style exercise videos on the market, so researchers reviewed a wide range of titles, eventually settling on *The Method: Cardio Boot Camp* with Tracey Mallett. "We chose that DVD because it has a good blend of aerobic movements and strength moves that you'd picture military guys doing at boot camp," notes Porcari. "Plus we wanted to pick one where people were taxed pretty hard because that's what you picture when you think of boot camp."

The study volunteers were given a copy of the DVD to take home and practice until they felt familiar enough with the choreography to be able to follow along easily with the workout. At that point, they were asked to return to the lab for testing. Each subject was then outfitted with the Cosmed portable analyzer, a backpack and facemask apparatus that measures oxygen consumption and caloric burn. Heart rate and perceived exertion were also tracked every three minutes throughout the 40-minute workout.

The Results

After analyzing the data, researchers found that the average exerciser burns approximately 9.8 calories per minute during a typical boot-camp workout, which equals nearly 400 calories during the entire 40-minute boot-camp video studied.

"The biggest benefit is you're burning an average of 600 calories per hour," says Porcari. "That's obviously going to help with weight loss, but you're also getting the muscle-building benefit from push-ups, arm curls, and squat thrusts that you wouldn't get just from going out for a fast walk or jog."

According to recommendations set by the American College of Sports Medicine (ACSM), to enhance cardiorespiratory endurance individuals need to exercise at 70% to 94% of HR max and 50% to 85% of VO2 max.

Based upon the data collected in this study, subjects were exercising well within those recommended intensity levels. "On average, people were working at 77% of heart-rate max, which is considered moderate intensity, but it also gets as high as 91%, meaning, all these boot-camp workouts have peaks and valleys," Porcari explains. Heart rate and oxygen consumption varied by the minute as the test subjects followed the video from high-intensity moves like kicking and punching, down to low-intensity moves with the dumbbells, and back up again to high-intensity moves.

"These workouts are designed to be cyclical like that," he explains. "Boot camp is a good form of interval training because you get periods of high intensity interspersed with moves that tend to be lower in aerobic intensity but they serve a whole different purpose—to build muscle strength."

The Bottom Line

Boot camp is an excellent way to enhance aerobic capacity and help control body weight. "I think it's a great workout with great variety," says Porcari. "It's a good combination of aerobic exercise and muscle conditioning and it's much more of a total-body workout than just going out for a run or bicycle ride."

But remember, not all boot-camp workouts are created equal, he warns. Some are heavy on cardio, while others emphasize martial arts–inspired movements or basic strength-training exercises. For best results, our researchers recommend picking a well-balanced program with equal helpings of aerobic movements and calisthenics. However, if you're looking to improve in a particular area, you might consider looking for a boot-camp class or video that caters to your particular fitness weaknesses. For example, if you'd prefer to build more upper-body strength and endurance, consider picking one with more push-ups, squat thrusts, and similar moves.

"If people are looking for something that's fun and variable that will increase their adherence to an exercise program, and, most importantly, burn a lot of calories," says Hendrickson, "boot camp would be a really great option."

Table 34.1. How Does Boot Camp Compare to Other Workouts

	% HR max	% VO2 max	kcal/min
Boot Camp	81	62	7.5
Cardio Kick Boxing	86	70	8.1
Spinning	89	75	9.6
Aerobic Dance	85	71	9.7
Curves	75	60	6.4
Power Yoga	62	46	5.9
Advanced Pilates	62	43	5.6

Chapter 35

Mind-Body Exercise

Chapter Contents

Section 35.1

Introduction to Mind-Body Exercise

Harnessing the Power of the Mind-Body Connection

The mind-body connection means that you can learn to use your thoughts to positively influence some of your body's physical responses, thereby decreasing stress. If you recall a time when you were happy, grateful, or calm, your body and mind tend to relax.

Research has shown that when you imagine an experience, you often have similar mental and physical responses to those you have when the event actually happens. For example, if you recall an upsetting or frightening experience, you may feel your heart beating faster, you may begin to sweat, and your hands may become cold and clammy.

Whether you have been diagnosed with an illness or need to prepare for a medical procedure such as surgery, it is very important to minimize the negative effects and maximize the healthy, healing aspects of your mind-body connection.

A variety of calming and empowering mind-body exercises have been proven to help people:

- decrease anxiety;
- decrease pain;
- enhance sleep;
- decrease the use of medication for post-surgical pain;
- decrease side effects of medical procedures;
- reduce recovery time and shorten hospital stays;
- strengthen the immune system and enhance the ability to heal;
- increase sense of control and well-being.

While the exercises described in this section are not alternatives to medical or surgical treatments, they provide a powerful way for you to actively participate in your own health care, minimize pain and insomnia, and promote recovery.

Calming/Relaxation Exercises

The goal of calming and relaxation exercises is to help change the way you perceive a situation and react to it—to help you feel more in control, more confident or secure, and to activate healing processes within the body. Become aware of any tension, anxiety, change in breathing, or symptoms that you recognize as being caused or worsened by stress. When you take about 15 minutes daily to practice these exercises to help "quiet" your mind and help your body become more relaxed, you can then call upon this ability with a shorter relaxation exercise at a stressful time.

Relaxation Breathing Practice

- Be aware of your current breathing pattern and learn how to change your breathing rate from fast, shallow chest breathing to slow, abdominal breathing.

- Focus on your breath while you place one hand on your chest, the other over your navel. Imagine there is a balloon in your abdomen. As you take a slow, deep breath, focus on inflating the balloon in your abdomen. You will notice that your abdomen will rise much more than your chest. As you exhale, just let your abdomen fall naturally.

- The goal is to learn how to breathe at six breaths a minute, about three or four seconds inhaling and six or seven seconds exhaling. Once you have the slow, deep breathing accomplished, don't worry about counting, and imagine breathing out any tension in the body or thoughts that get in the way of comfort and relaxation.

- If it helps, you can imagine a spot located on your abdomen, just below your navel. Breathe into and through that spot, filling your abdomen with air, allowing it to expand. Imagine the air filling you inside from your abdomen, and then let it out, like deflating a balloon. With every long, slow breath out, you should feel more relaxed.

Progressive Muscle Relaxation

- Progressive muscle relaxation involves sequentially tensing and then relaxing specific muscle groups in the body, one at a time, and progressing throughout the entire body.

- The key to this exercise is to tighten a specific muscle group for at least 5 seconds until you feel the tension, and then release the muscles for 10 seconds, noticing the difference in how the muscles feel before and after the exercise.

- You can start by relaxing the muscles in your legs and feet, working up through each muscle group to your neck, shoulders, and scalp. You should notice that during this process, the tension in your muscles will be reduced.

Note: Be careful not to tense muscles in areas that have incisions, devices, or tubes.

Mind Relaxation

Close your eyes. Breathe normally through your nose. As you exhale, silently say to yourself the word "one," or any other short word such as "peaceful," or a phrase such as "I feel quiet" or "I'm safe." Continue for 10 minutes. If your mind wanders, gently remind yourself to think about your breathing and your chosen word or phrase. Let your breathing become slow and steady. Recall and focus on a pleasant memory. Take another deep breath and exhale slowly. You should feel more relaxed.

Try this exercise that incorporates a few different relaxation techniques:

- Begin by interrupting your normal daily thoughts. Think about what is going on around you. Then switch your thoughts to yourself and your breathing. Take a few deep breaths, exhaling slowly.

- Mentally scan your body. Notice areas that feel tense or cramped, such as your neck or shoulders. Loosen up these areas. Let go of as much tension as you can.

- Slowly rotate your head to the left in a smooth, circular motion, leaning your left ear to your left shoulder. Rotate your head to the right in a smooth, circular motion, leaning your right ear to your right shoulder. (Stop any movements that cause pain.)

- Roll your shoulders forward and backward several times. Let all of your muscles completely relax.

Guided Imagery

Research shows that guided imagery and relaxation can decrease anxiety and pain and possibly shorten your hospital stay. Guided imagery is often presented on an audio program in which you are guided in using your imagination to induce peace, calm, strength, and control. The calming music accompanying guided imagery can be helpful in quieting the mind.

Massage Therapy

Massage can help reduce muscle tension, relieve stress, and soothe pain. A light, 10-minute massage (with your physician's approval) can assist your experience of well-being as you are healing.

Reiki

Reiki is a relaxing, nurturing energy therapy that uses gentle touch to help balance your physical, mental, emotional, and spiritual well-being to promote a deep sense of relaxation. Reiki works with your energy to support your natural ability to heal.

Mind-Body Coach

A mind-body coach is a trained professional who can teach you multiple ways to use your mind to reach a higher level of peace, calm, and comfort before surgery. You'll also learn the "tools" to help you during recovery, including guided imagery.

Spiritual Practices

Centering prayer and meditation are some of the oldest methods of relaxation involving a specific mental focus. These techniques induce a deep state of relaxation and well-being. Many people find spiritual practices helpful in achieving total mind-body relaxation.

Music Therapy

Under the supervision of a board-certified music therapist, music therapy combines music and therapeutic techniques and aids in the physiological, psychological, and emotional well-being of the individual during treatment of an illness.

Art Therapy

Art therapy uses art media and the creative process to help patients in their healing and recovery. Art therapy can help patients decrease anxiety, manage stress, and deal with emotional issues.

Self-Help Relaxation Techniques

These techniques will help you release muscle tension and relieve pain. Practice these techniques as often as necessary.

- **Fold and hold:** If a muscle in the shoulders or neck is tight, you can release it without rubbing it. Just bend toward the tight side and hold it for 90 seconds. The muscle should be soft after doing this. If this causes any strain on the incision site, stop immediately. Please do not use this method on the legs.

- **Chucking/Jostling:** If a muscle is tight, brush lightly over the muscle with your hand and it should release in 30 seconds. Do not rub over any muscles that are near or under an incision, tube, or if a medical device is implanted in the area.

Section 35.2

Yoga

What Is Yoga?

Yoga is an ancient Indian practice and type of mind-body exercise that has been in existence for thousands of years. The term yoga means "yoke" or "union," and yoga practice involves breath work (pranayama) to connect the mind and body, as well as to connect our thoughts and feelings with movement.

Yoga provides a number of well-documented physical, mental, and emotional benefits. These include reduced blood pressure, enhanced feelings of relaxation, stress reduction, improved digestion, better posture, increased strength and flexibility, and improved balance, among others. Yoga also has been shown to benefit individuals with chronic diseases and disabilities through improved body awareness and orientation, the development of focus and concentration, the encouragement of learning and creativity, and increased awareness of our connectedness to others.

Selecting a Yoga Class

You can choose from a wide variety of yoga classes offering different types of yoga and different teachers and styles. Selecting an appropriate class and teacher for your level of experience, health and/or fitness goals, and preferences can help yoga become an enjoyable experience that provides the benefits that you seek.

Types or styles of yoga vary in pace and emphasis from slower-paced practices that include breathing and meditation (Hatha yoga) to faster, flowing movement sequences combined with rhythmic breathing (Vinyasa-style yoga, such as Ashtanga and Power yoga). Short descriptions of some of the different styles are provided in the following:

- **Ananda:** Provides a tool for spiritual growth while releasing tension; uses silent affirmations while holding poses.

401

- **Ashtanga:** A vigorous practice incorporating a fast-paced series of sequential postures that increase in difficulty.

- **Bikram:** Designed by Bikram Choudhury as a method of staying healthy from the inside out; involves practicing a series of 26 traditional Hatha yoga postures (13 standing and 13 sitting) in a hot environment (near 100 ° Fahrenheit); guaranteed to make you sweat!

- **Hatha:** A more relaxed, slower-paced practice that includes breathing and meditation exercises; emphasizes breathing, strength, and flexibility; good for beginner exercisers or those new to yoga.

- **Iyengar:** Developed by B.K.S. Iyengar, one of the most influential yogis of his time; focuses on proper alignment with the use of props; poses are typically held much longer than in other styles of yoga.

- **Jivamukti:** A highly meditative yet physically challenging form of yoga that includes vinyasa-style sequences of poses, asanas, chanting, meditation, readings, music, and affirmations.

- **Kripalu:** Developed by Amrit Desai and the staff at the Kripalu Center for Yoga and Health in Massachusetts; three stages make up this practice: will practice, willful surrender, and meditation in motion; characterized by trusting the body's wisdom to move in a way needed to release tensions and enter more deeply into meditation.

- **Kundalini:** Incorporates postures with dynamic breathing techniques, chanting, and meditating to awaken the energy at the base of the spine and draw it upward through each of the seven energy centers of the body (chakras).

- **Power Yoga:** Developed by Bender Birch; a challenging and disciplined series of poses designed with the intention of creating heat and energy flow.

- **Sivananda:** Developed by Rama Berch, who created the yoga program from Dr. Deepak Chopra's Center for Well Being in La Jolla, California; geared toward aiding participants in their journeys toward self-discovery.

- **Svaroopa:** Incorporates proper breathing (pranayama), exercise, relaxation (Savasana), and vegetarian diet with positive thinking (Vedanta) and meditation (dhyana).

- **Therapeutic:** Addresses all levels—physical, emotional, and spiritual—of the healing process to promote health, function, and enhanced quality of life for special populations (e.g., heart patients, hypertensives, cancer survivors, or others with physical limitations).

- **Viniyoga:** A gentle yet powerful and transformative practice in which poses are synchronized with the breath in sequences determined by the practitioner.

- **Vinyasa:** A flow-style of yoga that melds breathing with movement, similar to Ashtanga but with less repetition or following of a set sequence.

- **Yoga for Fitness:** Based upon the Hatha yoga practice, this fitness-based approach is tailored for the mainstream health club member. It utilizes strength, flexibility, balance, and power to give you a full workout great for all levels.

Safety

There is an inherent safety partnership that exists between the participant and the instructor in yoga practice. The yoga instructor should be certified through or hold one or more credentials from an established and respected organization and have experience teaching yoga. Some certifications, such as Yoga Alliance's Registered Yoga Teacher —200 and 500 hours (RYT-200 and RYT-500, respectively), require completion of a certain number and type of trainings along with a specified number of hours of yoga teaching. Ideally, the yoga instructor should minimize risk of injury to participants as well as have CPR/first aid training in order to be prepared to respond appropriately in the event of an emergency.

With regard to minimizing risk of injury, the instructor should have and be able to demonstrate his/her ability to modify poses and flow sequences for different levels of ability and physical limitations. Your yoga instructor may ask at the beginning of a class or series of classes about physical injuries or parts of the body that are healing or need protection. If he/she doesn't inquire, it's helpful to you and the instructor and in your best interests to let him/her know about any physical issues so he/she can offer modifications of poses and flow sequences before or during class. These modifications are important not only from a safety standpoint, but from the perspective of helping each participant optimize the yoga experience and reap as many of the potential benefits of a yoga practice as possible.

Like other workouts and exercise classes, a safe yoga class should include a warm-up of low- to moderate-intensity movements designed to increase heart rate and respiration, increase blood flow to the muscles, and prepare the body for more intense activity. The warm-up may be followed by a work phase of more intense activity, which would be different from one yoga style to another. For example, the work phase might include a greater number of repetitions, holding poses for a longer period of time, and/or using more explosive movements such as jumping into or out of poses (e.g., forward fold to plank). A yoga class should end with some type of cool-down, which may include lower-intensity exercise, stretching, twisting poses, and a final relaxation.

For participants, it is vital we listen to our own bodies. We need to know our limits and respect them. Yoga often challenges us to find our "edge"—a place where we are "uncomfortably comfortable," where we feel challenged, yet able to hold a position or move safely through a flow sequence. It is important to remember that everyone brings a different body (with its unique anatomy, range of motion, function, and genetic potential), different histories with yoga and exercise in general, and different goals for his/her yoga practice. Thus, letting go of the need to compare ourselves to or compete with others helps us practice yoga in a way that is safe and appropriate for us as unique individuals. A good yoga teacher can help remind us of this and to listen to our bodies, but it's up to each of us to put these principles into practice as we do yoga. This might include modifying poses or movements so they are safe for our bodies or choosing to do different poses or movements that our bodies can handle safely, even when not prompted by the instructor.

Equipment and Clothing

The minimum equipment needed for yoga is a sticky mat (a mat your feet won't slide on, and that won't slide on the surface on which it's placed), or gloves and socks with rubber-like pads or dots on the palms and soles. These help participants hold their positions and move safely between poses without slipping and sliding. Mats come in different thicknesses, and participants can use two mats for extra cushioning for the knees and spine or other parts of the body when they are in contact with the mat and bearing body weight. Mats are also made of different materials, some of which are "eco-friendly." Some yoga mats are made especially for travel and fold up to take up minimal space in luggage. Mats vary in price, but can usually be purchased from a sporting goods store, a yoga or exercise studio or health/fitness facility, or online for $10–$40. Yoga mats should be cleaned regularly to prevent bacterial growth, either with a damp cloth or sponge and mild soap or detergent, or following the manufacturer's recommendations.

Additional types of equipment that may be used in yoga classes, or that can be purchased for home use, include blocks, straps, bolsters, and blankets for modifying poses to enhance technique and body position and/or increase safety and comfort for the participant.

Yoga clothing should be comfortable for the wearer and allow freedom of movement or full range of motion at all major joints of the body (e.g., shoulders, elbows, spine, hips, and knees.). Yoga clothing comes in a variety of colors and styles and at various prices and is designed for a variety of body types. Because the body is moved through a variety of positions and yoga classes are often co-ed, participants might wish to consider how their clothing fits and provides coverage as they move and bend.

Etiquette

When attending a yoga class in any setting, there are a few guidelines to follow to ensure that you and everyone in your class have a positive experience.

- **Arrive early:** Allow ample time for your mat and prop setup as well as personal preparation.

- **Enter quietly:** Enter the room/studio gently, so as not to disturb others.

- **Be free of distraction:** Do not bring a cell phone, pager, etc. to class. This can disrupt you and others around you.

- **Be considerate:** Allow plenty of room between you and your neighbor for free movement. Also, if you must leave the room during class, do so quietly and discretely.

Other Considerations

It is more comfortable to practice yoga on a somewhat empty or empty stomach, so participants might choose to eat lightly in the minutes or hour before practice, or have a bigger meal two or more hours before, depending on what is comfortable and allows the maintenance of appropriate blood sugar levels. Yoga participants may want to have a bottle of water at hand if they get thirsty during practice as well as to rehydrate themselves after practice.

A Home Yoga Practice

Establishing and maintaining a home yoga practice: You can establish a yoga practice at home with minimum equipment and little more space than that required for a yoga mat. Choose a time to practice yoga that works with your schedule (morning, afternoon, or evening), and practice for an amount of time that is appropriate for your schedule, your level of experience (shorter duration for beginners, perhaps longer duration for intermediate and advanced practitioners), your desire, your lifestyle, and the results you seek.

Yoga can be practiced in silence or with music of your choice. It can be practiced alone using poses and flow series of your own creation, or as guided by an instructor and participants on video or DVD. If using a video or DVD, choose one based on the type or style of yoga and the instructor's credentials and experience.

How to maximize benefits: You may experience benefits such as a greater sense of relaxation and connectedness with your body in as little as 5 to 10 minutes of yoga per day, or develop greater strength, flexibility, and balance in a longer yoga practice lasting 30–90 minutes or more.

Yoga practice can also be tailored to focus on strengthening and stretching specific muscle groups critical to performance in a given sport, such as running, golf, or tennis.

Consistency in your yoga practice, whether taking a yoga class and/or doing yoga at home, is key to experiencing the many benefits yoga has to offer. Yoga can comprise the whole of an individual's exercise program and be done daily or most days of the week. Alternatively, yoga can be practiced less frequently as part of a regular exercise program in conjunction with activity that is more specifically geared to develop various aspects of health-related fitness (i.e., cardiorespiratory endurance, muscular strength and endurance, and flexibility).

Yoga offers a great way to stay active when you are traveling. You can take a foldable yoga mat or yoga gloves and socks on the road and practice in your hotel room, or take a local drop-in class in your destination city.

Section 35.3

Pilates

Pilates (pronounced: puh-*lah*-teez) improves your mental and physical well-being, increases flexibility, and strengthens muscles. Pilates uses controlled movements in the form of mat exercises or equipment to tone and strengthen the body. For decades, it's been the exercise of choice for dancers and gymnasts (and now Hollywood actors), but it was originally used to rehabilitate bedridden or immobile patients during World War I.

What Is Pilates?

Pilates is a body conditioning routine that seeks to build flexibility, strength, endurance, and coordination without adding muscle bulk. In addition, Pilates increases circulation and helps to sculpt the body and strengthen the body's "core" or "powerhouse" (torso). People who do Pilates regularly feel they have better posture, are less prone to injury, and experience better overall health.

Joseph H. Pilates, the founder of the Pilates exercise method, was born in Germany. As a child he was frail, living with asthma in addition to other childhood conditions. To build his body and grow stronger, he took up several different sports, eventually becoming an accomplished athlete. As a nurse in Great Britain during World War I, he designed exercise methods and equipment for immobilized patients and soldiers.

In addition to his equipment, Pilates developed a series of mat exercises that focus on the torso. He based these on various exercise methods from around the world, among them the mind-body formats of yoga and Chinese martial arts.

Joseph Pilates believed that our physical and mental health are intertwined. He designed his exercise program around principles that support this philosophy, including concentration, precision, control, breathing, and flowing movements.

There are two ways to exercise in Pilates. Today, most people focus on the mat exercises, which require only a floor mat and training. These exercises are designed so that your body uses its own weight as resistance. The other method of Pilates uses a variety of machines to tone and strengthen the body, again using the principle of resistance.

Getting Started

The great thing about Pilates is that just about everyone—from couch potatoes to fitness buffs—can do it. Because Pilates has gained lots of attention recently, there are lots of classes available. You'll probably find that many fitness centers and YMCAs offer Pilates classes, mostly in mat work. Some Pilates instructors also offer private classes that can be purchased class by class or in blocks of classes; these may combine mat work with machine work. If your health club makes Pilates machines available to members, make sure there's a qualified Pilates instructor on duty to teach and supervise you during the exercises.

The fact that Pilates is hot and classes are springing up everywhere does have a downside, though: inadequate instruction. As with any form of exercise, it is possible to injure yourself if you have a health condition or don't know exactly how to do the moves. Some gyms send their personal trainers to weekend-long courses and then claim they're qualified to teach Pilates (they're not!), and this can lead to injury.

So look for an instructor who is certified by a group that has a rigorous training program. These instructors have completed several hundred hours of training just in Pilates and know the different ways to modify the exercises so new students don't get hurt.

The Pilates mat program follows a set sequence, with exercises following on from one another in a natural progression, just as Joseph Pilates designed them. Beginners start with basic exercises and build up to include additional exercises and more advanced positioning.

Keep these tips in mind so that you can get the most out of your Pilates workout.

- **Stay focused.** Pilates is designed to combine your breathing rhythm with your body movements. Qualified instructors teach ways to keep your breathing working in conjunction with the exercises. You will also be taught to concentrate on your muscles and what you are doing. The goal of Pilates is to unite your mind and body, which relieves stress and anxiety.

- **Be comfortable.** Wear comfortable clothes (as you would for yoga—shorts or tights and a T-shirt or tank top are good choices), and keep in mind that Pilates is usually done without shoes. If you start feeling uncomfortable, strained, or experience pain, you should stop.

- **Let it flow.** When you perform your exercises, avoid quick, jerky movements. Every movement should be slow, but still strong and flexible. Joseph Pilates worked with dancers and designed his movements to flow like a dance.

- **Don't leave out the heart.** The nice thing about Pilates is you don't have to break a sweat if you don't want to—but you can also work the exercises quickly (bearing in mind fluidity, of course!) to get your heart rate going. Or, because Pilates is primarily about strength and flexibility, pair your Pilates workout with a form of aerobic exercise like swimming or brisk walking.

Most fans of Pilates say they stick with the program because it's diverse and interesting. Joseph Pilates designed his program for variety—people do fewer repetitions of a number of exercises rather than lots of repetitions of only a few. He also intended his exercises to be something people could do on their own once they've had proper instruction, cutting down the need to remain dependent on a trainer.

Before you begin any type of exercise program, it's a good idea to talk to your doctor, especially if you have a health problem.

Section 35.4

Tai Chi

"Tai Chi: An Introduction," National Center for Complementary
and Alternative Medicine (nccam.nih.gov), April 2009.

Tai chi, which originated in China as a martial art, is a mind-body practice in complementary and alternative medicine (CAM). Tai chi is sometimes referred to as "moving meditation"—practitioners move their bodies slowly, gently, and with awareness, while breathing deeply.

Key Points

- Many people practice tai chi to improve their health and well-being.

- Scientific research is under way to learn more about how tai chi may work, its possible effects on health, and chronic diseases and conditions for which it may be helpful.

- Tell your health care providers about any complementary and alternative practices you use. Give them a full picture of what you do to manage your health. This will help ensure coordinated and safe care.

Overview

Tai chi developed in ancient China. It started as a martial art and a means of self-defense. Over time, people began to use it for health purposes as well.

Accounts of the history of tai chi vary. A popular legend credits its origins to Chang San-Feng, a Taoist monk, who developed a set of 13 exercises that imitate the movements of animals. He also emphasized meditation and the concept of internal force (in contrast to the external force emphasized in other martial arts, such as kung fu and tae kwon do).

The term "tai chi" (shortened from "tai chi chuan") has been translated in various ways, such as "internal martial art" and "supreme ultimate fist." It is sometimes called "taiji" or "taijiquan."

Tai chi incorporates the Chinese concepts of yin and yang (opposing forces within the body) and qi (a vital energy or life force). Practicing tai chi is said to support a healthy balance of yin and yang, thereby aiding the flow of qi.

People practice tai chi by themselves or in groups. In the Chinese community, people commonly practice tai chi in nearby parks—often in the early morning before going to work. There are many different styles, but all involve slow, relaxed, graceful movements, each flowing into the next. The body is in constant motion, and posture is important. The names of some of the movements evoke nature (e.g., "Embrace Tiger, Return to Mountain"). Individuals practicing tai chi must also concentrate, putting aside distracting thoughts, and they must breathe in a deep and relaxed but focused manner.

Use in the United States

A 2007 survey by the National Center for Health Statistics and the National Center for Complementary and Alternative Medicine (NCCAM) on Americans' use of CAM found that 1% of the more than 23,300 adults surveyed had used tai chi in the past 12 months. Adjusted to nationally representative numbers, this means more than 2.3 million adults.

People practice tai chi for various health-related purposes, such as the following:

- For benefits associated with low-impact, weight-bearing, aerobic exercise

- To improve physical condition, muscle strength, coordination, and flexibility

- To improve balance and decrease the risk of falls, especially in elderly people

- To ease pain and stiffness—for example, from osteoarthritis

- To improve sleep

- For overall wellness

The Status of Tai Chi Research

Scientific research on the health benefits of tai chi is ongoing. Several studies have focused on the elderly, including tai chi's potential for preventing falls and improving cardiovascular fitness and overall well-being. A 2007 NCCAM-funded study on the immune response to

411

varicella-zoster virus (the virus that causes shingles) suggested that tai chi may enhance the immune system and improve overall well-being in older adults. Tai chi has also been studied for improving functional capacity in breast cancer patients and quality of life in people with HIV infection. Studies have also looked at tai chi's possible benefits for a variety of other conditions, including cardiovascular disease, hypertension, and osteoarthritis. In 2008, a review of published research, also funded by NCCAM, found that tai chi reduced participants' blood pressure in 22 (of 26) studies.

In general, studies of tai chi have been small, or they have had design limitations that may limit their conclusions. The cumulative evidence suggests that additional research is warranted and needed before tai chi can be widely recommended as an effective therapy.

Side Effects and Risks

Tai chi is a relatively safe practice. However, there are some cautions:

- As with any exercise regimen, if you overdo practice, you may have sore muscles or sprains.

- Tai chi instructors often recommend that you do not practice tai chi right after a meal, or when you are very tired, or if you have an active infection.

- If you are pregnant, or if you have a hernia, joint problems, back pain, fractures, or severe osteoporosis, your health care provider may advise you to modify or avoid certain postures in tai chi.

Training, Licensing, and Certification

Tai chi instructors do not have to be licensed, and the practice is not regulated by the federal government or individual states. In traditional tai chi instruction, a student learns from a master teacher. To become an instructor, an experienced student of tai chi must obtain a master teacher's approval. Currently, training programs vary. Some training programs award certificates; some offer weekend workshops. There is no standard training for instructors.

If You Are Thinking about Practicing Tai Chi

- Do not use tai chi as a replacement for conventional care or to postpone seeing a doctor about a medical problem.

- If you have a medical condition or have not exercised in a while, consult with your health care provider before starting tai chi.

- Keep in mind that learning tai chi from a video or book does not ensure that you are doing the movements correctly and safely.

- If you are considering a tai chi instructor, ask about the individual's training and experience.

- Look for published research studies on tai chi for the health condition you are interested in.

- Tell your health care providers about any complementary and alternative practices you use. Give them a full picture of what you do to manage your health. This will help ensure coordinated and safe care. For tips about talking with your health care providers about CAM, see NCCAM's Time to Talk campaign (nccam .nih.gov/timetotalk/).

Selected References

Adler PA, Roberts BL. The use of tai chi to improve health in older adults. *Orthopaedic Nursing*. 2006;25(2):122–126.

Barnes PM, Bloom B, Nahin R. Complementary and alternative medicine use among adults and children: United States, 2007. *CDC National Health Statistics Report #12*. 2008.

Chu DA. Tai chi, qi gong, and Reiki. *Physical Medicine and Rehabilitation Clinics of North America*. 2004;15(4):773–781.

Farrell SJ, Ross AD, Sehgal KV. Eastern movement therapies. *Physical Medicine and Rehabilitation Clinics of North America*. 1999;10(3):617–629.

Irwin MR, Olmstead R, Oxman MN. Augmenting immune responses to varicella zoster virus in older adults: a randomized, controlled trial of tai chi. *Journal of the American Geriatrics Society*. 2007;55(4):511–517.

Lan C, Lai JS, Chen SY. Tai chi chuan: an ancient wisdom on exercise and health promotion. *Sports Medicine*. 2002;32(4):217–224.

Lewis D. T'ai chi ch'uan. *Complementary Therapies in Nursing & Midwifery*. 2000;6(4):204–206.

Robins JL, McCain NL, Gray DP, et al. Research on psychoneuroimmunology: tai chi as a stress management approach for individuals with HIV disease. *Applied Nursing Research*. 2006;19(1):2–9.

Tai chi. Natural Medicines Comprehensive Database. Accessed on August 4, 2008.

Tai chi. Natural Standard Database Web site. Accessed on January 9, 2008.

Wang C, Collet JP, Lau J. The effect of tai chi on health outcomes in patients with chronic conditions: a systemic review. *Archives of Internal Medicine.* 2004;164(5):493–501.

Yeh GY, Wang C, Wayne PM, et al. The effect of tai chi exercise on blood pressure: a systematic review. *Preventive Cardiology.* 2008;11(2):82–89.

Chapter 36

Power Training and Plyometrics for Athletes

Power is the ultimate combination of the two most fundamental human factors of survival: speed and strength. From the true warrior to the finest athlete to young children, power is quintessential to success. Power by its very definition suggests you cannot go without, yet it deceives many and is generally considered necessary for contact sport or weightlifting athletes. However, many forget about the positive impact that power has on endurance performance.

Power Defined

Physics defines power as the rate at which work is performed. Human physiology defines power as the ability to generate enough energy to accomplish a specific feat or task in the least amount of time possible. Simply put, if you want to perform better in a specific sport or in daily activities, you should incorporate some form of power training into your workouts. For the endurance athlete this is no exception. In fact, power training may considerably improve running times by enhancing both physiological and mental functions.

The very nature of the word endurance suggests that power is not a significant part of the equation. For power to truly exist, the duration of an activity must be quick in nature, but with endurance, the opposite is true. Since the endurance athlete focuses on many aspects of improving performance through cardiovascular adaptation and improving metabolic efficiency, the idea of being explosive eludes many of these athletes. Being more explosive gives the endurance athlete another tool they can utilize during training and competition, such as speed to burst at the end of a race, power to climb a hill, and confidence knowing that you have more in "the tank" if needed.

Why Power Training?

The obvious connection of explosive training to power sports makes its training for endurance sports seem counter intuitive. The endurance athlete typically spends time doing long slow duration (LSD) training mixed with interval training. Why do intervals? By comparison, it is relatively new to training since people have been running distances for centuries. They are performed in order to improve anaerobic threshold parameters as well as maximal aerobic power. Power training is also beneficial to the endurance athlete for the same reason but for a different application. Power training can improve an endurance athlete's submaximal strength as well as maximal power. This translates to an easier time running hills, applying quick bursts, or improving maximal speed.

When Do We Add Power Training?

Since intervals have become commonplace in the endurance athletes training program, it may seem wise to add explosive exercises to your daily routine as well. However, power training comes at a cost. High intensity exercise places greater stress on the soft tissue network (such as muscles, tendons, and ligaments) as well as a significantly higher neurological demand on the central nervous system.[1] To combat these stresses, power training should be done in cycles, allowing the athlete plenty of recovery time to focus on other aspects of endurance sports. When adding explosive exercises to your program, they should be done first after a good warm-up, last no more then about 20 minutes, incorporated no more then twice per week, and cycled off after three to four weeks of training. More importantly, explosive exercises should not be done right before a big event; rather, your power training should end two weeks before your major competition. For those who compete year round, power exercises should be included in the training program when training for less important events.

416

What Type of Explosive Exercises Should I Do?

If you have rarely lifted weights in the past, you should stick to the basics, but for those who are more experienced with weight training, power cleans and snatches, provided form is correct, are safe and effective. In general though, you do not want to lose focus of your ultimate goal, which is moving your body on the field or the course, so this author's recommendation is to focus on bodyweight plyometric applications, lighter medicine ball exercises, and faster pace rep schemes for your general exercises.

The set of workouts described in table 36.1 are for combining your power and strength exercises into one workout. Each day could be done once or twice per week. If you are looking for a three-day program, use the first workout, then the following two.

What Are Plyometrics and Do I Need to Do Them?

Plyometrics, often called "plyos," are a method of training which enhances muscle's natural ability to contract more forcefully and rapidly. By decreasing the time and increasing the magnitude of the eccentric to concentric action of muscle (known as the stretch shorten cycle), the athlete improves his or her ability to produce greater force more rapidly, thus improving the overall power of the movement. Plyometric activity utilizes muscle's inherent stretch-contract mechanism and over time improves the rate at which force is developed. So, yes, even an endurance athlete should perform plyometrics.

Power Training and Workout Pace

First and foremost, before you begin to train power you should make sure you have developed an adequate amount of strength to perform this type of training. While certain strength measures are not feasible, you should be able to perform deep barbell squats, bench presses, and basic pulling exercises. If you have never done these exercises before, power training is not recommended until after at least 8–12 weeks of solid strength training. For those who have established a base level of strength, workout pace will be a key. Although the idea of shorter rest, fast pace workouts are opposite to power training recommendations, for the endurance athlete, ultimate one-time power is not requested. Power training for the endurance athlete should emphasize more power-endurance, rather than maxing power. Endurance athletes will still perform short rep sets of no more then eight reps; however, rest time should be 60 seconds to no more then 90 seconds between sets (as opposed to the recommendation of three to five minutes for power athletes).

Table 36.1. Workouts for Combining Power and Strength Exercises

Upper Body Day

Exercise	Sets	Reps	Rest
Speed/Power/Plyometrics			
Medicine Ball Chest Pass	4	6	1 min
Medicine Ball Power Drop	4	6	1 min
Plyo Push Up	2	6	1 min
Basic Strength/Hypertrophy			
Flat Bench Press	3	12	90 sec
Incline Dumbbell Press	2	10	90 sec
Seated Row	3	12	90 sec
Lat Pulldown	2	10	90 sec
Overhead Press	3	10	90 sec

Lower Body Day

Exercise	Sets	Reps	Rest
Speed/Power/Plyometrics			
Box Jump	4	6	1 min
Split Jump	4	6	1 min
Lateral Hurdle Hops	3*	6	1 min
Leg Press (timed for speed)	3	10	90 sec
Leg Extension (timed for speed)	3	12	90 sec
Basic Strength/Hypertrophy			
Leg Curl	3	12	
Romanian Deadlift	4	8	
Standing Calf Raise	3	15	

* performed to each side

This resistance workout should be performed twice per week for three to four weeks provided that a good strength base already exists. To keep time in the gym to a minimum, alternate exercises between upper and lower body after plyometrics. Resistance sets are timed so that all lifts become "explosive" in nature. Rather then using a controlled slow rep speed, you should look to complete your reps in the time allotted.

Plyometrics and power training in general is beneficial to everyone, not just power athletes. Improving strength and speed, while maybe less important for the endurance athlete focusing on cardiovascular fitness, will improve overall performance. More importantly, the athlete will feel stronger and be more secure in his or her pacing knowing that they have the burst speed and strength when needed. Be careful not to overdo it, but also make sure to push yourself hard for more profound results.

1. Fleck, SJ, and WJ Kramer. *Designing Resistance Programs,* 2nd Edition. Champaign, IL: Human Kinetics, 1997. 135–142. 1997.

Table 36.2. Training Circuit

Exercise for Beginner	Time/Reps	Rest	Modified Exercise for Moderate to Advanced
Seated Row	15s/8	10s	Bench Pull
Leg Press	15s/6	30s	Speed Squats w/ Bar
Bench Press	15s/6	15s	Bench Press
Leg Curl	15s/6	10s	Glute Ham Raise or RDL [Romanian Deadlift]
Arm Curl	15s/10	10s	Arm Curl
Calf Raise	15s/15	10s	Calf Jumps for Speed
Overhead Press	15s/6	15s	Push Press or Push Jerk
Back Extension	15s/6	15s	Straight Leg Deadlift
Triceps Press	15s/10	10s	Dips or Triceps Press

Rest for two minutes then perform this workout for two more circuits.

Chapter 37

Wii

It all really started going downhill with TV remotes. Those little handheld devices saved us the trouble of getting off the sofa to change the channel and successfully sucked yet another tiny bit of movement from our daily lives. Then came video games, which gave Americans, especially our kids, more reason to keep their rear ends firmly planted on the couch. In fact, people in this country now spend an average of 19 to 25 hours per week watching TV and playing video games.

In the fall of 2006, a new video game system called the Nintendo Wii hit the streets. It became an instant hit and is now a full-fledged craze, selling more than 11 million consoles in the Americas alone since its release. At first blush, this would seem like another sad blow to the battle between fit and fat, but thankfully the Wii is actually an exergame. That is, it's a video game that requires players to use actual physical movements to manipulate the action.

Employing a wireless handheld controller (about the size of a TV remote, ironically) with acceleration sensors and an infrared camera built into the console, the Wii senses players' motions and translates them into on-screen movement. For instance, in Wii Tennis you swing the controller like a racket; for Wii Golf, the controller is your club.

"When my brother-in-law and sister first got Wii they were saying, 'Oh we're getting a workout from it.' I thought they were just being ridiculous, but then I played it," says Karel Schmidt, a graduate

---

student in clinical exercise physiology at the University of Wisconsin, La Crosse. "There were certain games that I could tell right away I was working harder than I would've been if I was playing a normal video game."

But just how hard was she really working? That very question is what motivated Schmidt and others to study the exercise benefits of Wii for this exclusive American Council on Exercise–sponsored research.

The Study

To test the potential fitness benefits of playing Wii, a team of exercise scientists at the University of Wisconsin, La Crosse Exercise and Health Program, led by John Porcari, Ph.D., and Schmidt, recruited 16 volunteers—8 men, 8 women—all between the ages of 20 to 29 years old.

First, all volunteers were given an exercise test on a motorized treadmill to determine each subject's maximal heart rate and maximal oxygen uptake (i.e., VO2 max). Once that fitness baseline was established, the subjects were given a quick demonstration on how to use the video game system. Researchers used the standard Nintendo Wii ($250; www.nintendo.com/wii) bundled with Wii Sports, which includes baseball, boxing, bowling, golf, and tennis games. Previous Wii experience was not required as subjects were given 15 minutes of practice time for each of the five sports and allowed to continue practicing until they felt they'd mastered the skills needed to play each one successfully.

Though it's possible to manipulate the onscreen players using minimal body movement, researchers instructed the subjects to simulate the body movements used in each actual sport. "With the tennis game, I could just stand in one spot and flick my wrist and the ball will go back. You can do minimal movement, but we tried to teach the participants to mimic the real game as closely as possible," says lead researcher John Porcari, Ph.D. "We told them when you hit a forehand, swing your arm the way you would swing a racket. When you're doing a backhand, change your stance and really use your body."

Actual testing on the Wii was conducted on a subsequent day. At that time, subjects played each of the five sports in random order. Each game lasted 10 minutes and researchers recorded heart rate and VO2 at one-minute intervals. Researchers also interviewed the subjects during the final minute of each sport to determine their perceived exertion levels using the Borg rating of perceived exertion (RPE). A five-minute break was given between each game to return the subjects' heart rates to within 10 beats of their normal resting heart rate prior to beginning testing for the next game.

The Results

Data compiled from all subjects showed that playing Wii Sports increases heart rate, VO2, and perceived exertion—and thus calorie burn. Specifically, playing the golf game burns approximately 3.1 calories per minute while eliciting 50% of HR max and 20% of VO2 max. The bowling game burns slightly more at 3.9 calories per minute with 52% of HR max and 23% of VO2 max. Calorie expenditure for the baseball game was recorded at 4.5 calories per minute with 55% of HR max and 28% of VO2 max. And finally, the energy expenditure for the tennis game (at 5.3 calories per minute, 59% of HR max, and 33% of VO2 max) was significantly greater than all of the other sports except boxing, which weighed in at 7.2 calories per minute, 74% of HR max, and 44% of VO2 max.

"When you play the lower-intensity games like bowling or golf you can see that you're not really doing that much," says Schmidt, "but then when you play tennis or boxing you really do feel like you're getting a workout, like you're getting breathy. And that's exactly what we found and that's what our subjects reported to us as well."

In fact, in addition to burning the most calories, boxing was the only Wii game tested that would be considered intense enough to maintain or improve cardiorespiratory endurance as defined by the American College of Sports Medicine (ACSM). "People were increasing their oxygen consumption, or how many calories they're burning, by five or six times above their normal resting values," notes Porcari. "Even the golf game was two or three times higher than resting rates."

To compare Wii Sports to the average calorie burn of playing the actual sports, researchers turned to values described in McArdle, Katch, and Katch's *Exercise Physiology*, a standard text for caloric expenditure information. Compared to golfing at a driving range (3.9 calories per minute), playing Wii Golf burned 0.8 calories less per minute. Actual bowling burns nearly twice as much (7.2 calories per minute) as Wii Bowling, while baseball burns 7.3 calories per minute and Wii Baseball burns 2.8 calories per minute less. Similarly, Wii Tennis burns 2.8 calories per minute less than the actual game (8.1 calories per minute). Finally, Wii Boxing burns about 3.0 calories per minute less than conventional sparring at 10.2 calories per minute.

The Bottom Line

"The take-home message is that it's better than sitting around," says Porcari. "While not as good as playing the real sport, Wii certainly does burn more calories and gets your energy expenditure up compared to sitting around playing a sedentary video game."

Of course participating in the actual sports themselves provides more cardiovascular and strength benefits than Wii because you're moving your entire body and swinging things with more weight like baseball bats, tennis racquets, and golf clubs. Even so, Wii can be a suitable workout and a great option for folks who can't find the time or motivation to get out of the house and exercise. For instance, playing 30 minutes of Wii Boxing burns 216 calories, which is 51 calories more than brisk walking, while a 30-minute Wii Tennis match burns a respectable 159 calories. Some people may also find that the natural competitiveness that comes with playing Wii against an opponent can help with their motivation and, thus, their ability to stick with a regular exercise regime. The convenience of exercising in one's own living room may also improve exercise adherence.

Wii can provide some fitness benefits and help with weight management, but the key comes down to simulating the movements used in the actual sports, says Porcari. "If you want to get as good a workout as you can with Wii Sports, you really need to mimic the real movements as closely as possible."

Too often people look at regular exercise as a chore. Our hope is that new exergames like Wii will entice non-exercisers to get up off the couch and realize that fitness can, in fact, be fun.

A Wii Bit More Exercise

The latest and most fitness-oriented addition to the Wii world is Wii Fit, a game that comes with a wired balance board and leads users through 40 different exercises, including everything from aerobic workouts to strength and balance training to yoga. The balance board acts as a game controller and body-weight scale, while also measuring balance and tracking users' fitness results. It was launched after this study was already completed, but an ACE-sponsored study examining Wii Fit is already underway ($90, requires standard Wii gaming system; www.nintendo.com/wiifit).

Web Sightings

exergamelab.blogspot.com: Hosted by Stephen Yang, co-director of the Physical Activity Research Laboratory at the State University of New York–Cortland, this blog explores the latest developments in the "exergame" trend.

www.gamesforhealth.org: An arm of the nonprofit Serious Games Initiative (founded at the Woodrow Wilson Center for International Scholars in Washington, D.C.), Games for Health offers news and hosts conferences based on how exergames and other computer-based games can best impact health care and policy.

Did You Know...

The American College of Sports Medicine and the American Cancer Society recently launched a specialty certification for fitness professionals, enabling to work with patients suffering or recovering from cancer. Visit www.acsm.org/certification for more details.

Part Five

Fitness Safety

Chapter 38

The Basics of Safe Physical Activity

Although physical activity has many health benefits, injuries and other adverse events do sometimes happen. The most common injuries affect the musculoskeletal system (the bones, joints, muscles, ligaments, and tendons). Other adverse events can also occur during activity, such as overheating and dehydration. On rare occasions, people have heart attacks during activity.

The good news is that scientific evidence strongly shows that physical activity is safe for almost everyone. Moreover, the health benefits of physical activity far outweigh the risks.

Still, people may hesitate to become physically active because of concern they'll get hurt. For these people, there is even more good news: they can take steps that are proven to reduce their risk of injury and adverse events.

The guidelines in this chapter provide advice to help people do physical activity safely. Most advice applies to people of all ages. Specific guidance for particular age groups and people with certain conditions is also provided.

Physical Activity Is Safe for Almost Everyone

Most people are not likely to be injured when doing moderate-intensity activities in amounts that meet the U.S. Department of

This chapter excerpted from "Chapter 6. Safe and Active," *Physical Activity Guidelines for Americans*, U.S. Department of Health and Human Services (www.hhs.gov), October 16, 2008.

Health and Human Services *Physical Activity Guidelines*. However, injuries and other adverse events do sometimes happen. The most common problems are musculoskeletal injuries. Even so, studies show that only one such injury occurs for every 1,000 hours of walking for exercise, and fewer than four injuries occur for every 1,000 hours of running.

Both physical fitness and total amount of physical activity affect risk of musculoskeletal injuries. People who are physically fit have a lower risk of injury than people who are not. People who do more activity generally have a higher risk of injury than people who do less activity. So what should people do if they want to be active and safe? The best strategies are the following:

- Be regularly physically active to increase physical fitness.

- Follow the other guidance in this chapter (especially increasing physical activity gradually over time) to minimize the injury risk from doing medium to high amounts of activity.

Following these strategies may reduce overall injury risk. Active people are more likely to have an activity-related injury than inactive people. But they appear less likely to have non-activity-related injuries, such as work-related injuries or injuries that occur around the home or from motor vehicle crashes.

Key Guidelines for Safe Physical Activity

To do physical activity safely and reduce risk of injuries and other adverse events, people should do the following:

- Understand the risks and yet be confident that physical activity is safe for almost everyone

- Choose to do types of physical activity that are appropriate for their current fitness level and health goals, because some activities are safer than others

- Increase physical activity gradually over time whenever more activity is necessary to meet guidelines or health goals; inactive people should "start low and go slow" by gradually increasing how often and how long activities are done

- Protect themselves by using appropriate gear and sports equipment, looking for safe environments, following rules and policies, and making sensible choices about when, where, and how to be active

- Be under the care of a health care provider if they have chronic conditions or symptoms (people with chronic conditions and symptoms should consult their health care provider about the types and amounts of activity appropriate for them)

Choose Appropriate Types and Amounts of Activity

People can reduce their risk of injury by choosing appropriate types of activity. As the following table shows, the safest activities are moderate intensity and low impact and don't involve purposeful collision or contact.

Walking for exercise, gardening or yard work, bicycling or exercise cycling, dancing, swimming, and golf are activities with the lowest injury rates. In the amounts commonly done by adults, walking (a moderate-intensity and low-impact activity) has a third or less of the injury risk of running (a vigorous-intensity and higher impact activity).

The risk of injury for a type of physical activity can also differ according to the purpose of the activity. For example, recreational bicycling or bicycling for transportation leads to fewer injuries than training for and competing in bicycle races.

People who have had a past injury are at risk of injuring that body part again. The risk of injury can be reduced by performing appropriate amounts of activity and setting appropriate personal goals. Performing a variety of different physical activities may also reduce the risk of overuse injury.

Table 38.1. The Continuum of Injury Risk Associated with Different Types of Activity

Injury Risk Level (Risk Level from Lower to Higher)	Activity Type	Examples
Lowest risk	Commuting	Walking, bicycling
Lower risk	Lifestyle	Home repair, gardening/yard work
Medium risk	Recreation/sports (no contact)	Walking for exercise, golf, dancing, swimming, running, tennis
Higher risk	Recreation/sports (limited contact)	Bicycling, aerobics, skiing, volleyball, baseball, softball
Highest risk	Recreation/sports (collision/contact)	Football, hockey, soccer, basketball

Note: The same activity done for different purposes and with different frequency, intensity, and duration leads to different injury rates. Competitive activities tend to have higher injury rates than noncompetitive activities, likely due to different degrees of intensity of participation.

The risk of injury to bones, muscles, and joints is directly related to the gap between a person's usual level of activity and a new level of activity.

Increase Physical Activity Gradually over Time

Scientific studies indicate that the risk of injury to bones, muscles, and joints is directly related to the gap between a person's usual level of activity and a new level of activity. The size of this gap is called the amount of overload. Creating a small overload and waiting for the body to adapt and recover reduces the risk of injury. When amounts of physical activity need to be increased to meet the guidelines or personal goals, physical activity should be increased gradually over time, no matter what the person's current level of physical activity.

Scientists have not established a standard for how to gradually increase physical activity over time. The following recommendations give general guidance for inactive people and those with low levels of physical activity on how to increase physical activity:

- Use relative intensity (intensity of the activity relative to a person's fitness) to guide the level of effort for aerobic activity.

- Generally start with relatively moderate-intensity aerobic activity. Avoid relatively vigorous-intensity activity, such as shoveling snow or running. Adults with a low level of fitness may need to start with light activity, or a mix of light- to moderate-intensity activity.

- First, increase the number of minutes per session (duration) and the number of days per week (frequency) of moderate-intensity activity. Later, if desired, increase the intensity.

- Pay attention to the relative size of the increase in physical activity each week, as this is related to injury risk. For example, a 20-minute increase each week is safer for a person who does 200 minutes a week of walking (a 10% increase) than for a person who does 40 minutes a week (a 50% increase).

The available scientific evidence suggests that adding a small and comfortable amount of light- to moderate-intensity activity, such as 5 to 15 minutes of walking per session, two to three times a week, to one's usual activities has a low risk of musculoskeletal injury and no known risk of severe cardiac events. Because this range is rather wide, people should consider three factors in individualizing their rate of increase: age, level of fitness, and prior experience.

Age: The amount of time required to adapt to a new level of activity probably depends on age. Youth and young adults probably can safely increase activity by small amounts every week or two. Older adults appear to require more time to adapt to a new level of activity, in the range of two to four weeks.

Level of fitness: Less fit adults are at higher risk of injury when doing a given amount of activity, compared to fitter adults. Slower rates of increase over time may reduce injury risk. This guidance applies to overweight and obese adults, as they are commonly less physically fit.

Prior experience: People can use their experience to learn to increase physical activity over time in ways that minimize the risk of overuse injury. Generally, if an overuse injury occurred in the past with a certain rate of progression, a person should increase activity more slowly the next time.

Take Appropriate Precautions

Taking appropriate precautions means using the right gear and equipment, choosing safe environments in which to be active, following rules and policies, and making sensible choices about how, when, and where to be active.

Use protective gear and appropriate equipment. Using personal protective gear can reduce the frequency of injury. Personal protective gear is something worn by a person to protect a specific body part. Examples include helmets, eyewear and goggles, shin guards, elbow and knee pads, and mouth guards.

Using appropriate sports equipment can also reduce risk of injury. Sports equipment refers to sport or activity-specific tools, such as balls, bats, sticks, and shoes.

For the most benefit, protective equipment and gear should be the following:

- The right equipment for the activity
- Appropriately fitted
- Appropriately maintained
- Used consistently and correctly

Be active in safe environments. People can reduce their injury risks by paying attention to the places they choose to be active. To help themselves stay safe, people can look for the following:

- Physical separation from motor vehicles, such as sidewalks, walking paths, or bike lanes

- Neighborhoods with traffic-calming measures that slow down traffic

- Places to be active that are well-lighted, where other people are present, and that are well-maintained (no litter or broken windows)

- Shock-absorbing surfaces on playgrounds

- Well-maintained playing fields and courts without holes or obstacles

- Breakaway bases at baseball and softball fields

- Padded and anchored goals and goal posts at soccer and football fields

Follow rules and policies that promote safety. Rules, policies, legislation, and laws are potentially the most effective and wide-reaching way to reduce activity-related injuries. To get the benefit, individuals should look for and follow these rules, policies, and laws. For example, policies that promote the use of bicycle helmets reduce the risk of head injury among cyclists. Rules against diving into shallow water at swimming pools prevent head and neck injuries.

Make sensible choices about how, when, and where to be active. A person's choices can obviously influence the risk of adverse events. By making sensible choices, injuries and adverse events can be prevented. Consider weather conditions, such as extremes of heat and cold. For example, during very hot and humid weather, people lessen the chances of dehydration and heat stress by taking these precautions:

- Exercising in the cool of early morning as opposed to midday heat

- Switching to indoor activities (playing basketball in the gym rather than on the playground)

- Changing the type of activity (swimming rather than playing soccer)

- Lowering the intensity of activity (walking rather than running)

- Paying close attention to rest, shade, drinking enough fluids, and other ways to minimize effects of heat

Inactive people who gradually progress over time to relatively moderate-intensity activity have no known risk of sudden cardiac events and very low risk of bone, muscle, or joint injuries.

Exposure to air pollution is associated with several adverse health outcomes, including asthma attacks and abnormal heart rhythms. People who can modify the location or time of exercise may wish to reduce these risks by exercising away from heavy traffic and industrial sites, especially during rush hour or times when pollution is known to be high. However, current evidence indicates that the benefits of being active, even in polluted air, outweigh the risk of being inactive.

Advice from Health Care Providers

The protective value of a medical consultation for persons with or without chronic diseases who are interested in increasing their physical activity level is not established. People without diagnosed chronic conditions (such as diabetes, heart disease, or osteoarthritis) and who do not have symptoms (such as chest pain or pressure, dizziness, or joint pain) do not need to consult a health care provider about physical activity.

Inactive people who gradually progress over time to relatively moderate-intensity activity have no known risk of sudden cardiac events and very low risk of bone, muscle, or joint injuries. A person who is habitually active with moderate-intensity activity can gradually increase to vigorous intensity without needing to consult a health care provider. People who develop new symptoms when increasing their levels of activity should consult a health care provider.

The choice of appropriate types and amounts of physical activity can be affected by chronic conditions. People with symptoms or known chronic conditions should be under the regular care of a health care provider. In consultation with their provider, they can develop a physical activity plan that is appropriate for them. People with chronic conditions typically find that moderate-intensity activity is safe and beneficial. However, they may need to take special precautions. For example, people with diabetes need to pay special attention to blood sugar control and proper footwear during activity.

Chapter 39

Workout Safety

Chapter Contents

Section 39.1

Warming Up

"Exercise Right: Proper Warm-Up and Cool-Down," by Melissa Burgemeister, ATC. © 2005. Reprinted with permission of the American College of Sports Medicine, ACSM Fit Society® Page, Winter 2005, pp 4–5. Reviewed by David A. Cooke, MD, FACP, May 2010.

Adequate warm-up prior to physical activity is important to ensure a safe and effective exercise session. A simple warm-up will increase blood flow throughout the body, especially to muscles, and will begin to raise the internal body temperature. Warm muscles and tendons are less prone to injury and may improve physical performance. A proper warm-up also helps to mentally prepare for exercise. The warm-up can be divided into a simple three-step process: 1) general warm-up, 2) stretching, and 3) specific warm-up.

General Warm-Up

The warm-up routine should begin with a low-intensity exercise which slightly increases your heart rate. The general warm-up can be personalized to include equipment you may access. If your exercise is jogging, begin your warm-up with a steady walk. If you are in for a game of basketball, begin with some free throws and relaxed shooting. Remember, start slow and don't wear yourself out during the warm-up.

Stretching

Once your muscles are warm, take time to stretch. Muscles are much more flexible when they have been warmed compared to when they are cold. Focus on stretching large muscle groups such as the hamstrings and quadriceps. Specifically, stretch the muscles that you will be using to perform your activity. To maximize the benefit received from the stretch and to help improve flexibility, hold each stretch for 20 to 60 seconds. Be sure not to stretch so far that you induce pain, and maintain proper breathing during each stretch. Hamstring, calf, and quadriceps stretching is essentially for lower body activities. Pectoralis major, deltoid, and neck stretches should be included for upper-body activities.

Specific Warm-Up

The final stage of the warm-up is to do exercises specific to the activity you will be completing. If you plan to lift weights, begin with a light weight and perform a few reps before increasing the weight and repetitions. Run up and down the sidelines prior to a basketball or soccer game. The warm-up should last at least 5 to 10 minutes, although more time may be necessary if preparing for more intense exercise. If you are exercising in cold weather, take additional time to ensure that your body is adequately warmed-up. Once you are sufficiently warm and flexible, your body is ready for exercise.

Cool Down

The cool-down period following a workout is just as important as the warm-up. This time is used to reduce your heart rate and breathing rate, and to help with recovery following exercise. Performing a cool-down has been shown to decrease light-headedness and prevent pooling of the blood within the muscles, which can lead to fainting and soreness. A cool-down also allows waste products to be removed from your muscles, possibly minimizing soreness after activity.

Begin the cool-down by decreasing the intensity of the activity you were performing or by walking or jogging at a lower intensity than the exercise. Remaining active is an important component of the cool-down. The cool-down should last 5 to 10 minutes and be followed by light stretching to help relax the muscles. The stretching should focus on the muscles used during the activity. Upon completion of your exercise routine, be sure to drink plenty of water and replenish lost nutrients.

Section 39.2

Avoiding Mistakes in the Gym

"The Top 10 Mistakes People Make in the Gym,"
© American Council on Exercise. Reprinted with permission
from the American Council on Exercise (www.acefitness.org).

This survey of 3,000 ACE [American Council on Exercise]-certified
fitness professionals points out the biggest mistakes in the gym.

In some cases, these mistakes may simply mean the difference
between an effective and an ineffective workout. Other mistakes, however, can be more costly, leading to strain and injury.

ACE, America's Authority on Fitness, shares the following mistakes
commonly made in the gym and offers tips to help individuals stay
safe during their workout.

Not stretching enough: Stretch immediately following an aerobic
activity while your muscles are warm and pliable to prevent injuries.

Lifting too much weight: Never lift more than your muscles can
handle. Gradual, progressive resistance is a far more effective—and
safe—way to increase muscle strength.

Not warming up prior to activity: Muscles need time to adjust
to the new demands aerobic activity places on them. Start slowly and
gradually increase intensity.

Not cooling down after any type of workout: Take a few minutes to lower your heart rate and stretch your muscles. This improves
flexibility and helps prepare the body for your next workout.

Exercising too intensely: It's more effective to sustain a moderate workout for longer periods of time than to exercise intensely for
only a few minutes.

Not drinking enough water: Don't wait until you're thirsty to
drink water—you're already on your way to dehydration. Keep a water
bottle close at hand during exercise and throughout the day.

Leaning heavily on a stair stepper: Leaning on the stair stepper is hard on both the wrists and the back. Lower the intensity to

the point at which you can maintain good posture while lightly resting your hands on the rails for balance.

Not exercising intensely enough: Exercise intensely enough to work up a light sweat and get your heart beating in your training zone.

Jerking while lifting weights: When you have to jerk the weight, it's likely you're jerking other muscles as well. This can lead to strain and injury, with the muscles of the back being particularly vulnerable. Control the weight, don't let it control you.

Consuming energy bars and sports drinks during moderate workouts: Unless you're working out for longer than two hours per day, you don't need to supplement with high-energy bars and drinks. (High-energy is often a code word for high-calorie.)

Section 39.3

Choosing an Athletic Shoe

"Selecting Athletic Shoes," © 2008 American Orthopaedic Foot and Ankle Society (www.aofas.org). Reprinted with permission.

Proper-fitting sports shoes can enhance performance and prevent injuries. Follow these specially designed fitting facts when purchasing a new pair of athletic shoes.

- Try on athletic shoes after a workout or run and at the end of the day. Your feet will be at their largest.

- Wear the same type of sock that you will wear for that sport.

- When the shoe is on your foot, you should be able to freely wiggle all of your toes.

- The shoes should be comfortable as soon as you try them on. There is no break-in period.

- Walk or run a few steps in your shoes. They should be comfortable.

- Always relace the shoes you are trying on. You should begin at the farthest eyelets and apply even pressure as you crisscross a lacing pattern to the top of the shoe.

- There should be a firm grip of the shoe to your heel. Your heel should not slip as you walk or run.

- If you participate in a sport three or more times a week, you need a sports specific shoe.

- It can be hard to choose from the many different types of athletic shoes available. There are differences in design and variations in material and weight. These differences have been developed to protect the areas of the feet that encounter the most stress in a particular athletic activity.

Athletic shoes are grouped into seven categories:

Running, training, and walking. Includes shoes for hiking, jogging, and exercise walking. Look for a good walking shoe to have a comfortable soft upper, good shock absorption, smooth tread, and a rocker sole design that encourages the natural roll of the foot during the walking motion. The features of a good jogging shoe include cushioning, flexibility, control and stability in the heel counter area, lightness, and good traction.

Court sports. Includes shoes for tennis, basketball, and volleyball. Most court sports require the body to move forward, backward, and side-to-side. As a result, most athletic shoes used for court sports are subjected to heavy abuse. The key to finding a good court shoe is its sole. Ask a coach or shoes salesman to help you select the best type of sole for the sport you plan on participating in.

Field sports. Includes shoes for soccer, football, and baseball. These shoes are cleated, studded, or spiked. The spike and stud formations vary from sport to sport, but generally are replaceable or detachable cleats, spikes, or studs affixed into nylon soles.

Winter sports. Includes footwear for figure skating, ice hockey, alpine skiing, and cross-country skiing. The key to a good winter sports shoe is its ability to provide ample ankle support.

Track and field sport shoes. Because of the specific needs of individual runners, athletic shoe companies produce many models for various foot types, gait patterns, and training styles. It is always best to ask your coach about the type of shoe that should be selected for the event you are participating in.

Specialty sports. Includes shoes for golf, aerobic dancing, and bicycling.

Outdoor sports. Includes shoes used for recreational activities such as hunting, fishing, and boating.

Section 39.4

Helmets

"Which Helmet for Which Activity?" Consumer
Product Safety Commission (www.cpsc.gov), 2006.

Why are helmets so important?

For many recreational activities, wearing a helmet can reduce the
risk of a serious head injury and even save your life.

How can a helmet protect my head?

During a fall or collision, most of the impact energy is absorbed by
the helmet, rather than your head and brain.

Are all helmets the same?

No. There are different helmets for different activities. Each type
of helmet is made to protect your head from the impacts common to
a particular activity or sport. Be sure to wear a helmet that is appropriate for the particular activity you're involved in. (See the table in
this chapter for guidance). Other helmets may not protect your head
as effectively.

How can I tell which helmet is the right one to use?

Bicycle and motorcycle helmets must comply with mandatory federal safety standards. Many other recreational helmets are subject to
voluntary safety standards.

Helmets certified to a safety standard are designed and tested to
protect the user from serious head injury while wearing the helmet.
For example, all bicycle helmets manufactured after 1999 must meet
the U.S. Consumer Product Safety Commission (CPSC) bicycle helmet
standard. Helmets meeting this standard provide substantial head
protection when the helmet is used properly. The standard requires
that chin straps be strong enough to keep the helmet on the head and
in the proper position during a fall or collision.

Table 39.1. Matching Activities and Helmets

1. Activity	2. Helmet Type	3. Applicable Standard(s)
Individual Activities—Wheeled		
Bicycling (including low speed, motor assisted); Roller and Inline Skating—Recreational; Scooter Riding (including low speed, motor assisted)	Bicycle	CPSC, ASTM F1447, Snell B-90/95, Snell N-94†
BMX Cycling	BMX	CPSC, ASTM F2032
Downhill Mountain Bike Racing	Downhill	CPSC, ASTM F1952
Roller and Inline Skating—Aggressive/Trick; Skateboarding	Skateboard	ASTM F1492†, Snell N-94†
Individual Activities—Wheeled Large Motor		
ATV Riding; Dirt-, and Mini-Bike Riding; Motocrossing	Motocross or Motorcycle	DOT FMVSS 218, Snell M-2005
Karting/Go-Karting	Karting or Motorcycle	DOT FMVSS 218, Snell K-98, Snell M-2005
Moped Riding; Powered Scooter Riding	Moped or Motorcycle	DOT FMVSS 218, Snell L-98, Snell M-2005
Individual Activities—Non-Wheeled		
Horseback Riding	Equestrian	ASTM F1163, Snell E-2001
Rock and Wall Climbing	Mountaineering	EN 12492†, Snell N-94†

The federal CPSC Safety Standard for Bicycle Helmets is mandatory for those helmets indicated by CPSC.

† This helmet is designed to withstand more than one moderate impact, but protection is provided for only a limited number of impacts. Replace if visibly damaged (e.g., a cracked shell or crushed liner) and/or when directed by the manufacturer.

Helmets specifically marketed for exclusive use in an activity other than bicycling (for example, go-karting, horseback riding, lacrosse, and skiing) do not have to meet the requirements of the CPSC bicycle helmet standard. However, these helmets should meet other federal and/or voluntary safety standards.

Don't rely on the helmet's name or claims made on the packaging (unless the packaging specifies compliance with an appropriate standard) to determine if the helmet meets the appropriate requirements for your activity. Most helmets that meet a particular standard will contain a special label that indicates compliance (usually found on the liner inside of the helmet).

Are there helmets that I can wear for more than one activity?

Yes, but only a few. You can wear a CPSC-compliant bicycle helmet while bicycling, recreational roller or in-line skating, and riding a

Table 39.1. Matching Activities and Helmets, continued

1. Activity	2. Helmet Type	3. Applicable Standard(s)
Team Sport Activities ‡		
Baseball, Softball, and T-Ball	Baseball Batter's	NOCSAE ND022
	Baseball Catcher's	NOCSAE ND024
Football	Football	NOCSAE ND002, ASTM F717
Ice Hockey	Hockey	NOCSAE ND030, ASTM F1045
Lacrosse	Lacrosse	NOCSAE ND041
Winter Activities		
Skiing; Snowboarding	Ski	ASTM F2040, CEN 1077, Snell RS-98 or S-98
Snowmobiling	Snowmobile	DOT FMVSS 218, Snell M-2000

Although a helmet has not yet been designed for the following two activities, until such helmets exist, wearing one of the three listed types of helmets may be preferable to wearing no helmet at all.

Ice Skating; Sledding	Bicycle	CPSC, ASTM F1447, Snell B-90/95 or N-94†
	Skateboard	ASTM F1492†, Snell N-94†
	Ski	ASTM F2040, CEN 1077, Snell RS-98 or S-98

‡ Team sport helmets are designed to protect against multiple head impacts typically occurring in the sport (e.g., ball, puck, or stick impacts; player contact; etc.), and, generally, can continue to be used after such impacts. Follow manufacturer's recommendations for replacement or reconditioning.

Definitions: ASTM—ASTM International; CEN—European Committee for Standardization, DOT Dept. of Transportation; EN—Euro-norm or European Standard; NOCSAE—National Operating Committee on Standards in Athletic Equipment; Snell—Snell Memorial Foundation.

nonpowered scooter. Look at the table for other activities that may share a common helmet.

Are there any activities for which one shouldn't wear a helmet?

Yes. Make sure your child takes off his/her helmet before playing on playgrounds or climbing trees. If a child wears a helmet during these activities, the helmet's chin strap can get caught on the equipment or tree and pose a risk of strangulation. The helmet itself may present an entrapment hazard.

How can I tell if my helmet fits properly?

A helmet should be both comfortable and snug. Be sure that it is level on your head—not tilted back on the top of the head or pulled too low over your forehead. It should not move in any direction, back-to-front or side-to-side. The chin strap should be securely buckled so that the helmet doesn't move or fall off during a fall or collision.

If you buy a helmet for a child, bring the child with you so that the helmet can be tested for a good fit. Carefully examine the helmet and accompanying instructions and safety literature.

What can I do if I have trouble fitting the helmet?

You may have to apply the foam padding that comes with the helmet and/or adjust the straps. If this doesn't work, consult with the store where you bought the helmet or with the helmet manufacturer. Don't wear a helmet that doesn't fit correctly.

Will I need to replace a helmet after an impact?

That depends on the severity of the impact and whether the helmet can withstand one impact (a single-impact helmet) or more than one impact (a multiple-impact helmet). For example, bicycle helmets are designed to protect against a single severe impact, such as a bicyclist's fall onto the pavement. The foam material in the helmet will crush to absorb the impact energy during a fall or collision and can't protect you again from an additional impact. Even if there are no visible signs of damage to the helmet, you must replace it.

Other helmets are designed to protect against multiple moderate impacts. Two examples are football and ice hockey helmets. These helmets are designed to withstand multiple impacts of the type associated with the respective activities. However, you may still have to replace the helmet after one severe impact, or if it has visible signs of damage, such as a cracked shell or permanent dent in the shell or liner. Consult the manufacturer's instructions for guidance on when the helmet should be replaced.

Where can I find specific information about which helmet to use?

Refer to table 39.1. Look at the information in columns 1 to 3 of the table and follow these easy steps:

Find the activity of interest in the first column (1).

Read across the row to find the appropriate helmet type for that activity listed in the second column (2).

Once you've found the right helmet, look for a label or other marking stating that it complies with an applicable standard listed in the third column (3).

Chapter 40

Nutrition and Exercise

Chapter Contents

Section 40.1

Healthy Hydration

"American College of Sports Medicine (ACSM) Offers Guidance to Athletes on Preventing Hyponatremia and Dehydration during Upcoming Races." News release, © 2005. Reprinted with permission of the American College of Sports Medicine (www.acsm.org). Reviewed by David A. Cooke, MD, FACP, March 2010.

A new report, which appears in the June [2005] issue of *Current Sports Medicine Reports*, addresses key issues and reviews research findings on the topics of hyponatremia and dehydration for endurance athletes—a subject that has generated significant media attention this year. The published report, "ACSM Roundtable Series: Hydration and Physical Activity," is based on findings from an international panel of hydration experts who conducted an evidence-based analysis on numerous past published studies.

Based on the findings of this report as well as previously published statements, ACSM [American College of Sports Medicine] is issuing the following guidelines to the endurance community:

Work to minimize risk of both hyponatremia and dehydration. Hyponatremia is a dangerous condition that occurs when an athlete consumes too much fluid (either water or other fluids), diluting the body's sodium levels. Despite heightened media attention to this issue this year, the international ACSM panel concluded that exertional hyponatremia is relatively rare and appears to occur most often in slow-paced athletes (running events lasting longer than 4 hours or triathlons lasting longer than 9–13 hours). The incidence of symptomatic hyponatremia during endurance exercise events such as the marathon and triathlon is generally low (probably less than one in 1,000 finishers).

The panel also concluded that especially during hot-weather training, dehydration occurs more frequently and has severe consequences, increasing the risk of heat exhaustion and heat stroke during and immediately after activity. Fluid deficits in athletes can affect physical and mental performance, increase cardiovascular strain, and decrease heat tolerance.

"While hyponatremia has gotten more attention lately, far more athletes are affected by dehydration," said W. Larry Kenney, PhD, FACSM, past president of ACSM and co-chair of the ACSM roundtable. "However, there are dangers associated with both extremes of behavior—severe under-drinking and severe over-drinking. Not drinking at all is not a safe option for preventing hyponatremia. The key is 'drinking intelligently, not drinking maximally,'" he added.

Drink to match fluid loss and on a schedule. The experts concluded that appropriate fluid intake (before, during, and after exercise) is important to help regulate body temperature and replace fluids lost in sweat. Since fluid and electrolyte needs are widely variable based on the athlete's genetics and environmental conditions, athletes should know their bodies' hourly sweat rate (weight lost during exercise per hour + fluid consumed during exercise per hour = hourly sweat rate) and aim to replace the total amount lost during that time.

According to the previously published "ACSM Exercise and Fluid Replacement Position Stand," athletes are encouraged to drink early and at regular intervals rather than rapid fluid replacement. It is noted that perception of thirst, an imperfect index of the magnitude of fluid deficit, cannot be used to provide complete restoration of water lost by sweating. As such, individuals participating in prolonged intense exercise must rely on strategies such as monitoring body weight loss and ingesting volumes of fluid during exercise at a rate equal to that lost from sweating to ensure complete fluid replacement. Drinking over a set period of time is more effective for complete rehydration as rapid replacement of fluid stimulates increased urine production, reducing body water retention. If athletes are not sweating heavily (such as slow runners) and are not thirsty then their fluid replacement needs are probably modest.

Consume salty foods and beverages. According to the published roundtable report, research shows foods and beverages with sodium help promote fluid retention and stimulate fluid intake. The report also notes that athletes performing prolonged exercise should ingest snacks or fluids containing sodium to help offset the loss of salt in sweat in an effort to prevent hyponatremia.

Section 40.2

Sports Nutrition

"Fast Facts about Sports Nutrition," President's Council on
Physical Fitness and Sports (www.fitness.gov), April 23, 2008.
Reviewed by David A. Cooke, MD, FACP, March 2010.

Water, Water Everywhere

- You can survive for a month without food, but only a few days without water.

- Water is the most important nutrient for active people.

- When you sweat, you lose water, which must be replaced. Drink fluids before, during, and after workouts.

- Water is a fine choice for most workouts. However; during continuous workouts of greater than 90 minutes, your body may benefit from a sports drink.

- Sports drinks have two very important ingredients—electrolytes and carbohydrates.

- Sports drinks replace electrolytes lost through sweat during workouts lasting several hours.

- Carbohydrates in sports drinks provide extra energy. The most effective sports drinks contain 15 to 18 grams of carbohydrate in every eight ounces of fluid.

Rev up Your Engine with Carbohydrates

- Carbohydrates are your body's main source of energy.

- Carbohydrates are sugars and starches, and they are found in foods such as breads, cereals, fruits, vegetables, pasta, milk, honey, syrups, and table sugar.

- Sugars and starches are broken down by your body into glucose, which is used by your muscles for energy.

- For health and peak performance, more than half your daily calories should come from carbohydrates.

- Sugars and starches have four calories per gram, while fat has nine calories per gram. In other words, carbohydrates have less than half the calories of fat.

- If you regularly eat a carbohydrate-rich diet you probably have enough carbohydrate stored to fuel activity. Even so, be sure to eat a precompetition meal for fluid and additional energy. What you eat as well as when you eat your precompetition meal will be entirely individual.

Flexing Your Options to Build Bigger Muscles

- It is a myth that eating lots of protein and/or taking protein supplements and exercising vigorously will definitely turn you into a big, muscular person.

- Building muscle depends on your genes, how hard you train, and whether you get enough calories.

- The average American diet has more than enough protein for muscle building. Extra protein is eliminated from the body or stored as fat.

Score with Vitamins and Minerals

- Eating a varied diet will give you all the vitamins and minerals you need for health and peak performance.

- Exceptions include active people who follow strict vegetarian diets, avoid an entire group of foods, or eat less than 1,800 calories a day. If you fall into any of these categories, a multivitamin and mineral pill may provide the vitamins and minerals missing in your diet.

- Taking large doses of vitamins and minerals will not help your performance and may be bad for your health. Vitamins and minerals do not supply the body with energy and, therefore, are not a substitute for carbohydrates.

Popeye and All That Spinach

- Iron supplies working muscles with oxygen.

- If your iron level is low, you may tire easily and not have enough stamina for activity.

- The best sources of iron are animal products, but plant foods such as fortified breads, cereals, beans, and green leafy vegetables also contain iron.

- Iron supplements may have side effects, so take them only if your doctor tells you to.

No Bones about It, You Need Calcium Every Day

- Many people do not get enough of the calcium needed for strong bones and proper muscle function.

- Lack of calcium can contribute to stress fractures and the bone disease osteoporosis.

- The best sources of calcium are dairy products, but many other foods such as salmon with bones, sardines, collard greens, and okra also contain calcium. Additionally, some brands of bread, tofu, and orange juice are fortified with calcium.

A Weighty Matter

- Your calorie needs depend on your age, body size, sport, and training program.

- The best way to make sure you are not getting too many or too few calories is to check your weight from time to time.

- If you're keeping within your ideal weight range, you're probably getting the right amount of calories.

Section 40.3

Top Sports Nutrition Myths

The field of sports nutrition is filled with myths that people follow blindly. This section looks at the top sports nutrition myths, and what science has to say about them.

Myth: The more protein I eat, the better.

Truth: While protein is necessary to support increased protein oxidation during endurance training as well as muscle growth for athletes participating in strength training activities, there is insufficient evidence to support the notion that "the more I exercise, the more protein I need." Athletes should consume between 1.2–1.8 grams per kg of body weight or 10–35% of total calories.[4,7,8]

Myth: It is not possible to drink too much water.

Truth: Headache, vomiting, swollen hands and feet, confusion, edema, respiratory arrest, and even death can occur in athletes who drink too much water.[7] Hyponatremia, low sodium in the blood stream, is more likely to occur in smaller, less lean individuals who run slowly, sweat less, and drink water (as opposed to fluids with electrolytes) before, during, and after exercise.[7] Weigh yourself before and after a "typical" exercise session to make sure you have not put on weight (which is a sign that you're drinking too much).

Myth: An eight-ounce serving is the right amount of fluid to drink.

Truth: There is a large range in sweat rates and total sweat losses of individuals between and within activities making individual recommendations difficult.[7] Individuals should strive to consume between 72 ounces and 100 ounces for men, and let thirst be their guide according to the Institute of Medicine's recent report on Dietary Reference Intakes.[5]

Myth: All athletes need supplements.

Truth: According to the joint ACSM/ADA [American Dietetic Association] position statement "...no vitamin and mineral supplements are required if an athlete is consuming adequate energy from a variety of foods to maintain body weight." Athletes who are consuming too few calories (such as in dieting), ill, recovering from injury, or with a specific medical/nutritional reason to supplement may benefit from a single supplement to correct that specific condition.[6] Always remember, food first, supplement if needed. Speak to an MD or RD about your specific situation.

Myth: Vitamin C will prevent me from getting sick during my training season.

Truth: While vitamin C has been shown to lessen the symptoms and severity of a cold, research to date does not show that vitamin C supplements help individuals ward off colds.[3] The best method to avoid getting sick is regular hand washing and a healthy diet. Vitamin C does play a role in respiratory defense mechanisms, so taking in additional vitamin C when you first feel a cold coming on may help.

Myth: Diluting sport drinks is a good idea to reduce my calorie intake.

Truth: Sport drinks are designed to provide a 6–8% carbohydrate solution and a reference amount of electrolytes to replace both fluids and electrolytes for athletes who lose these through sweat. For exercises lasting 60 minutes or longer, taking in a sport drink, without diluting it, is appropriate for optimal hydration.[6]

Myth: If I'm thin, I don't need to worry about what I eat.

Truth: Low energy intake compromises performance and negates the benefits of training. With a hypocaloric diet, fat and lean tissue will be used for fuel by the body leading to loss of strength and endurance, as well as compromised immune, endocrine, and musculoskeletal function. A poor nutrient intake may also result in metabolic dysfunctions associated with nutrient deficiencies as well as a lowered resting metabolic rate (RMR).[6]

Myth: I need to watch my weight because my BMI [body mass index] is too high.

Truth: Trained athletes typically have more skeletal muscle and less body fat than sedentary individuals. Therefore, BMI is not an appropriate disease risk screening tool for athletes.[2] The Centers for Disease Control and Prevention (CDC) recommends that athletes use methods other than BMI to assess body composition.[1] Waist circumference is a good indicator of risk, as abdominal fat is a strong predictor of obesity-related diseases.[1] The CDC also recommends using bioelectric impedance (BIA), underwater weighing, or dual-energy X-ray absorptiometry (DXA) to determine body fat percentage.[1]

Myth: Eliminating carbs will help me lose weight.

Truth: While taking in fewer calories than your body requires (through a decrease in any macronutrient—carbs, protein, or fats) will lead to weight loss, eliminating (or severely restricting) carbohydrates can lead to fatigue and poor performance as carbohydrates fuel your working muscles (even during high intensity activities such as strength training).[4,8] According to the Institute of Medicine, individuals should consume between 45–65% of total calories from carbohydrates,[4,8] with athletes requiring the higher end of that recommendation.[6]

The bottom line is do not believe everything you hear. Always consider the source and check to make sure your information comes from credible sources such as nationally recognized medical and research organizations.

References

1. Centers for Disease Control and Prevention. BMI for Adults. Retrieved July 21, 2008, from www.cdc.gov/nccdphp/dnpa/bmi/adult_BMI/ about_adult_BMI.htm, n.d.

2. Dunford, M, and Doyle J. Nutrition for Sport and Exercise. Belmont, CA: Thomson Wadsworth. 2008.

3. Hemilä H, Chalker E, Treacy B, Douglas B. Vitamin C for preventing and treating the common cold. Cochrane Database of Systematic Reviews. 2007.

4. Institute Of Medicine. Dietary Reference Intakes for Energy, Carbohydrate, Fiber, Fat, Fatty Acids, Cholesterol, Protein, and Amino Acids (Macronutrients), Sodium, Chloride, Potassium, and Sulfate, Washington, D.C: National Academy Press, 2005.

5. Institute of Medicine. Dietary Reference Intakes for Water, Sodium, Chloride, Potassium, and Sulfate, Washington, D.C: National Academy Press, 2005.

6. Rodriguez NR, Di Marco NM, and Langley S. American Dietetic Association; Dietitians of Canada; American College of Sports Medicine position stand. Nutrition and athletic performance. *Med Sci Sports Exerc.* Mar;41(3):709–31. 2009.

7. Sawka MN, Burke LM, Eichner ER, Maughan RJ, Montain SJ, Stachenfeld NS. Exercise and Fluid Replacement. *Medicine and Science in Sports and Exercise*, 39(2):377–390, 2007.

8. Zello, G. Dietary Reference Intakes for the macronutrients and energy: considerations for physical activity. *Appl Physiol Nutr Metab,* 31 (1): 74–9, 2006.

Chapter 41

Preventing Sports Injuries

Chapter Contents

Section 41.1

Common Sports Injuries and Their Prevention

"Sports Injuries," National Institute of Arthritis and
Musculoskeletal and Skin Diases (www.niams.nih.gov), April 2009.

What Are Sports Injuries?

The term sports injury, in the broadest sense, refers to the kinds
of injuries that most commonly occur during sports or exercise. Some
sports injuries result from accidents; others are due to poor training
practices, improper equipment, lack of conditioning, or insufficient
warm-up and stretching.

Although virtually any part of your body can be injured during
sports or exercise, the term is usually reserved for injuries that involve
the musculoskeletal system, which includes the muscles, bones, and
associated tissues like cartilage. Following are some of the most common sports injuries.

Sprains and Strains

A sprain is a stretch or tear of a ligament, the band of connective tissues that joins the end of one bone with another. Sprains are
caused by trauma such as a fall or blow to the body that knocks a
joint out of position and, in the worst case, ruptures the supporting
ligaments. Sprains can range from first degree (minimally stretched
ligament) to third degree (a complete tear). Areas of the body most
vulnerable to sprains are ankles, knees, and wrists. Signs of a sprain
include varying degrees of tenderness or pain; bruising; inflammation; swelling; inability to move a limb or joint; or joint looseness,
laxity, or instability.

A strain is a twist, pull, or tear of a muscle or tendon, a cord of tissue connecting muscle to bone. It is an acute, noncontact injury that
results from overstretching or overcontraction. Symptoms of a strain
include pain, muscle spasm, and loss of strength. Although it's hard to
tell the difference between mild and moderate strains, severe strains
not treated professionally can cause damage and loss of function.

Knee Injuries

Because of its complex structure and weight-bearing capacity, the knee is the most commonly injured joint. Each year, more than 5.5 million people visit doctors for knee problems.

Knee injuries can range from mild to severe. Some of the less severe, yet still painful and functionally limiting, knee problems are runner's knee (pain or tenderness close to or under the knee cap at the front or side of the knee), iliotibial band syndrome (pain on the outer side of the knee), and tendinitis, also called tendinosis (marked by degeneration within a tendon, usually where it joins the bone).

More severe injuries include bone bruises or damage to the cartilage or ligaments. There are two types of cartilage in the knee. One is the meniscus, a crescent-shaped disc that absorbs shock between the thigh (femur) and lower leg bones (tibia and fibula). The other is a surface-coating (or articular) cartilage. It covers the ends of the bones where they meet, allowing them to glide against one another. The four major ligaments that support the knee are the anterior cruciate ligament (ACL), the posterior cruciate ligament (PCL), the medial collateral ligament (MCL), and the lateral collateral ligament (LCL).

Knee injuries can result from a blow to or twist of the knee; from improper landing after a jump; or from running too hard, too much, or without proper warm-up.

Compartment Syndrome

In many parts of the body, muscles (along with the nerves and blood vessels that run alongside and through them) are enclosed in a "compartment" formed of a tough membrane called fascia. When muscles become swollen, they can fill the compartment to capacity, causing interference with nerves and blood vessels as well as damage to the muscles themselves. The resulting painful condition is referred to as compartment syndrome.

Compartment syndrome may be caused by a one-time traumatic injury (acute compartment syndrome), such as a fractured bone or a hard blow to the thigh, by repeated hard blows (depending upon the sport), or by ongoing overuse (chronic exertional compartment syndrome), which may occur, for example, in long-distance running.

Shin Splints

Although the term "shin splints" has been widely used to describe any sort of leg pain associated with exercise, the term actually refers to pain along the tibia or shin bone, the large bone in the front of the lower leg. This pain can occur at the front outside part of the lower leg, including the foot and ankle (anterior shin splints), or at the inner edge of the bone where it meets the calf muscles (medial shin splints).

Shin splints are primarily seen in runners, particularly those just starting a running program. Risk factors for shin splints include overuse or incorrect use of the lower leg; improper stretching, warm-up, or exercise technique; overtraining; running or jumping on hard surfaces; and running in shoes that don't have enough support. These injuries are often associated with flat (overpronated) feet.

Achilles Tendon Injuries

An Achilles tendon injury results from a stretch, tear, or irritation to the tendon connecting the calf muscle to the back of the heel. These injuries can be so sudden and agonizing that they have been known to bring down charging professional football players in shocking fashion.

The most common cause of Achilles tendon tears is a problem called tendinitis, a degenerative condition caused by aging or overuse. When a tendon is weakened, trauma can cause it to rupture.

Achilles tendon injuries are common in middle-aged "weekend warriors" who may not exercise regularly or take time to stretch properly before an activity. Among professional athletes, most Achilles injuries seem to occur in quick-acceleration, jumping sports like football and basketball, and almost always end the season's competition for the athlete.

Fractures

A fracture is a break in the bone that can occur from either a quick, one-time injury to the bone (acute fracture) or from repeated stress to the bone over time (stress fracture).

Acute fractures: Acute fractures can be simple (a clean break with little damage to the surrounding tissue) or compound (a break in which the bone pierces the skin with little damage to the surrounding tissue). Most acute fractures are emergencies. One that breaks the skin is especially dangerous because there is a high risk of infection.

Stress fractures: Stress fractures occur largely in the feet and legs and are common in sports that require repetitive impact, primarily running/jumping sports such as gymnastics or track and field. Running creates forces two to three times a person's body weight on the lower limbs.

The most common symptom of a stress fracture is pain at the site that worsens with weight-bearing activity. Tenderness and swelling often accompany the pain.

Dislocations

When the two bones that come together to form a joint become separated, the joint is described as being dislocated. Contact sports such as football and basketball, as well as high-impact sports and sports that can result in excessive stretching or falling, cause the majority of dislocations. A dislocated joint is an emergency situation that requires medical treatment.

The joints most likely to be dislocated are some of the hand joints. Aside from these joints, the joint most frequently dislocated is the shoulder. Dislocations of the knees, hips, and elbows are uncommon.

What's the Difference Between Acute and Chronic Injuries?

Regardless of the specific structure affected, sports injuries can generally be classified in one of two ways: acute or chronic.

Acute Injuries

Acute injuries, such as a sprained ankle, strained back, or fractured hand, occur suddenly during activity. Signs of an acute injury include the following:

- Sudden, severe pain
- Swelling
- Inability to place weight on a lower limb
- Extreme tenderness in an upper limb
- Inability to move a joint through its full range of motion
- Extreme limb weakness
- Visible dislocation or break of a bone

Chronic Injuries

Chronic injuries usually result from overusing one area of the body while playing a sport or exercising over a long period. The following are signs of a chronic injury:

- Pain when performing an activity
- A dull ache when at rest
- Swelling

What Should I Do if I Suffer an Injury?

Whether an injury is acute or chronic, there is never a good reason to try to "work through" the pain of an injury. When you have pain from a particular movement or activity, *stop!* Continuing the activity only causes further harm.

Some injuries require prompt medical attention, while others can be self-treated. Here's what you need to know about both types:

When to Seek Medical Treatment

You should call a health professional if you have the following symptoms:

- The injury causes severe pain, swelling, or numbness.
- You can't tolerate any weight on the area.
- The pain or dull ache of an old injury is accompanied by increased swelling or joint abnormality or instability.

When and How to Treat at Home

If you don't have any of these symptoms, it's probably safe to treat the injury at home—at least at first. If pain or other symptoms worsen, it's best to check with your health care provider. Use the RICE method to relieve pain and inflammation and speed healing. Follow these four steps immediately after injury and continue for at least 48 hours.

- **Rest:** Reduce regular exercise or activities of daily living as needed. If you cannot put weight on an ankle or knee, crutches may help. If you use a cane or one crutch for an ankle injury, use it on the uninjured side to help you lean away and relieve weight on the injured ankle.

- **Ice:** Apply an ice pack to the injured area for 20 minutes at a time, four to eight times a day. A cold pack, ice bag, or plastic bag filled with crushed ice and wrapped in a towel can be used. To avoid cold injury and frostbite, do not apply the ice for more than 20 minutes. (Note: Do not use heat immediately after an injury. This tends to increase internal bleeding or swelling. Heat can be used later on to relieve muscle tension and promote relaxation.)

- **Compression:** Compression of the injured area may help reduce swelling. Compression can be achieved with elastic wraps, special boots, air casts, and splints. Ask your health care provider for advice on which one to use.

- **Elevation:** If possible, keep the injured ankle, knee, elbow, or wrist elevated on a pillow, above the level of the heart, to help decrease swelling.

Who Should I See for My Injury?

Although severe injuries will need to be seen immediately in an emergency room, particularly if they occur on the weekend or after office hours, most sports injuries can be evaluated and, in many cases, treated by your primary health care provider.

Depending on your preference and the severity of your injury or the likelihood that your injury may cause ongoing, long-term problems, you may want to see, or have your primary health care professional refer you to, one of the following:

- **Orthopedic surgeon:** A doctor specializing in the diagnosis and treatment of the musculoskeletal system, which includes bones, joints, ligaments, tendons, muscles, and nerves.

- **Physical therapist/physiotherapist:** A health care professional who can develop a rehabilitation program. Your primary care physician may refer you to a physical therapist after you begin to recover from your injury to help strengthen muscles and joints and prevent further injury.

How Are Sports Injuries Treated?

Although using the RICE technique described previously can be helpful for any sports injury, RICE is often just a starting point. Here are some other treatments your doctor or other health care provider may administer, recommend, or prescribe to help your injury heal.

Nonsteroidal Anti-Inflammatory Drugs (NSAIDs)

The moment you are injured, chemicals are released from damaged tissue cells. This triggers the first stage of healing: inflammation. Inflammation causes tissues to become swollen, tender, and painful. Although inflammation is needed for healing, it can actually slow the healing process if left unchecked.

463

To reduce inflammation and pain, doctors and other health care providers often recommend taking an over-the-counter (OTC) NSAID such as aspirin, ibuprofen (Advil,[1] Motrin IB, Nuprin), ketoprofen (Actron, Orudis KT), or naproxen sodium (Aleve). For more severe pain and inflammation, doctors may prescribe one of several dozen NSAIDs available in prescription strength.[2]

Though not an NSAID, another commonly used OTC medication, acetaminophen (Tylenol), may relieve pain. It has no effect on inflammation, however.

Immobilization

Immobilization is a common treatment for sports injuries that may be done immediately by a trainer or paramedic. Immobilization involves reducing movement in the area to prevent further damage. By enabling the blood supply to flow more directly to the injury (or the site of surgery to repair damage from an injury), immobilization reduces pain, swelling, and muscle spasm and helps the healing process begin. Following are some devices used for immobilization:

- **Slings**, to immobilize the upper body, including the arms and shoulders.

- **Splints and casts**, to support and protect injured bones and soft tissue. Casts can be made from plaster or fiberglass. Splints can be custom made or ready made. Standard splints come in a variety of shapes and sizes and have Velcro straps that make them easy to put on and take off or adjust. Splints generally offer less support and protection than a cast and, therefore, may not always be a treatment option.

- **Leg immobilizers**, to keep the knee from bending after injury or surgery. Made from foam rubber covered with fabric, leg immobilizers enclose the entire leg, fastening with Velcro straps.

Surgery

In some cases, surgery is needed to repair torn connective tissues or to realign bones with compound fractures. The vast majority of sports injuries, however, do not require surgery.

Rehabilitation (Exercise)

A key part of rehabilitation from sports injuries is a graduated exercise program designed to return the injured body part to a normal level of function.

With most injuries, early mobilization—getting the part moving as soon as possible—will speed healing. Generally, early mobilization starts with gentle range-of-motion exercises and then moves on to stretching and strengthening exercise when you can without increasing pain. For example, if you have a sprained ankle, you may be able to work on range of motion for the first day or two after the sprain by gently tracing letters with your big toe. Once your range of motion is fairly good, you can start doing gentle stretching and strengthening exercises. When you are ready, weights may be added to your exercise routine to further strengthen the injured area. The key is to avoid movement that causes pain.

As damaged tissue heals, scar tissue forms, which shrinks and brings torn or separated tissues back together. As a result, the injury site becomes tight or stiff, and damaged tissues are at risk of reinjury. That's why stretching and strengthening exercises are so important. You should continue to stretch the muscles daily and as the first part of your warm-up before exercising.

When planning your rehabilitation program with a health care professional, remember that progression is the key principle. Start with just a few exercises, do them often, and then gradually increase how much you do. A complete rehabilitation program should include exercises for flexibility, endurance, and strength; instruction in balance and proper body mechanics related to the sport; and a planned return to full participation.

Throughout the rehabilitation process, avoid painful activities and concentrate on those exercises that will improve function in the injured part. Don't resume your sport until you are sure you can stretch the injured tissues without any pain, swelling, or restricted movement, and monitor any other symptoms. When you do return to your sport, start slowly and gradually build up to full participation.

Rest

Although it is important to get moving as soon as possible, you must also take time to rest following an injury. All injuries need time to heal; proper rest will help the process. Your health care professional can guide you regarding the proper balance between rest and rehabilitation.

1. Brand names included in this booklet are provided as examples only, and their inclusion does not mean that these products are endorsed by the National Institutes of Health or any other government agency. Also, if a particular brand name is not mentioned, this does not mean or imply that the product is unsatisfactory.

465

2. Like all medications, NSAIDs can have side effects. The list of possible adverse effects is long, but major problems are few. The intestinal tract heads the list with nausea, abdominal pain, vomiting, and diarrhea. Changes in liver function frequently occur in children (but not in adults) who use aspirin. Changes in liver function are rare in children using the other NSAIDs. Questions about the appropriate use of NSAIDs should be directed toward your health care provider or pharmacist.

Section 41.2

Sports-Related Concussions: What You Need to Know to Be Safe

"Sport-Related Concussions" by Tracey Covassin, PhD, ATC, and Robert Elbin, MA. © 2009. Reprinted with permission of the American College of Sports Medicine, ACSM Fit Society ® Page, Summer 2009, p 4–5.

Sport-related concussions continue to be a serious public health concern, as approximately 1.6 to 3 million concussions occur annually in the United States. Recent studies have shown increases in the prevalence and incidence of concussion in both high school and college athletes. Approximately 8.9% of all high school athletic injuries are concussions, while incidence rates for college athletes range from 5 to 7.9%. This section will provide a general overview of the signs, symptoms, management, and treatment of sport-related concussion.

Definition of a Concussion

A concussion occurs when an athlete's skull contacts another object (i.e., an opponent, the ball, or the ground) or comes to an abrupt halt (as in whiplash), causing the brain to rebound off of, or twist up against, the inside of the skull. These shearing forces can damage blood vessels that cause swelling and bleeding in the brain. Neurons can also be damaged, which impairs the brain's ability to transmit important information from one area of the brain to another. This damage causes the concussed athlete to experience a wide variety of symptoms and cognitive difficulties.

Signs and Symptoms of a Concussion

A concussed athlete may present a wide variety of symptoms and impairments (see table). A common misconception regarding concussive injury is that an athlete must experience loss of consciousness in order for a concussion to be diagnosed. However, several studies suggest that fewer than 10% of athletes who sustain a concussion actually experience loss of consciousness, whereas headache, dizziness, confusion, and disorientation are reported more often by concussed athletes.

Table 41.1. Signs and Symptoms of Concussion

Amnesia	Confusion
Headache	Decreased appetite
Loss of consciousness	Tinnitus
Nausea	Slurred speech
Poor attention	Double vision
Dizziness	Fatigue
Irritability	Anxiety/depression
Intolerance to loud noise	Sleep disturbances
Intolerance to bright light	Emotional disturbances

How to Prevent a Concussion

Unfortunately, there is no surefire way to prevent a concussion from occurring; however, steps can be taken to reduce the chances of sustaining this injury. First, athletic equipment should meet recommended standards for safety. All helmets should be thoroughly inspected, re-conditioned, or replaced every year to ensure they meet safety standards set by the National Operating Committee for Safety in Athletic Equipment.

Second, athletes need to be taught proper tackling and heading techniques used in sports such as football and soccer, as both these sports have high incidence of concussion. Football players must be taught the dangers of the "spear" tackle (i.e., using the helmet as a battering ram). The National Athletic Trainers' Association recommends football coaches mandate two educational sessions each year (e.g., preseason and midseason) for proper tackling techniques. Soccer players should make sure they use proper form to head a soccer ball as improper heading may increase the chances of sustaining a concussion.

Third, athletes, coaches, and parents need to be educated on the signs and symptoms of concussion. Sports medicine professionals often rely on athletes to tell them if they are experiencing concussion symptoms. However, many athletes do not know the signs and symptoms of concussion, which cause many concussions to go undetected. Athletes who continue to play while concussed are at risk for more catastrophic injury (e.g., second-impact syndrome) if they sustain another concussion before recovering from the first one. This second injury can lead to persisting symptoms that can last for months, and can even be fatal in rare cases. Therefore, coaches, athletes, and parents should not underestimate the seriousness of concussion, as athletes may often feel pressured to return to play prematurely.

Concussion Management

The initial management of concussion begins by addressing the ABCs (airway, breathing, circulation) of life support. If the athlete is unconscious, one must assume a neck or spine injury until proven otherwise. When a spinal injury has been ruled out, the extent of symptoms such as head and neck pain, dizziness, confusion, and amnesia must be determined. If the athlete has any signs and symptoms of a concussion, he or she should not return to play and should be referred to a physician. If you are not sure if an athlete has suffered a concussion, follow this motto: "When in doubt, sit them out!"

Concussion Treatment

Concussed athletes should also be regularly monitored for any signs of deterioration and receive a full medical evaluation following injury. The recommended return-to-play process includes:

1. no activity, complete rest;
2. light aerobic exercise such as walking or stationary cycling, no resistance training;
3. sport-specific exercise and progressive addition of resistance training;
4. non-contact training drills;
5. full-contact training after medical clearance;
6. game play.

If concussion symptoms reappear, the athlete should revert back to the previous asymptomatic stage and resume the progression after 24 hours. These guidelines allow for a more individualized approach when returning an athlete back to competition from concussion.

Conclusion

In summary, each sport-related concussion should be treated individually. Concussions can be a serious injury if mismanaged, but with proper education and precautionary measures, concussed athletes can experience a full recovery and return to participation.

Chapter 42

Preventing Sports Injuries for Child Athletes

Causes of Sports Injuries

Participation in any sport, whether it's recreational bike riding or Pee-Wee football, can teach kids to stretch their limits and learn sportsmanship and discipline. But any sport also carries the potential for injury.

By knowing the causes of sports injuries and how to prevent them, you can help make athletics a positive experience for your child.

Kids can be particularly susceptible to sports injuries for a variety of reasons. Kids, particularly those younger than eight years old, are less coordinated and have slower reaction times than adults because they are still growing and developing.

In addition, kids mature at different rates. Often there's a substantial difference in height and weight between kids of the same age. And when kids of varying sizes play sports together, there may be an increased risk of injury.

As kids grow bigger and stronger, the potential for injury increases, largely because of the amount of force involved. For example, a collision between two 8-year-old Pee-Wee football players who weigh 65 or 70 pounds each does not produce as much force as that produced by two 16-year-old high school football players who may each weigh up to 200 pounds.

Also, kids may not assess the risks of certain activities as fully as adults might. So they might unknowingly take risks that can result in injuries.

Preventing Sports Injuries

You can help prevent your child from being injured by following some simple guidelines:

Use of Proper Equipment

It's important for kids to use proper equipment and safety gear that is the correct size and fits well. For example, kids should wear helmets for baseball, softball, bicycle riding, and hockey. They also should wear helmets while they're inline skating or riding scooters and skateboards.

For racquet sports and basketball, ask about any protective eyewear, like shatterproof goggles. Ask your child's coach about the appropriate helmets, shoes, mouth guards, athletic cups and supporters, and padding.

Protective equipment should be approved by the organizations that govern each of the sports. Hockey facemasks, for example, should be approved by the Hockey Equipment Certification Council (HECC) or the Canadian Standards Association (CSA). Bicycle helmets should have a safety certification sticker from the Consumer Product Safety Commission (CPSC).

Also, all equipment should be properly maintained to ensure its effectiveness. In the United States, the National Operating Committee on Standards for Athletic Equipment (NOCSAE) sets many of the standards for helmets, facemasks, and shin guards. In addition to meeting the NOCSAE standards, all equipment should be properly maintained to ensure its effectiveness over time.

Maintenance and Appropriateness of Playing Surfaces

Check that playing fields are not full of holes and ruts that might cause kids to fall or trip. Kids doing high-impact sports, like basketball and running, should do them on surfaces like tracks and wooden basketball courts, which can be more forgiving than surfaces like concrete.

Adequate Adult Supervision and Commitment to Safety

Any team sport or activity that kids participate in should be supervised by qualified adults. Select leagues and teams that have the same commitment to safety and injury prevention that you do.

The team coach should have training in first aid and CPR, and the coach's philosophy should promote players' well-being. A coach with a win-at-all-costs attitude may encourage kids to play through injury and may not foster good sportsmanship. Be sure that the coach enforces playing rules and requires that safety equipment be used at all times.

Additionally, make sure your kids are matched for sports according to their skill level, size, and physical and emotional maturity.

Proper Preparation

Just as you wouldn't send a child who can't swim to a swimming pool, it's important not to send kids to play a sport that they're unprepared to play. Make sure that your child knows how to play the sport before going out on the field.

Your child should be adequately prepared with warm-ups and training sessions before practices as well as before games. This will help ensure that your child has fun and reduce the chances of an injury.

In addition, your child should drink plenty of fluids and be allowed to rest during practices and games.

Common Types of Sports Injuries

Three common types of sports injuries in children are acute injuries, overuse injuries, and reinjuries:

Acute Injuries

Acute injuries occur suddenly and are usually associated with some form of trauma. In younger children, acute injuries typically include minor bruises, sprains, and strains. Teen athletes are more likely to sustain more severe injuries, including broken bones and torn ligaments.

More severe acute injuries that can occur, regardless of age, include: eye injuries, including scratched corneas, detached retinas, and blood in the eye; broken bones or ligament injuries; brain injuries, including concussions, skull fractures, brain hemorrhages; and spinal cord injuries.

Acute injuries often occur because of a lack of proper equipment or the use of improper equipment. For example, without protective eyewear, eye injuries are extremely common in basketball and racquet sports. In addition, many kids playing baseball and softball have suffered broken legs or ankles from sliding into immobile bases.

473

Overuse Injuries

Overuse injuries occur from repetitive actions that put too much stress on the bones and muscles. Although these injuries can occur in adults as well as kids, they're more problematic in a child athlete because of the effect they may have on bone growth.

All kids who play sports can develop an overuse injury, but the likelihood increases with the amount of time a child spends on the sport.

Some of the most common types of overuse injuries are:

- **Anterior knee pain:** Anterior knee pain is pain in the front of the knee under the kneecap. The knee will be sore and swollen due to tendon or cartilage inflammation. The cause is usually muscle tightness in the hamstrings or quadriceps, the major muscle groups around the thigh.

- **Little League elbow:** Repetitive throwing sometimes results in pain and tenderness in the elbow. The ability to flex and extend the arm may be affected, but the pain typically occurs after the follow-through of the throw. In addition to pain, pitchers sometimes complain of loss of velocity or decreased endurance.

- **Swimmer's shoulder:** Swimmer's shoulder is an inflammation (swelling) of the shoulder caused by the repeated stress of the overhead motion associated with swimming or throwing a ball. The pain typically begins intermittently but may progress to continuous pain in the back of the shoulder.

- **Shin splints:** Shin splints are characterized by pain and discomfort on the front of the lower parts of the legs. They are often caused by repeated running on a hard surface or overtraining at the beginning of a season.

- **Spondylolysis:** Spondylolysis often results from trauma or from repetitive flexing, then overextension, twisting, or compression of the back muscles. This can cause persistent lower back pain. Spondylolysis is commonly seen in kids who participate in soccer, football, weight lifting, gymnastics, wrestling, and diving.

Overuse injuries can be caused or aggravated by:

- growth spurts or an imbalance between strength and flexibility;

- inadequate warm-up;

- excessive activity (for example, increased intensity, duration, or frequency of playing and/or training);

- playing the same sport year-round or multiple sports during the same season;

- improper technique (for example, overextending on a pitch);

- unsuitable equipment (for example, nonsupportive athletic shoes).

Reinjuries

Reinjury occurs when an athlete returns to the sport before a previous injury has sufficiently healed. Athletes are at a much greater risk for reinjury when they return to the game before recovering fully. Doing so places stress upon the injury and forces the body to compensate for the weakness, which can put the athlete at greater risk for injuring another body part.

Reinjury can be avoided by allowing an injury to completely heal. Once the doctor has approved a return to the sport, make sure that your child properly warms up and cools down before and after exercise.

Sudden exertion can also cause reinjury, so your child should re enter the sport gradually. Explain that easing back into the game at a sensible pace is better than returning to the hospital!

Treating Sports Injuries

Treatment of sports injuries varies by the type of injury.

For acute injuries, many pediatric sports medicine specialists usually take a "better safe than sorry" approach. If an injury appears to affect basic functioning in any way—for example, if your child can't bend a finger, is limping, or has had a change in consciousness—first aid should be administered immediately. A doctor should then see the child. If the injury seems to be more serious, it's important to take your child to the nearest hospital emergency department.

For overuse injuries, the philosophy is similar. If a child begins complaining of pain, it's the body's way of saying there's a problem. Have the child examined by a doctor who can then determine whether it's necessary to see a sports medicine specialist. A doctor can usually diagnose many of these conditions by taking a medical history, examining the child, and ordering some routine tests.

It's important to get overuse injuries diagnosed and treated to prevent them from developing into larger chronic problems. The doctor may advise the child to temporarily modify or eliminate an activity to limit stress on the body.

In some cases, the child may not be able to resume the sport without risking further injury. Because overuse injuries are characterized by swelling, the doctor may prescribe rest, medications to help reduce inflammation, and physical therapy. When recovery is complete, your child's technique or training schedule may need to be adjusted to prevent the injury from flaring up again.

Chapter 43

Fitness and Your Feet

Fitness Planning

Striving for physical fitness is not to be taken lightly. The President's Council on Physical Fitness and Sports cautions that unless you are convinced of the benefits of fitness and the risks of unfitness, you will not succeed. Patience is essential. Don't try to do too much too soon; give yourself a chance to improve.

As you exercise, pay attention to what your body, including your feet, tells you. If you feel discomfort, you may be trying to do too much too fast. Ease up a bit or take a break and start again at another time. Drink fluids on hot days or during very strenuous activities to avoid heat stroke and heat exhaustion.

First Step—See Your Doctor

Before you start a fitness program, you should consult a physician for a complete physical and a podiatric physician for a foot exam. This is especially so if you are over 60, haven't had a physical checkup in the last year, have a disease or disability, or are taking medication. It is recommended that if you are 35–60, substantially overweight, easily fatigued, smoke excessively, have been physically inactive, or have a family history of heart disease, you should consult a physician.

"Fitness and Your Feet," © 1999 American Podiatric Medical Association (www .apma.org). Reprinted with permission. Despite the older date of this document, the guidelines presented are still helpful for people concerned about foot health.

Once you have been cleared to begin exercise, your first goal is to make physical activity a habit. The goals for your activity program, at whatever level of fitness you presently have, are (a) 30 minutes of exercise, (b) four times a week, (c) at a comfortable pace. Stay true to these goals, and you will become fit.

Suiting Up and Shoe Up

For your fitness success, you should wear the right clothes and the proper shoes. Wear loose-fitting, light-colored, and loosely woven clothing in hot weather and several layers of warm clothing in cold weather.

In planning for your equipment needs, don't ignore the part of your body that takes the biggest beating—your feet. Podiatric physicians recommend sturdy, properly fitted athletic shoes of proper width, with leather or canvas uppers, soles that are flexible (but only at the ball of the foot), cushioning, arch supports, and room for your toes. They also suggest a well-cushioned sock for reinforcement, preferably one with an acrylic fiber content so that some perspiration moisture is "wicked" away.

Because of the many athletic shoe brands, and styles within those brands, you may want to ask a podiatrist to help you select the shoe you need. Generally speaking, athletic shoes are available in sport-specific styles or cross-training models.

Foot Care for Fitness

The importance of foot care in exercising is stressed by the American Podiatric Medical Association [APMA]. According to the American Academy of Podiatric Sports Medicine, an APMA affiliate, people don't realize the tremendous pressure that is put on their feet while exercising. For example, when a 150-pound jogger runs three miles, the cumulative impact on each foot is more than 150 tons.

Even without exercising, foot problems contribute to pain in knees, hips, and lower back, and also diminish work efficiency and leisure enjoyment. It is clear, however, that healthy feet are critical to a successful fitness program.

Further evidence for the necessity of proper foot care is the fact that there are more than 300 foot ailments. Although some are hereditary, many stem from the cumulative impact of a lifetime of abuse and neglect and, if left untreated, these foot ailments can prevent the successful establishment of fitness programs.

The Human Foot—A Biological Masterpiece

The human foot is a biological masterpiece. Like a finely tuned race car or a space shuttle, it is complex, containing within its relatively small size 26 bones (the two feet contain a quarter of all the bones in the body), 33 joints, and a network of more than 100 tendons, muscles, and ligaments, to say nothing of blood vessels and nerves.

Foot problems are among the most common health ills. Studies show that at least three-quarters of the American populace experiences foot problems of some degree of seriousness at some time in their lives; only a small percentage of them seek medical treatment, apparently because most mistakenly believe that discomfort and pain are normal.

To keep your feet healthy for daily pursuits or for fitness, you should be familiar with the most common ills that affect them. Remember, though, that self treatment can often turn a minor problem into a major one and is generally not advisable. If the conditions persist, you should see a podiatrist.

These conditions may also occur because of the impact of exercise on your feet:

Athlete's foot: A skin disease, frequently starts between the toes, and can spread to other parts of the foot and body. It is caused by a fungus that commonly attacks the feet because the warm, dark climate of shoes and such places as public locker rooms fosters fungus growth. You can prevent infection by washing your feet daily in soap and water; drying carefully, especially between the toes; changing shoes and hose regularly to decrease moisture; and using foot powder on your feet and in your shoes on a daily basis.

Blisters: Caused by skin friction and moisture, often from active exercising in poorly fitting shoes. There are different schools of thought about whether to pop them. If the blister isn't large, apply an antiseptic and cover with a bandage, and leave it on until it falls off naturally in the bath or shower. If it is large, it may be appropriate to pop the blister with a sterile needle by piercing it several times at its roof, then to drain the fluid as thoroughly as possible before applying an antiseptic, and bandaging. If the area appears infected or excessively inflamed, see your podiatrist. Keep your feet dry and wear a layer of socks as a cushion.

Corns and calluses: Protective layers of compacted, dead skin cells. They are caused by repeated friction and pressure from skin rubbing against bony areas or against an irregularity in a shoe (another reason to have your shoes properly fitted). Corns ordinarily form on the toes and calluses on the soles of the feet, but both can occur on either surface. Never cut corns or calluses with any instrument, and never apply home remedies, except under a podiatrist's instructions.

Heel pain: Generally traced to faulty biomechanics which place too much stress on the heel bone. Stress also can result from a bruise incurred while walking or jumping on hard surfaces or from poorly made or excessively worn footwear. Inserts designed to take the pressure off the heel are generally successful. Heel spurs are bony growths on the underside, forepart of the heel bone. Pain may result when inflammation develops at the point where the spur forms. Spurs can also occur without pain. Both heel pain and heel spurs are often associated with plantar fasciitis, an inflammation of the long band of supportive connective tissue running from the heel to the ball of the foot. There are many excellent treatments for heel pain and heel spurs. However, some general health conditions—arthritis and gout, for example—also cause heel pain.

Fitness and Your Podiatrist

A doctor of podiatric medicine can make an important contribution to your total health and to the success of your fitness program. While podiatrists focus on foot care, they are aware of total health needs and should be seen as part of your annual medical checkup. If your foot ailments are related to a more generalized health problem, your podiatrist will consult with your primary physician or refer you to an appropriate specialist.

For more foot health information, visit the American Podiatric Medical Association's website, www.apma.org. The American Academy of Podiatric Sports Medicine, an affiliate of APMA, may be reached at 800-438-3355.

Chapter 44

Overtraining and Compulsive Exercise

Chapter Contents

Section 44.1

Overtraining in Women and the Risk to Bone Health

This section excerpted from "Exercise and Bone Health," National Institute of Arthritis and Musculoskeletal and Skin Diseases (www.niams.nih.gov), May 2009.

Are you exercising too much? Eating too little? Have your menstrual periods stopped or become irregular? If so, you may be putting yourself at high risk for several serious problems that could affect your health, your ability to remain active, and your risk for injuries. You also may be putting yourself at risk for developing osteoporosis, a disease in which bone density is decreased, leaving your bones vulnerable to fracture (breaking).

Why is missing my period such a big deal?

Some athletes see amenorrhea (the absence of menstrual periods) as a sign of successful training. Others see it as a great answer to a monthly inconvenience. And some young women accept it blindly, not stopping to think of the consequences. But missing your periods is often a sign of decreased estrogen levels. And lower estrogen levels can lead to osteoporosis, a disease in which your bones become brittle and more likely to break.

Usually, bones don't become brittle and break until women are much older. But some young women, especially those who exercise so much that their periods stop, develop brittle bones and may start to have fractures at a very early age. Some 20-year-old female athletes have been said to have the bones of 80-year-old women. Even if bones don't break when you're young, low estrogen levels during the peak years of bone building, the preteen and teen years, can affect bone density for the rest of your life. And studies show that bone growth lost during these years may never be regained.

Broken bones don't just hurt—they can cause lasting physical malformations. Have you noticed that some older women and men have stooped postures? This is not a normal sign of aging. Fractures from osteoporosis have left their spines permanently altered.

Overtraining can cause other problems besides missed periods. If you don't take in enough calcium and vitamin D (among other nutrients), bone loss may result. This may lead to decreased athletic performance, decreased ability to exercise or train at desired levels of intensity or duration, and increased risk of injury.

Who is at risk for these problems?

Girls and women who engage in rigorous exercise regimens or who try to lose weight by restricting their eating are at risk for these health problems. They may include serious athletes, "gym rats" (who spend considerable time and energy working out), and girls and women who believe "you can never be too thin."

How can I tell if someone I know, train with, or coach may be at risk for bone loss, fracture, and other health problems?

Here are some signs to look for:

- Missed or irregular menstrual periods
- Extreme or "unhealthy-looking" thinness
- Extreme or rapid weight loss
- Behaviors that reflect frequent dieting, such as eating very little, not eating in front of others, trips to the bathroom following meals, preoccupation with thinness or weight, focus on low-calorie and diet foods, possible increase in the consumption of water and other no- and low-calorie foods and beverages, possible increase in gum chewing, limiting diet to one food group, or eliminating a food group
- Frequent intense bouts of exercise (e.g., taking an aerobics class, then running five miles, then swimming for an hour, followed by weight-lifting)
- An "I can't miss a day of exercise/practice" attitude
- An overly anxious preoccupation with an injury
- Exercising despite illness, inclement weather, injury, and other conditions that might lead someone else to take the day off
- An unusual amount of self-criticism or self-dissatisfaction
- Indications of significant psychological or physical stress, including depression, anxiety or nervousness, inability to concentrate,

low levels of self-esteem, feeling cold all the time, problems sleeping, fatigue, injuries, and constantly talking about weight

How can I make needed changes to improve my bone health?

If you recognize some of these signs in yourself, the best thing you can do is to make your diet more healthful. That includes consuming enough calories to support your activity level. If you've missed periods, it's best to check with a doctor to make sure it's not a sign of some other problem and to get his or her help as you work toward a more healthy balance of food and exercise. Also, a doctor can help you take steps to protect your bones from further damage.

What can I do if I suspect a friend may have some of these signs?

First, be supportive. Approach your friend or teammate carefully and be sensitive. She probably won't appreciate a lecture about how she should be taking better care of herself. But maybe you could suggest that she talk to a trainer, coach, or doctor about the symptoms she's experiencing.

My friend drinks a lot of diet sodas. She says this helps keep her trim.

Girls and women who may be dieting often drink diet sodas rather than milk. Yet, milk and other dairy products are a good source of calcium, an essential ingredient for healthy bones. Drinking sodas instead of milk can be a problem, especially during the teen years when rapid bone growth occurs. If you (or your friend) find yourself drinking a lot of sodas, try drinking half as many sodas each day, and gradually add more milk and dairy products to your diet. A frozen yogurt shake can be an occasional low-fat, tasty treat. Or try a fruit smoothie made with frozen yogurt, fruit, or calcium-enriched orange juice.

What do fitness instructors and trainers need to know?

It's important for you to be aware of problems associated with bone loss in today's active young women. As an instructor or trainer, you are the one who sees, leads, and perhaps even evaluates the training sessions and performances of your clients. You may know best when something seems to be amiss. You also may be the best person to help a zealous female exerciser recognize that she is putting herself at risk for bone loss and other health problems and that she should establish new goals.

Trainers and instructors also should be aware of the implicit or explicit messages they send. Health, strength, and fitness should be emphasized, rather than thinness. Use caution when advising female clients to lose weight. And, if such a recommendation is deemed necessary, knowledgeable personnel should offer education and assistance about proper and safe weight management. As an instructor or trainer, it's best to maintain a professional rapport with your clients so they can feel comfortable approaching you with concerns about their exercise training programs, appropriate exercise goals and time lines, body image and nutrition issues, as well as more personal problems regarding eating practices and menstruation.

My coach and I think I should lose just a little more weight. I want to be able to excel at my sport!

Years ago, it was not unusual for coaches to encourage athletes to be as thin as possible for many sports (e.g., dancing, gymnastics, figure skating, swimming, diving, and running). However, many coaches now realize that being too thin is unhealthy and can negatively affect performance. It's important to exercise and watch what you eat. However, it's also important to develop and maintain healthy bones and bodies. Without these, it will not matter how fast you can run, how thin you are, or how long you exercise each day. Balance is the key!

I'm still not convinced. If my bones become brittle, so what? What's the worst thing that could happen to me?

Brittle bones may not sound as scary as a fatal or rare disease. The fact is that osteoporosis can lead to fractures. It can cause disability.

Imagine having so many spine fractures that you've lost inches in height and walk bent over. Imagine looking down at the ground everywhere you go because you can't straighten your back. Imagine not being able to find clothes that fit you. Imagine having difficulty breathing and eating because your lungs and stomach are compressed into a smaller space. Imagine having difficulty walking, let alone exercising, because of pain and misshapen bones. Imagine constantly having to be aware of what you are doing and having to do things so slowly and carefully because of a very real fear and dread of a fracture—a fracture that could lead to a drastic change in your life, including pain, loss of independence, loss of mobility, loss of freedom, and more.

485

Osteoporosis isn't just an "older person's" disease. Young women also experience fractures. Imagine being sidelined because of a broken bone and not being able to get those good feelings you get from regular activity.

Section 44.2

Compulsive Exercise

Melissa has been a track fanatic since she was 12 years old. She has run the mile in meets in junior high and high school, constantly improving her times and winning several medals. Best of all, Melissa truly loves her sport.

Recently, however, Melissa's parents have noticed a change in their daughter. She used to return tired but happy from practice and relax with her family, but now she's hardly home for 15 minutes before she heads out for another run on her own. On many days, she gets up to run before school. When she's unable to squeeze in extra runs, she becomes irritable and anxious. And she no longer talks about how much fun track is, just how many miles she has to run today and how many more she should run tomorrow.

Melissa is living proof that even though exercise has many positive benefits, too much can be harmful. Teens, like Melissa, who exercise compulsively are at risk for both physical and psychological problems.

What Is Compulsive Exercise?

Compulsive exercise (also called obligatory exercise and anorexia athletica) is best defined by an exercise addict's frame of mind: he or she no longer chooses to exercise but feels compelled to do so and struggles with guilt and anxiety if he or she doesn't work out. Injury, illness, an outing with friends, bad weather—none of these will deter those who compulsively exercise. In a sense, exercising takes over a compulsive exerciser's life because he or she plans life around it.

Of course, it's nearly impossible to draw a clear line dividing a healthy amount of exercise from too much. The government's 2005 dietary guidelines, published by the U.S. Department of Agriculture (USDA) and the U.S. Department of Health and Human Services (HHS), recommend at least 60 minutes of physical activity for kids and teens on most—if not all—days of the week.

Experts say that repeatedly exercising beyond the requirements for good health is an indicator of compulsive behavior, but because different amounts of exercise are appropriate for different people, this definition covers a range of activity levels. However, several workouts a day, every day, is overdoing it for almost anyone.

Much like with eating disorders, many people who engage in compulsive exercise do so to feel more in control of their lives, and the majority of them are female. They often define their self-worth through their athletic performance and try to deal with emotions like anger or depression by pushing their bodies to the limit. In sticking to a rigorous workout schedule, they seek a sense of power to help them cope with low self-esteem.

Although compulsive exercising doesn't have to accompany an eating disorder, the two often go hand in hand. In anorexia nervosa, the excessive workouts usually begin as a means to control weight and become more and more extreme. As the person's rate of activity increases, the amount he or she eats may also decrease. A person with bulimia may also use exercise as a way to compensate for binge eating.

Compulsive exercise behavior can also grow out of student athletes' demanding practice schedules and their quest to excel. Pressure, both external (from coaches, peers, or parents) and internal, can drive the athlete to go too far to be the best. He or she ends up believing that just one more workout will make the difference between first and second place . . . then keeps adding more workouts.

Eventually, compulsive exercising can breed other compulsive behavior, from strict dieting to obsessive thoughts about perceived flaws. Exercise addicts may keep detailed journals about their exercise schedules and obsess about improving themselves. Unfortunately, these behaviors often compound each other, trapping the person in a downward spiral of negative thinking and low self-esteem.

Why Is Exercising Too Much a Bad Thing?

We all know that regular exercise is an important part of a healthy lifestyle. But few people realize that too much can cause physical and psychological harm:

- Excessive exercise can damage tendons, ligaments, bones, cartilage, and joints, and when minor injuries aren't allowed to heal, they often result in long-term damage. Instead of building muscle, too much exercise actually destroys muscle mass, especially if the body isn't getting enough nutrition, forcing it to break down muscle for energy.

- Girls who exercise compulsively may disrupt the balance of hormones in their bodies. This can change their menstrual cycles (some girls lose their periods altogether, a condition known as amenorrhea) and increase the risk of premature bone loss (a condition known as osteoporosis). And of course, working their bodies so hard leads to exhaustion and constant fatigue.

- An even more serious risk is the stress that excessive exercise can place on the heart, particularly when someone is also engaging in unhealthy weight loss behaviors such as restricting intake, vomiting, and using diet pills or supplements. In extreme cases, the combination of anorexia and compulsive exercise can be fatal.

- Psychologically, exercise addicts are often plagued by anxiety and depression. They may have a negative image of themselves and feel worthless. Their social and academic lives may suffer as they withdraw from friends and family to fixate on exercise. Even if they want to succeed in school or in relationships, working out always comes first, so they end up skipping homework or missing out on time spent with friends.

Warning Signs

A child may be exercising compulsively if he or she:

- won't skip a workout, even if tired, sick, or injured;
- doesn't enjoy exercise sessions, but feels obligated to do them;
- seems anxious or guilty when missing even one workout;
- does miss one workout and exercises twice as long the next time;
- is constantly preoccupied with his or her weight and exercise routine;

- doesn't like to sit still or relax because of worry that not enough calories are being burnt;

- has lost a significant amount of weight;

- exercises more after eating more;

- skips seeing friends, gives up activities, and abandons responsibilities to make more time for exercise;

- seems to base self-worth on the number of workouts completed and the effort put into training;

- is never satisfied with his or her own physical achievements.

It's important, too, to recognize the types of athletes who are more prone to compulsive exercise because their sports place a particular emphasis on being thin. Ice skaters, gymnasts, wrestlers, and dancers can feel even more pressure than most athletes to keep their weight down and their body toned. Runners also frequently fall into a cycle of obsessive workouts.

Getting Professional Help

If you recognize two or more warning signs of compulsive exercise in your child, call your doctor to discuss your concerns. After evaluating your child, the doctor may recommend medical treatment and/or other therapy. Because compulsive exercise is so often linked to an eating disorder, a community agency that focuses on treating these disorders might be able to offer advice or referrals. Extreme cases may require hospitalization to get a child's weight back up to a safe range.

Treating a compulsion to exercise is never a quick-fix process—it may take several months or even years. But with time and effort, kids can get back on the road to good health. Therapy can help improve self-esteem and body image, as well as teach them how to deal with emotions. Sessions with a nutritionist can help develop healthy eating habits. Once they know what to watch out for, kids will be better equipped to steer clear of unsafe exercise and eating patterns.

Ways to Help at Home

Parents can do a lot to help a child overcome a compulsion to exercise:

- Involve kids in preparing nutritious meals.

489

- Combine activity and fun by going for a hike or a bike ride together as a family.

- Be a good body-image role model. In other words, don't fixate on your own physical flaws, as that just teaches kids that it's normal to dislike what they see in the mirror.

- Never criticize another family member's weight or body shape, even if you're just kidding around. Such remarks might seem harmless, but they can leave a lasting impression on kids or teens struggling to define and accept themselves.

- Examine whether you're putting too much pressure on your kids to excel, particularly in a sport (because some teens turn to exercise to cope with pressure). Take a look at where kids might be feeling too much pressure. Help them put it in perspective and find other ways to cope.

Most important, just be there with constant support. Point out all of your child's great qualities that have nothing to do with how much he or she works out—small daily doses of encouragement and praise can help improve self-esteem. If you teach kids to be proud of the challenges they've faced and not just the first-place ribbons they've won, they will likely be much happier and healthier kids now and in the long run.

Chapter 45

Exercising Safely Outdoors

Chapter Contents

Section 45.1

Outdoor Exercise Safety

This section excerpted from "Your Guide to Physical Activity and Your Heart,"
National Heart, Lung, and Blood Institute (www.nhlbi.nih.gov), June 2006.

Avoid Injury

- It can't be said too often: Start your activity program gradually, and work up slowly. Be sure to warm up, cool down, and stretch each and every time you are physically active. Exercising too much, too fast, can cause injuries.

- A certain amount of stiffness is normal at first. But if you do hurt a joint or pull a muscle, stop the activity for several days to avoid more serious injury. Rest and over-the-counter painkillers can heal most minor muscle and joint problems.

- Use proper equipment. Wear good shoes with adequate cushioning in the soles for jogging or walking. Use goggles to protect your eyes for sports such as handball or racquetball.

- Joggers should run on soft, even surfaces such as a level grass field, a dirt path, or a track. Hard or uneven surfaces, such as cement or rough fields, are more likely to cause injuries. Also, try to land on your heels, rather than on the balls of your feet, to minimize strain on your feet and lower legs.

- If you jog or walk on the street, watch for cars. Wear light-colored clothing with a reflecting band at night so that drivers can see you more easily. Always face oncoming traffic. Remember, drivers can't see you as well as you can see their cars.

- If you bicycle, always wear a helmet. Ride in the direction of traffic and try to avoid busy streets. At night, use lights and wheel-mounted reflectors.

Eat Right

- If you've just eaten a meal, avoid strenuous physical activity for at least two hours.

- If you've just been vigorously active, wait about 20 minutes before eating.

- If you plan to be continuously active for more than 60 minutes, you may want to take a snack along to keep up your energy level. Good choices are light foods and drinks that are high in carbohydrates, such as bananas, raisins, bagels, or sport drinks.

Check the Weather Report

Take the following precautions on hot, humid days:

- Try to be physically active during the cooler and less humid parts of the day, such as early morning or early evening.

- Wear light, loose-fitting, "breathable" clothing. Never wear rubberized or plastic suits. Such clothing won't help you lose weight by making you sweat more, but it can cause dangerously high body temperatures.

- Drink adequate fluids—particularly water—before, during, and after your physical activity.

- Watch for symptoms of heat exhaustion and heat stroke.

When you're active outdoors in hot, humid weather, be alert for signs of heat exhaustion and heat stroke. Although many of their symptoms are similar, heat stroke is the more serious condition.

Heat stroke occurs when the body temperature increases too much, causing stress on the body that may harm tissues. The rise in temperature occurs when the heat produced during exercise exceeds the heat that leaves the body. Table 45.1 lists the main symptoms of each type of heat problem.

Table 45.1. Main Symptoms of Heat Problems

Heat Exhaustion	Heat Stroke
Dizziness	Dizziness
Headache	Headache
Nausea	Nausea
Confusion	Confusion
Body temperature below normal	Muscle cramps
	Sweating stops
	High body temperature

Both heat exhaustion and heat stroke can be avoided by drinking enough water to replace fluids lost during physical activity. Drink water regularly throughout your activity, but don't "over water" yourself. Drink no more than three cups of water per hour.

Take the following precautions on cold days:

- When dressing for outdoor activity, wear one layer less than you'd wear if you were outside but not physically active. Ideally wear several layers of clothing rather than one heavy jacket so you can remove a layer if you get too warm.

- Use mittens, gloves, or cotton socks to protect your hands.

- Wear a hat, since up to 40% of your body heat is lost through your head and neck.

Be cautious on rainy, icy, or snowy days:

- Be aware of reduced visibility—for both yourself and for drivers—and reduced traction on roadways.

Seek Company

- If you're concerned about the safety of your surroundings, pair up with a buddy for outdoor activities. If possible, walk, bike, or jog during daylight hours.

- Check out the hours of nearby shopping malls. Many malls are open early and late for people who prefer to walk or jog at those times of day, but in a safe, well-lit area. (Indoor malls also make it possible to stay active during summer heat, winter cold, and allergy seasons.)

Know the Signs of a Heart Problem

While physical activity can strengthen your heart, some types of activity may worsen existing heart problems. Warning signals include sudden dizziness, cold sweat, paleness, fainting, extreme breathlessness, or pain or pressure in your upper body. These symptoms may occur during, or just after, an activity. Ignoring these signals and continuing your activity may lead to serious heart problems. Instead, call your doctor right away.

Get Back in the Swing

If you have to miss a few sessions of physical activity because of illness or injury, don't be discouraged. Once you recover, you can get right back on the "activity track." But do wait until you recover.

If you come down with a minor illness, such as a cold, wait until you feel normal before you resume your activity. If you suffer a minor injury, wait until the pain disappears before continuing. When you do resume your fitness sessions, start at one-half to two-thirds of your previous level, depending on the number of days you've missed and how you feel while moving.

If your activity program has been interrupted by a major illness or injury, consult your doctor about the best time—and pace—for resuming your fitness program. Whatever your reasons for missing sessions, don't worry about the skipped days or weeks. Just get back into your routine and focus on the progress you'll be making toward your fitness goals.

Section 45.2

Air Pollution and Exercise

"Smog Matters: Physical exercise and smog don't mix. Protect your health when air quality is poor," Government of Ontario Ministry of the Environment. © Queen's Printer for Ontario, 2008. Reproduced with permission.

Air pollution is a year-round problem, but smog levels are generally highest during hot, sunny days from May to September—when we most spend time outdoors.

Staying healthy is important, but you should be aware of some of the risks of exercising outdoors when air quality is poor and plan accordingly.

Smog Affects Your Body

Smog can affect everyone's health, but health risks may increase during high smog levels for:

- those who play sports or exercise outdoors;
- cyclists;
- runners.

When you exercise outdoors, you breathe harder than normal, inhaling more polluted air into your lungs. This can lead to the following symptoms even in healthy, active people:

- Difficulty breathing

- Chest tightness and coughing

- Headache

- Eye, nose, and throat irritation

- Aggravation of respiratory diseases (such as asthma)

- Low energy

For more information on the impacts of smog on your health, visit: www.health.gov.on.ca/english/public/pub/pubhealth/smog.html

In addition to those who play sports or exercise outdoors, other groups may experience health problems at lower levels of air pollution:

- People with lung diseases and heart conditions

- Children

- Pregnant women

- People with asthma

- Seniors

- Smokers

Staying Active during Smog Days

Listen and watch for smog alerts on the news especially during traditional smog season—from May to September.

If a Smog Advisory is issued in your community, consider tailoring your activities accordingly:

- Avoid or reduce strenuous physical outdoor activities when smog levels are high, especially during the late afternoon.

- Shift from vigorous activity levels (i.e., jogging outdoors) to moderate or light activity levels (e.g., brisk or slow pace walking).

- Consider exercising indoors.

- Avoid congested streets and rush hour traffic, sources of air pollution.

- Anyone experiencing respiratory symptoms should reduce their level of activity.

- If you experience any breathing difficulties or respiratory complications, contact your physician or go to the nearest hospital.

If you have a heart or lung condition, talk to your health care professional about additional ways to protect your health when smog levels are high.

To find the current air quality in your community go to www.airqualityontario.com or call 800-387-7768 (English); 800-221-8852 (French).

Reduce Smog, Reduce the Risk

Whenever we burn fuel, we create the pollutants necessary to form smog. We burn oil and gas to power our cars and to heat and cool our homes.

Actions You Can Take to Reduce Smog

At Home

- Conserve electricity by turning off lights and the air conditioner when not in use.

- Limit the amount of wood you burn in your fireplace or wood stove and use only the dry, seasoned variety.

- Try manual instead of gasoline-powered equipment.

- Reduce your use of oil-based products such as paints, solvents, or cleaners if you can avoid them. They contain volatile organic compounds (VOCs), which contribute to smog.

- Ensure you schedule regular car maintenance.

At Work

- Take public transit or walk to work.

- Encourage and facilitate carpooling.

- Avoid traffic congestion.

- Consider teleconferencing instead of traveling to meetings.

Part Six

Physical Fitness for People with Health Conditions

Chapter 46

Introduction to Exercise with a Health Condition

Exercise can increase longevity and quality of life; improve energy, strength, balance, and coordination; and act as a potent pain reliever and antidepressant. Its benefits can reach all people, perhaps especially those with health conditions. But many people don't know what exercise guidelines to follow for optimal health and management of their disease or disorder. If this sounds like you, look no further than your physician and local ACE [American Council on Exercise]-certified Advanced Health & Fitness Specialist.

Start with Your Health Care Practitioner

Before beginning an exercise program, talk with your physician. Inquire about special limitations you need to be aware of and ask your physician if he or she can refer you to a fitness professional who is experienced in training clients with your condition.

Certified Fitness Professionals Make a Difference

A certified fitness professional with experience working with individuals with your medical condition can help you jumpstart a fitness program and ensure that your program is safe, effective, and enjoyable. The key is to find the right person to meet your needs. Do this by asking questions, such as:

"Exercising with a Health Challenge," reprinted with permission from the American Council on Exercise (www.acefitness.org), © 2009. All rights reserved.

- Where did you receive your exercise science education and experience? What certifications do you have? (Be sure that he or she has received certification from an accredited and reputable organization.)

- What is your experience training individuals with my health condition?

- Do you have any concerns about training me? If you do not feel comfortable training me, can you refer me to another experienced trainer?

- What knowledge do you have of my medical condition? (Beyond present knowledge, try to determine if the trainer is motivated to learn more about your condition to provide you the best care.)

- What can I expect to achieve with an exercise program?

- May I contact other clients of yours and ask them about their experiences working with you? (When you talk to these clients, ask them if they were pleased with their workouts, if the trainer was punctual and prepared, if they felt their individual needs were addressed, and any other questions that you have.)

Tell the fitness professional about your general health, your specific illness or injury, and your physical-activity history. He or she may administer fitness assessments, such as a range-of-motion test for a certain joint or cardiorespiratory testing to measure heart rate during aerobic exercise. This information will help you and your trainer establish realistic goals and design a safe and effective exercise program.

Your trainer also may request to speak with your health care provider. (These conversations about your personal health information should only occur with your consent.) The trainer may want to ask the physician for specific guidance, clarify your physical-activity program goals, or simply introduce him- or herself as a member of the health care team that is helping you to achieve your goals.

Your Exercise Program

With few exceptions, a quality exercise program includes cardiovascular training, resistance training, and flexibility exercises. And whether you exercise one-on-one or in a group, training should progress from an initial, easy effort to a challenging workout. Also make sure that you are offered exercise modifications and exercise recommendations tailored to your fitness level and abilities.

Exercise can be an important, fulfilling part of coping with a chronic disease or recovering from injury. Coordinate with your health care provider and fitness professional to make the most of your exercise experience, and to improve your health and quality of life.

Additional Resources

- **The National Center on Physical Fitness and Disability:** www.ncpad.org.

- **Mayo Clinic—Exercise and Disability: Physical Activity Is within Your Reach:** www.cnn.com/HEALTH/library/SM/0042.html.

- **American Academy of Physical Medicine and Rehabilitation:** www.aapmr.org.

Conditions That May Require Special Exercise Guidelines

Cardiovascular Disease and Risk Factors

- Hypertension
- Elevated blood cholesterol
- Diabetes
- Angina
- Post–heart attack or post-bypass
- Heart valve disease
- Peripheral circulatory disease

Breathing Conditions

- Asthma
- Emphysema

Bone or Joint Conditions

- Low-back pain
- Osteoporosis
- Post-surgical/rehabilitation
- Arthritis

Other Conditions

- Neuromuscular (stroke, Parkinson's disease, epilepsy, fibromyalgia)
- Breast cancer
- Vision or hearing impairments
- Pregnancy
- Psychological disorders
- Mental handicaps

Note: This list is not exhaustive, so speak with your health practitioner about exercise-program modifications or limitations specific to your condition.

Chapter 47

Physical Activity for People with Disabilities

Chapter Contents

505

Section 47.1

Increasing Physical Activity for People with Disabilities

"Increasing Physical Activity in People with Disabilities," President's Council on Physical Fitness and Sports (www.fitness.gov), 2008.

Why Be Active?

Children and adults who have a disability can gain numerous mental and physical benefits from being physically active on a regular basis. These benefits include the following:

- Reduced risk of developing a chronic condition, such as diabetes, stroke, or heart disease

- Reduced risk of developing a secondary condition related to the primary disability (for example, an individual who has a lower limb paralysis and utilizes a wheelchair may become overweight due to inactivity; over time, chronic shoulder pain or a rotator cuff tear may develop due to overuse or poor muscle development in the shoulders and arms, continuing the cycle of inactivity)

- Improved self-esteem

- Greater social interaction

- Ability to maintain a higher level of independence

Increasing Physical Activity, Fitness, and Sports Participation

People with disabilities face multiple barriers to being active. Lack of programming or knowledge on how to adapt activities, inaccessible or unwelcoming facilities, financial constraints, and the disability itself are just a few of these barriers.

A few things to keep in mind:

- The activity doesn't have to be strenuous to provide physical and emotional benefits.

- Be positive and encouraging. Remember that a person with a disability is just as capable and worthy of being active as someone without a disability.

- Seek out opportunities to be active. Look for programs that may already be in place that include people with disabilities. Places to start are public agencies; health care, fitness, or recreational centers; sports clubs; and parks departments. Including people with disabilities in existing programs does not require major adaptations. Inclusion can be as simple as knowing alternative movements or techniques for engaging in the activity and ways to adapt existing equipment using readily available materials. With a little training, it's easy for program or facility staff to make adaptations.

- Find enjoyable activities. Having fun is key! Some options include team or individual sports, a gym-based exercise program, outdoor recreational activities, or running, biking, or swimming in area races.

- Set goals prior to enrolling in a program or starting a routine. This may help identify the activities or programs that will lead to success. Goals may range from making a new friend to learning the rules of a game or increasing muscle strength or stamina.

Some Things to Consider

Nearly one-in-five Americans aged five years and older have at least one disability. Only 12% of adults with a disability meet the minimum physical activity recommendation of 30 minutes of moderate physical activity five or more days a week or 20 minutes of vigorous activity at least three days a week.[1] Physical inactivity "among people who have a disability has been linked to an increase in the severity of disability" and a decreased involvement in the community. This is particularly concerning as individuals age and the natural effects of the aging process become more problematic due to years of being inactive.[2]

A Tool to Help: The Pedometer[3]

Although the original intent of the pedometer was to measure walking by wearing the device on the waist, it will measure any general movement. The most important things are that the device be worn at the same location on the body and kept parallel to the ground. Some alternative locations include the arm, wrist, ankle, or attached to a shoe. A safety strap, arm band, or piece of clothing can help secure the pedometer and keep it from rubbing against the skin. To track activity, start with a baseline count. Wear the pedometer (in the same location) every day for one week. At the end of each day, record the number. Find the baseline number by adding the counts from each day together and dividing by the total number of days (seven).

Establish a goal that is challenging yet achievable. For example, increase the average daily count by 10% each week for six weeks. The President's Challenge program, www.presidentschallenge.org, has a free Web- and paper-based activity log that can help track progress.

Resources

U.S. Department of Health and Human Services, Office on Disability: Links to a variety of Web-based resources on topics ranging from health and wellness to education, employment, and information technology, www.hhs.gov/od/index.html.

Adaptive Information Resource Center: Provides information on recreational and sports programs for adults and children. Website allows user to search by state or program type, www.adaptiveirc.org.

Disabled Sports USA: Information on sports rehabilitation programs nationwide. Programs are open to anyone with a permanent disability and range from water and snow skiing to rafting and tennis, www.dsusa.org.

References

1.   National Center for Health Statistics. DATA2010. Regular physical activity: moderate or vigorous, 2005. Available at: http://wonder.cdc.gov/scripts/broker.exe. Accessed June 21, 2007.

2.   Rimmer J. (2005). The conspicuous absence of people with disabilities in public fitness and recreation facilities: lack of interest or lack of access? *Am Jrnl Health Promotion*, 19(5), 327–329.

3.   What is a pedometer and how can I benefit from using one? [Electronic fact sheet]. (2006). Chicago, IL: National Center on Physical Activity and Disability [Producer and Distributor]. Available from: http:// www.ncpad.org/exercise/fact_sheet.php?sheet=420&view=all. Accessed June 15, 2007.

Section 47.2

Promoting Inclusive Physical Activity Communities for People with Disabilities

This section excerpted from "Promoting Inclusive Physical Activity Communities for People with Disabilities," President's Council on Physical Fitness and Sports (www.fitness.gov), June/July 2008. The full text of this document, including references, is available at www.fitness.gov/publications/digests/digest-junejuly2008-508version.pdf.pdf.

It is estimated that there are 40 to 50 million people in the United States who have a disability. This number is expected to increase over the next several decades as the baby boom generation reaches retirement age. An aging population brings with it a host of physical, cognitive, and sensory impairments that will increase the number of adults who are disabled in this nation and throughout the world. In addition to the growing number of people with disabilities over age 65, millions of children and younger people also have a disability. Thus, increased effective strategies are needed to improve and maintain function and quality of life among individuals with disabilities, older and younger alike.

Increasing physical activity participation among people with disabilities is an important goal for the health and fitness profession. Despite the enormous health benefits that can be attained from regular physical activity, most people with disabilities are not achieving the U.S. recommended goal of 30 minutes a day five or more days of the week. This low level of physical activity participation could be an even greater issue for people with disabilities compared to a relatively sedentary population without existing comorbidity because people with disabilities are often having to deal with other health issues related to their disability such as secondary (e.g., pain, fatigue, deconditioning, depression, and weight gain) and associated conditions (e.g., spasticity, autonomic dysfunction, incontinence, seizures, balance, and thermoregulatory alterations). When these conditions overlay chronic conditions (e.g., cancer, type 2 diabetes, asthma, and heart disease), health becomes a front-and-center issue for millions of people with disabilities because it threatens their ability to work effectively, shop, participate in leisure and social activities, and live independently.

Many health disparities observed in people with disabilities aren't necessarily a direct result of having a disability and may occur directly or indirectly from a lack of good health promotion practices. While regular physical activity has the potential to offset some of the decline in health and function observed in people with disabilities, barriers to promoting increased physical activity must first be addressed. Health and fitness professionals have a unique opportunity to impact a large and substantial segment of the population (i.e., people with disabilities) who are underutilizing fitness and recreation facilities in their community.

Health Status and Physical Activity Levels of People with Disabilities

People with disabilities report substantially poorer health profiles compared to the general population. Disabled individuals tend to have more physical and cognitive impairments, greater functional limitations, more chronic health conditions, less access to community activities, and poorer health behaviors. People with disabilities have a substantially higher rating of poor health compared to people without disabilities and report less frequently that they are in excellent health.

People with disabilities also report a higher incidence of obesity, smoking, and physical inactivity. The median proportion of adults who smoke is 30.5% among those with disabilities compared to 21.7% among those without disabilities. Disabled individuals are more likely to be obese (median: 31.2% vs. 19.6%) and physically inactive (median: 22.4% vs. 11.9%) compared to people without disabilities (median: 11.9%).

The higher incidence of obesity observed in people with disabilities is particularly troublesome as activities of daily living (ADL) and instrumental activities of daily living (IADL) are more difficult to perform, and the excess weight may reduce or limit opportunities for various types of community participation including employment and leisure activities.

Lower Physical Activity Participation Reported in People with Disabilities

National data indicate that approximately twice as many adults with a disability (25.6%) were physically inactive during the preceding week than adults without a disability (12.8%). Patterns of low physical activity reported among people with disabilities raise serious concerns regarding their health and well-being, particularly as they enter their later years when the effects of the natural aging process are compounded by years of sedentary living. The interaction between the natural aging process and secondary conditions associated with various types of disabilities (i.e., weight gain, deconditioning, fatigue, pain) creates greater physical demands in getting around the home or community. Tasks that could be accomplished in younger adulthood often become significantly more difficult in middle and later life. Climbing stairs; walking with a cane or walker; carrying packages; transferring from a wheelchair to a bed, commode, chair, or car; pushing a wheelchair up a ramp or over a curb; and standing for long periods each require adequate levels of physical fitness (i.e., cardiorespiratory endurance, strength, flexibility, balance). Low physical fitness, in combination with functional impairments (i.e., spasticity) and secondary conditions associated with the disability (e.g., obesity, peripheral artery disease), may limit physical independence among individuals with disability and may preclude participation in activities that require moderate to high levels of energy expenditure (i.e., community ambulation, pushing a wheelchair up a ramp or curb, etc.).

Physical Activity Is Also Lower among Youth with Disabilities

Children and adolescents with disabilities also have significantly lower levels of physical activity compared to their nondisabled peers. Data from a national study conducted in Canada comparing health risk behaviors of 319 adolescents with physical disabilities to 7,020 nondisabled adolescents found that physical inactivity was 4.5 times higher among disabled compared to nondisabled youth. Adolescents with physical disabilities were also twice as likely as nondisabled youth to report watching television for more than four hours a day.

Data from the 2005 Youth Risk Behavior Survey (YRBS) also indicated that the proportion of students who engaged in sedentary activities (i.e., playing video/computer games) three or more hours per school day was significantly higher in those with physical disabilities (26.6%) compared to those without disabilities (20.4%). In contrast, the percentage of students who were members of a sports team was significantly lower for youth with physical disabilities compared to youth without disabilities. Researchers have suggested that barriers to participation in recreational sports programs by youth with disabilities may result in further avoidance of other physically demanding activities (i.e., soccer, basketball) and greater time spent in sedentary behaviors after school and on the weekends.

The low levels of physical activity participation reported among youth with disabilities is of great concern because this adverse behavior generally tracks into adulthood. In theory, higher levels of physical inactivity during childhood and adolescence are likely to contribute to an increased risk of obesity and other adverse health conditions in adulthood.

Barriers to Physical Activity Participation

People with disabilities experience many different types of barriers to regular physical activity that can be similar (e.g., time, lack of interest) or different from the general population. Barriers that have been reported in people with disabilities include cost of memberships, lack of transportation to fitness centers, lack of information on available and accessible facilities and programs, lack of accessible exercise equipment that can be purchased for home use, and the perception that fitness facilities are unfriendly environments for those with a disability. Such barriers can result in insufficient physical activity participation and a decline in physical function, each of which may increase the risk of developing secondary health conditions.

Many disabilities are accompanied by various impairments including loss of balance, vision, hearing, pain, fatigue, decreased cognition, paralysis, and others. Environmental hazards such as narrow paths of travel, low lighting, loud noise, and minimal space between exercise machines can limit the person's ability to exercise. Group exercise classes or sports competition often isolate individuals with disabilities because the equipment used in the class is not accessible, the pace of the class is too fast, or possible adaptations to accommodate the person (e.g., slower tempo, adaptive equipment) are not available. Collectively, these barriers can make it extremely difficult for people with disabilities to engage in regular, sustainable exercise.

To a large extent, the primary barrier, lack of time, that prevents many people without disabilities from engaging in regular physical activity may not be as big an issue as other barriers, since the employment rate among people with disabilities is significantly lower than in the general population, leaving them with more time for leisure activity. However, other more substantial barriers can make it extremely difficult to exercise among individuals with disabilities. These barriers must be identified and strategies to overcome these barriers must be developed to facilitate greater participation in physical activity by youth, adults, and seniors with disabilities living in communities across America.

A Framework for Promoting Physical Activity Participation among People with Disabilities

Health/fitness professionals must recognize that many physical activity programs, facilities, and services offered in their communities have an element of inaccessibility. From sports and recreation programs for youth to fitness equipment and swim classes for adults and seniors, accessibility is an inherent problem for many people with disabilities. When concentrating efforts on removing these environmental barriers to participation, a critical feature is to understand the type and nature of the barrier(s) that may prevent individuals with disabilities from engaging in physical activity.

J.H. Rimmer and W.J. Schiller ("Future directions in exercise and recreational technology for people with spinal cord injury and other disabilities," *Top Spinal Cord Injury Rehabil*, 2006; 11:82–993) developed a framework for systematically addressing barriers in the built environment experienced by people with disabilities. The model uses the acronym RAMP—Restoring Activity, Mobility, and Participation—to reflect the broad need to create a barrier-free environment. The RAMP model consists of four components—Access, Participation, Adherence, and Health and Function—each building on the previous component and reflecting the interconnectedness between components in achieving optimal health and well-being among people with disabilities. The metaphor also reflects the logical sequencing of the four components: access is necessary for participation, and regular participation and adherence are necessary to obtain benefits in health and function.

The first component in the RAMP model is access. Within the context of physical activity, access refers to offering the individual an opportunity to experience typical use of the environment or exercise product (i.e., equipment). The most common access issues for people with disabilities involve physical access—getting the person into the building, allowing full use of available facilities, and allowing access on and off the equipment. A more subtle aspect of access is information on the availability of facilities, services, programs, and equipment. Without at least awareness of the options available, the options are functionally unavailable.

One way that health and fitness professionals can make their facilities more accessible is when purchasing new equipment, they could consider universal design features such as swivel-away seats that allow wheelchair users to access the machine from their wheelchair; easy reach to changing weight on various resistance machines; easy transfer onto cardiovascular exercise equipment such as seen on recumbent steppers; good color contrasts so that users with visual impairments can operate equipment and reduce the risk of injury; wide enough space between machines to allow a wheelchair user to transfer onto and off of the machine; and similar changes that can make the equipment much more user friendly. Other features of access include entranceways and exits that are wide enough for wheelchairs; paths of travel that are free of temporary or permanent obstacles; firm surfaces for supporting people with balance impairments and those who use wheelchairs; locker rooms that contain wide, padded benches to allow individuals to transfer from their wheelchair to allow for dressing and changing; a few lockers that can be reached from the height of a wheelchair; swimming pools with transfer walls, lifts, or sloped entries to allow easy entrance and exit for individuals who are unable to climb stairs; and many other features that make the facility accessible to people with disabilities.

The second component focuses on promoting participation in healthful levels of physical activity by people with disabilities. Participation goes beyond physical access and use of universal design and refers to developing modalities of physical activity that are both beneficial and satisfactory for people with disabilities. While access is primarily concerned with availability of opportunities for recreation, leisure, and exercise, participation is primarily concerned with the usability or stage of readiness to use available physical activity opportunities. For a person with a disability, simply having access to a facility (e.g., swimming pool, weight training room, or exercise equipment) is necessary but not sufficient for a successful outcome. For example, someone who has a disability may be able to get into an exercise room (i.e., weight room) but have little or no success with participating in programs that are available with the existing equipment (e.g., circuit training class). A pool lift allows someone to enter the water (access) but is of little utility if the person is unable to participate in the aqua-aerobics class due to a lack of adaptive equipment. Group exercise classes (e.g., tai chi, Pilates, yoga, aerobics), team sports (e.g., basketball, or softball), exercise rooms (e.g., cardio and strength equipment), and outdoor recreation activities (e.g., cycling, climbing) often must be modified for people with disabilities to allow them to have satisfying and beneficial experiences.

The second component in the RAMP model is participation. The emphasis of the participation component in the RAMP model is to ensure that the experiences of people with disabilities are not diminished relative to the experiences of other participants. If people with disabilities are able to participate in more forms of physical activity with reasonable accommodations and adaptations, there is an increased likelihood that they will meet the U.S. recommended guidelines of 30 minutes or more a day of moderate to vigorous intensity levels of physical activity most days of the week. The participation component also stands for education and training of professionals who have little or no background in working with people with disabilities. Many people with disabilities find that the lack of knowledge about disability, poor professional behavior, and negative attitudes limits their opportunity to participate in a much wider variety of physical activity programs.

Adapted physical activity and therapeutic professionals can play a major role in enhancing participation by children, adults, and seniors with disabilities in all areas of indoor and outdoor physical activity. These professionals have training and experience in adapting sports, recreation, and physical activity programs to allow people with disabilities to obtain a much more enriching experience. Health and fitness professionals with little background in working with people with disabilities should determine if there are any local professionals with this specialty certification who can assist them in making their programs more accommodating for people with disabilities. Many of these professionals work in public schools, hospitals, and long-term-care facilities and maybe available to conduct a workshop or provide consultation on an as-needed basis.

The third component of the RAMP model addresses the issue of adherence, which presents the greatest challenge in securing the health benefits of physical activity. To achieve the full benefits of physical activity on health, the individual must participate in moderate physical activity on most days throughout the lifespan. While some of the health benefits associated with moderate physical activity can be realized in the short-term, others continue to accrue over the long-term. Further, most of these health benefits lessen and fade if the individual relapses into a sedentary lifestyle.

While adherence to a physically active lifestyle is a chronic problem for most people, it presents substantially greater difficulties for people with disabilities because of limited opportunities with regard to access and participation. One of the great challenges facing health and fitness professionals is to find effective adherence strategies for people with disabilities. Possible strategies for increasing adherence to beneficial recreation and exercise programs involve varying the types of activities or activity locations and developing social support networks that connect people and make the physical activity part of a socially engaging experience.

When any new member with a disability joins a facility program, it is important for the health/fitness professional to learn more about their social history and determine a good match with another member or members who have similar interests and levels of health and function.

At the top of the RAMP model, the fourth component addresses health and function. The ultimate goal for health/fitness professionals is to improve quality of life and help lower the risk of various health conditions. One important element of health and function is identifying effective methods for measuring and monitoring physical activity in people with disabilities. For example, movement of upper extremities may account for only a small portion of total energy expenditure in the ambulatory population. However, wheelchair users use their upper body for all activities of daily living and for exercise such as arm cranking and wheelchair propulsion. Consequently, quantifying upper-extremity movement is necessary for an adequate measure of physical activity among wheelchair users.

Another issue associated with the health and function domain is avoiding an overuse injury resulting from recreation repetitive motions associated with a certain exercise. For example, while walking is widely promoted as a safe and beneficial form of physical activity for the general population, this modality is not applicable to people who rely on wheelchairs for mobility or have severe orthopedic impairments (e.g., rheumatoid arthritis, osteoarthritis). Further, inferring an equivalent benefit for "wheeling" a manual wheelchair or walking for an extended period with a significant mobility limitation may predispose the participant to increased risk of overuse injuries and pain. Therefore, health and fitness professionals must establish good monitoring strategies to ensure that the modalities chosen are safe and effective for the participant.

Building a program for individuals with disabilities based on the four interconnected components of the RAMP model will assist health and fitness professionals in restoring activity, mobility, and participation in the lives of people with disabilities. Three of the components in the RAMP model reflect key elements of the physical activity guidelines as follows:

- Participation = the equivalent of at least 30 minutes of moderate physical activity

- Adherence = most days of the week

- Health and Function = achievements in beneficial health outcomes (e.g., musculoskeletal, cardiorespiratory, functional, metabolic, and mental health)

The first component, access, defined as opportunities and options to participate in healthful physical activity, is added because people with disabilities have significantly less access to the types of areas, structures, fixtures, and equipment needed to participate in regular physical activity.

Conclusion

Health and fitness professionals have a unique opportunity to improve the health and well-being of millions of people with disabilities who are not engaging in moderate, health-enhancing physical activity. Physical, programmatic, and attitudinal barriers that affect the ability of many people with disabilities to become physically active must be eliminated if we are going to achieve higher levels of physical activity in this underserved segment of the population. Increased participation in physical activity and improved fitness levels could have substantial health benefits for this underserved audience. Small increments in physical activity could pay substantial dividends in reducing health care expenditures and caregiver burden. Lowering the incidence of chronic conditions, minimizing or eliminating secondary conditions directly or indirectly resulting from the disability, and reducing the need for personal assistance in performing ADL and IADL are important outcomes of regular physical activity. The focus of this effort should be on offering programs, services, and facilities that are universally designed and fully accessible to all people with and without disabilities.

Public health programs and professionals who work in local and state health departments, fitness and recreation centers, and rehabilitation facilities must recognize the low rates of physical activity reported among people with disabilities and begin to develop effective and cohesive strategies that address this problem. While most of the financial resources in public health have been directed at prevention of disease, injury, and disability, there is growing recognition among public policy experts that prevention of secondary conditions is an equally important issue among people with disabilities. Health promotion activities, especially increased participation in physical activity, can have an enormous positive impact on reducing secondary conditions and improving health, function, and quality of life in people with disabilities.

Chapter 48

Physical Fitness for People Who Are Overweight

Chapter Contents

Section 48.1

Physical Fitness at Any Size

"Active at Any Size," National Institute of Diabetes and
Digestive and Kidney Diseases (www.niddk.nih.gov), October 2006.

Would you like to be more physically active, but are not sure if you can do it? Good news—if you are a very large person, you can be physically active—and you can have fun and feel good doing it.

There may be special challenges for very large people who are physically active. You may not be able to bend or move in the same way that other people can. It may be hard to find clothes and equipment for exercising. You may feel self-conscious being physically active around other people.

Facing these challenges is hard—but it can be done! The information in this chapter may help you start being more active and healthier—no matter what your size.

Why should I be active?

Being physically active may help you live longer and protect you from the following diseases:

- Type 2 diabetes
- Heart disease
- Stroke
- High blood pressure

If you have any of these health problems, being physically active may help improve your symptoms. Regular physical activity helps you feel better because it has the following effects:

- Lowers your stress and boosts your mood
- Increases your strength, movement, balance, and flexibility
- Helps control blood pressure and blood sugar
- Helps build healthy bones, muscles, and joints

- Helps your heart and lungs work better

- Improves your self-esteem

- Boosts energy during the day and may aid in sleep at night

How do I get started?

Think about your barriers to being active. Then try to come up with creative ways to solve them. The following examples may help you overcome barriers.

- **Barrier: I don't have enough time.** Solution: Be active for a few minutes at a time throughout the day. Sit less. Try to walk more while doing your errands, or schedule lunchtime workouts to boost your overall activity. Plan ahead and be creative!

- **Barrier: I feel self-conscious when I'm active.** Solution: Be active at home while doing household chores and find ways to move during your day-to-day activities. Try walking with a group of friends with whom you feel comfortable.

- **Barrier: I'm worried about my health or injury.** Solution: You might feel better if you talk to a health care professional first. Find a fitness provider to guide you, or sign up for a class so you feel safe. Remember that activity does not have to be difficult. Gentle activity is good, too.

- **Barrier: I just don't like exercise.** Solution: Good news— you do not have to run or do push-ups to get the benefits of being physically active. Try dancing to the radio, walking outdoors, or being active with friends to spice things up.

- **Barrier: I can't stay motivated!** Solution: Try to add variety to your activities and rely on friends to stay focused on being active. Try activity videos for extra encouragement. Set realistic goals, track your progress, and be sure to celebrate your achievements.

To start being more active, try these tips:

- Start slowly. Your body needs time to get used to your new activity.

- Warm up. Warm-ups get your body ready for action. Shrug your shoulders, tap your toes, swing your arms, or march in place. You should spend a few minutes warming up for any physical activity—even walking. Walk slowly for the first few minutes.

- Cool down. Slow down little by little. If you have been walking fast, walk slowly or stretch for a few minutes to cool down. Cooling down may protect your heart, relax your muscles, and keep you from getting hurt.

If you cannot do an activity, do not be hard on yourself. Feel good about what you can do. Be proud of pushing yourself up out of a chair or walking a short distance.

Pat yourself on the back for trying even if you cannot do it the first time. It may be easier the next time!

How do I continue to be active?

To maintain your active lifestyle, try these suggestions:

- Set goals. Set short-term and long-term goals. A short-term goal may be to walk 5 to 10 minutes, five days a week. It may not seem like a lot, but any activity is better than none. A long-term goal should be to do at least 30 minutes of moderate-intensity physical activity on most days of the week. You can accumulate your physical activity in shorter segments of 10 minutes or more. An example of a long-term goal is to walk briskly on five days of the week by the end of six months.

- Set rewards. Whether your goal was to be active for 15 minutes a day, to walk farther than you did last week, or simply to stay positive, you deserve recognition for your efforts. Some ideas for rewards include a new CD to motivate you, new walking shoes, or a new outfit.

- Get support. Get a family member or friend to be physically active with you. It may be more fun, and your buddy can cheer you on and help you stick with it.

- Track progress. Keep a journal of your physical activity. You may not feel like you are making progress but when you look back at where you started, you may be pleasantly surprised!

- Build up to it. Any physical activity is better than none, so start where you can and gradually increase the amount. The government recommends 30 minutes of moderate-intensity physical activity on most days of the week. Do not worry if that sounds like a lot! It does not have to be done all at once. Try breaking this into three 10-minute slots. A few minutes of activity here and there can really add up.

- Have fun! Try different activities to find the ones you really enjoy.

Do I need to see my health care provider before I start being physically active?

You should talk to your health care provider if any of the following apply to you:

- You have a chronic disease or have risk factors for a chronic disease, such as asthma or diabetes

- You have high blood pressure, high cholesterol, or a personal or family history of heart disease

- You are pregnant

- You are a smoker

- You are unsure of your health status or have any concerns that exercise might be unsafe for you

Chances are your health care provider will be pleased with your decision to start an activity program. It is unlikely that you will need a complete medical exam before you go out for a short walk.

What physical activities can a very large person do?

Most very large people can do some or all of the physical activities in this section. You do not need special skills or a lot of equipment. You can try the following:

- Weight-bearing activities, like walking, climbing stairs, and golfing, which involve lifting or pushing your own body weight

- Non-weight-bearing activities, like swimming and water workouts, which put less stress on your joints because you do not have to lift or push your own weight; if your feet or joints hurt when you stand, non-weight-bearing activities may be best for you

- Lifestyle activities, like gardening or washing the car, which are great ways to get moving (lifestyle activities do not have to be planned out ahead of time)

Remember that physical activity does not have to be hard or boring to be good for you. Anything that gets you moving around—even for only a few minutes a day—is a healthy start to getting more fit.

Walking (weight bearing): The walking that you do during the day (like doing chores around the house or in the yard) can help you become more fit. But regular, steady walking that makes you breathe heavier can help you to be healthier. It will give your heart and lungs—as well as your leg muscles—a good workout.

If you are not active now, start slowly. Try to walk 5 minutes a day for the first week. Walk 8 minutes the next week. Stay at 8-minute walks until you feel comfortable. Then increase your walks to 11 minutes. Slowly lengthen each walk by 3 minutes—or walk faster.

- Wear comfortable walking shoes with a lot of support. If you walk frequently, you may need to buy new shoes often. You may wish to speak with a podiatrist about when you need to purchase new walking shoes.

- Wear garments that prevent inner-thigh chafing, such as tights or spandex shorts.

- Make walking fun. Walk with a friend or pet. Walk in places you enjoy, like a park or shopping mall.

Dancing (weight bearing or non-weight bearing): Dancing may help in the following ways:

- Tone your muscles

- Improve your flexibility

- Make your heart stronger

- Make your lungs work better

You can dance in a health club, in a nightclub, or at home. To dance at home, just move your body to some lively music!

Dancing on your feet is a weight-bearing activity. Dancing while seated lets you move your arms and legs to music while taking the weight off your feet. This may be a good choice if you cannot stand on your feet for a long time.

Water workouts (non-weight bearing): Exercising in water offers the following benefits:

- Helps flexibility: You can bend and move your body in water in ways you cannot on land.

- Reduces risk of injury: Water makes your body float, which keeps your joints from being pounded or jarred and helps prevent sore muscles and injury.

- Keeps you refreshed: You can keep cool in water—even when you are working hard.

You do not need to know how to swim to work out in water—you can do shallow-water or deep-water exercises without swimming.

For shallow-water workouts, the water level should be between your waist and your chest. If the water is too shallow, it will be hard to move your arms underwater. If the water is deeper than chest height, it will be hard to keep your feet on the pool bottom.

For deep-water workouts, most of your body is underwater. This means that your whole body will get a good workout. For safety and comfort, wear a foam belt or life jacket.

Many swim centers offer classes in water workouts. Check with the pools in your area to find the best water workout for you.

Weight training (weight bearing or non-weight bearing): Weight training builds strong muscles and bones. Getting stronger may also help prepare you for other kinds of physical activity. You can weight train at home or at a fitness center.

You do not need benches or bars to begin weight training at home. You can use a pair of hand weights or even two soup cans.

Make sure you know the correct posture and that your movements are slow and controlled.

If you decide to buy a home gym, check its weight rating (the number of pounds it can support) to make sure it is safe for your size. If you want to join a fitness center where you can use weights, shop around for one where you feel at ease.

If you cannot lift a weight six times in a row, the weight you are lifting is too heavy. If you can easily lift a weight 15 times in a row, your weight is too light.

Bicycling (non-weight bearing): You can bicycle indoors on a stationary bike or outdoors on a road bike. Biking does not stress any one part of the body—your weight is spread among your arms, back, and hips.

You may want to use a recumbent bike. On this type of bike, you sit low to the ground with your legs reaching forward to the pedals. This may feel better than sitting upright. The seat on a recumbent bike is also wider than the seat on an upright bike.

For biking outdoors, you may want to try a mountain bike. These bikes have wider tires and are heavy. You can also buy a larger seat to put on your bike.

Make sure the bike you buy has a weight rating at least as high as your own weight.

Stretching (weight bearing or non-weight bearing): Stretching may help you in the following ways:

- Be more flexible
- Feel more relaxed
- Improve posture
- Keep your muscles from getting tight after doing other physical activities

You do not have to set aside a special time or place to stretch. At home or at work, stand up, push your arms toward the ceiling, and stretch. Stretch slowly and only enough to feel tightness—not until you feel pain. Hold the stretch, without bouncing, for about 30 seconds. Do not stretch cold muscles.

Yoga and tai chi are two types of stretching. They help you breathe deeply, relax, and get rid of stress. Your local fitness center may offer yoga, tai chi, or other stretching classes. You may want to start with "gentle" classes, like those aimed at seniors.

Lifestyle activities: Lifestyle physical activities do not have to be planned. You can make small changes to make your day more physically active and improve your health.

- Take two- to three-minute walking breaks at work a few times a day.
- Put away the TV remote control—get up to change the channel.
- March in place during TV commercials.
- Take the stairs instead of the elevator.
- Stand or walk, rather than sit, while talking on the phone.
- Play with your family—kids, grandchildren, nieces and nephews, and so forth.
- Walk to your co-worker's office rather than use the phone or email.

Even a shopping trip can be exercise: it is a chance to walk and carry your bags. In addition, doing chores like lawn mowing, leaf raking, gardening, and housework can count as activity.

Where should I work out?

You can do many activities in your home. But there are other fun places to be active, including health clubs, recreation centers, or outdoors. It may be hard to be physically active around other people. Keep in mind that you have just as much right to be healthy and active as anyone else.

What questions should I ask when choosing a fitness center?

- Can the treadmills or benches support people who are large?

- Does the fitness staff know how to work with people of larger sizes?

- Can I take time to see how I like the center before I sign up?

- Is the aim to have fun and get healthy—not to lose weight?

- What are the hours, and what time of day is it crowded?

Are there safety tips I should follow?

- Slow down if you feel out of breath. You should be able to talk during your activity, without gasping for breath.

- Drink water when you are thirsty to replace the water you lose by sweating.

- Wear suitable clothes.

    - Wear lightweight, loose-fitting tops so you can move easily.

    - Wear clothes made of fabrics that absorb sweat and remove it from your skin.

    - Never wear rubber or plastic suits. Plastic suits could hold the sweat on your skin and make your body overheat.

    - Women should wear a good support bra.

    - Wear supportive athletic shoes for weight-bearing activities.

    - Wear a knit hat to keep you warm when you are physically active outdoors in cold weather. Wear a tightly woven, wide-brimmed hat in hot weather to help keep you cool and protect you from the sun.

    - Wear sunscreen when you are physically active outdoors.

    - Wear garments that prevent inner-thigh chafing, such as tights or spandex shorts.

- Drink water when you are thirsty (water helps every cell and organ in your body work; it cushions your joints, helps keep you regular, keeps your body cool, and prevents dehydration when you are sweating).

- Stop your activity right away and talk to your health care provider if you experience any of these symptoms:

  - Have pain, tightness, or pressure in your chest or neck, shoulder, or arm

  - Feel dizzy or sick

  - Break out in a cold sweat

  - Have muscle cramps

  - Are extremely short of breath

  - Feel pain in your joints, feet, ankles, or legs (you could hurt yourself if you ignore the pain)

Healthy, fit bodies come in all sizes. Whatever your size or shape, get physically active now and keep moving for a healthier life!

Section 48.2

Fat Loss and Weight Training Myths

Spot Reduction Myth

Contrary to what the infomercials suggest there is no such thing as spot reduction. Fat is lost throughout the body in a pattern dependent upon genetics, sex (hormones), and age. Overall body fat must be reduced to lose fat in any particular area. Although fat is lost or gained throughout the body it seems the first area to get fat, or the last area to become lean, is the midsection (in men and some women, especially after menopause) and hips and thighs (in women and few men). Sit-ups, crunches, leg-hip raises, leg raises, hip adduction, hip abduction, etc. will only exercise the muscles under the fat.

Lower Abdominal Myth

It is widely believed the lower abs are exercised during the leg raise or other hip flexor exercises. However, it can be misleading to judge the mechanics of an exercise based on localized muscular fatigue. The primary muscle used in hip flexion is actually the iliopsoas, one of many hip flexors. The iliopsoas, particularly the psoas portion, happens to lie deep below the lower portion of the rectus abdominis. During the leg raise, the entire abdominal musculature isometrically contracts (contracts with no significant movement) to:

- posture the spine and pelvis;
  - supports the weight of the lower body so the lumbar spine does not hyperextend excessively;
  - maintains optimal biomechanics of the iliopsoas;
  - hips are kept from prematurely flexing if the lumbar spine and pelvis does not hyperextend excessively;

- iliopsoas can contract more forcefully in a relatively slight stretched position;

- bent knee (and hip) sit-ups actually place iliopsoas at a mechanical disadvantage.

- counteracts iliopsoas's pull on spine;

  - many people with weak abdominal muscles are not able to perform hip flexor exercises without acute lower back pain or discomfort.

The combination of the local muscular fatigue, or a burning sensation from the isometrically contracted abdominal muscles, and from the working hip flexors produces fatigue in the pelvis area which we mistakenly interpret as the lower portion of the rectus abdominis being exercised. In movements where the rectus abdominis does isotonically contract (contracts with movement), it flexes the spine by contracting the entire muscle from origin to insertion. The spine is not significantly flexed during the leg raise. Incidentally, both the spine and hip flexes during the full range of motion in sit-ups and leg-hip raises. See aforementioned spot reduction myth.

High Repetitions Burn More Fat Myth

Performing lighter weight with more repetitions (15–20 reps, 20–30 reps, or 20–50 reps) does not burn more fat or tone (simultaneous decrease of fat and increase muscle) better than a heaver weight with moderate repetitions (8–12 reps). Weight training utilizes carbohydrates after the initial ATP [adenosine triphosphate] and CP [creatine phosphate] stores have been exhausted after the first few seconds of intense muscular contraction. Typically a set's duration is 20 to 30 seconds. For the average fit person, it requires 20 to 30 minutes of continuous aerobic activity with large muscle groups (e.g. gluteus maximus and quadriceps) to burn even 50% fat; fat requires oxygen to burn. Performing a few extra repetitions on a weight-training exercise is not significant enough to burn extra fat and may in effect burn less fat. If intensity is compromised, less fat may be burned when light weight is used with high repetitions. The burning sensation associated with high repetition training seems to be the primary deterrent for achieving higher intensities.

Higher volume weight training (i.e., three sets versus one set of each exercise) with short rest periods of approximately one minute can stimulate a greater acute growth hormone release (Kraemer 1991,

1993; Mulligan 1996). Growth hormone is lipolytic in adults. It is hypothesized that maximal effort is necessary for optimizing exercise induced secretion of growth hormone. Growth hormone release is related to the magnitude of exertion (Pyka 1992) and is attenuated with greater lactic acidosis (Gordon 1994).

Intense weight training utilizing multiple large muscles with longer rest between sets may also accentuate body lipid deficit by increasing post training epinephrine. Intramuscular triacylglycerol is thought to be an important energy substrate following repeated 30 second maximal exercise with four minute recovery intervals (McCartney 1996, Tremblay 1994). Rest periods lasting approximately four minutes between maximal exercise of very short duration is required for almost complete creatine phosphate recovery required for repeated maximal bouts (McCartney 1986). Insufficient recovery may compromise the intensity of the exercise and in turn, possibly decrease intramuscular triacylglycerol utilization following anaerobic exercise with significantly shorter rest periods.

For individuals attempting to achieve fat loss for aesthetics, the intensity of weight training can be a double-edged sword. When beginning an exercise program, muscle mass increases may outpace fat losses, resulting in a small initial weight gain. Significant fat loss requires a certain intensity, duration, and frequency that novice exercisers may not be able to achieve until they develop greater tolerance to exercise. If an exercise and nutrition program is not adequate for significant fat loss, a lighter weight with higher repetitions may be recommended to minimize any bulking effects, although less fat may be utilized hours later. If an aerobic exercise and nutrition program is sufficient enough to lose fat, a moderate repetition range with a progressively heavier weight will accelerate fat loss with a toning effect. If a muscle group ever outpaces fat loss, the slight bulking effect is only temporary. For a toning effect, fat can be lost later when aerobic exercise can be significantly increased or the weight training exercise(s) for that particular muscle can be ceased altogether. The muscle will atrophy to a pre-exercise girth within months. Higher repetitions training may be later implemented and assessed.

It still may be recommended to perform high repetitions (e.g., 20–30) for abdominal and oblique training. It has been theorized muscular endurance may be more beneficial for lower back health than for muscular strength. Furthermore, moderate repetitions with a greater resistance can increase muscular girth under the subcutaneous fat, particularly in men, who have greater potential for muscular hypertrophy. Increasing the thickness around the waist with existing abdominal fat may further increase bulk, particularly in men who typically have greater intra-abdominal and subcutaneous fat in this area. The abdominal musculature is composed of relatively small muscle mass as compared to the glutes, quadriceps, hamstrings, chest, and upper back. Performing high reps with a lighter resistance should not compromise metabolism or muscle increases, as would performing high reps with light resistance on other, larger muscle groups. See aforementioned spot reduction myth.

It is plausible that the high repetition myth was originated and later propagated by bodybuilders that used calorie restrictive diets to shed fat before a contest. Because of their weakened state from dieting, they were unable to use their usual heavier weights. When asked about their use of lighter weights, they explained they were "cutting up" for a contest. This is merely a theory, but it is easy to see how it may have been misunderstood that the lighter weight was used to reduce fat instead of actually being a result of their dietary regime.

Typically with weight training alone, the fat loss is equal to the muscle gain, give or take a few pounds. Certain dietary modification can have much greater impact on fat loss than with weight training alone. The ideal program for fat loss would include the combination of proper diet, weight training, and cardio exercise. Also see study summaries: Weight Training and Diet (www.exrx.net/FatLoss/WTCalLBWStudy .html) and Endurance and Weight Training (www.exrx.net/FatLoss/ WT%26End.html).

Section 48.3

Abdominal Fat and Your Health

"Abdominal Obesity and Your Health," reprinted from the Harvard Medical School Family Health Guide, March 2009 update. © 2009 Harvard University. For additional information, visit www.health.harvard.edu/FHG.

Excess body weight has serious consequences for health. Obesity is responsible for high levels of LDL ("bad") cholesterol and triglycerides. At the same time, it lowers HDL ("good") cholesterol. It impairs the body's responsiveness to insulin, raising blood sugar and insulin levels. Obesity contributes to major causes of death and disability, including heart attacks, strokes, high blood pressure, cancer, diabetes, osteoarthritis, fatty liver, and depression.

Faced with these risks, it's no wonder that you want to know how much you should weigh. But this common and important question is actually the wrong question. For health, the issue is not how much you weigh, but how much abdominal fat you have.

Evaluating Obesity

Methods have changed over the years. But when scientists recognized that what matters is not body weight but body fat, standards began to change. The body mass index (BMI) remains enshrined as the standard way to diagnose overweight and obesity.

Beyond the BMI

The BMI provides a good estimate of body fat, and it's more accurate than skinfold measurements. Although the BMI is the official standard, it has several flaws. For one thing, highly trained athletes with big muscles can have BMIs of 30, with little body fat. At the other extreme, the BMI may fail to accurately reflect body fatness in adults who have lost substantial amounts of muscle mass. But the most important problem is that the BMI reflects total body fat without regard to how the fat is distributed. And although no excess fat is good, one type of excess fat is much more dangerous than the others. Research shows that abdominal fat is the worst of the worst.

The Inside Story

What makes abdominal fat so harmful? Scientists don't know for sure, but research is providing strong clues. To understand these clues, you must first understand that abdominal fat comes in two different forms. Some of it is located in the fatty tissue just beneath the skin. This *subcutaneous fat* behaves like the fat elsewhere in the body; it's no friend to health, but it's no special threat either.

Fat *inside* the abdomen is another story. This *visceral fat* is located around the internal organs, and it's the true villain of the piece. One of the earliest explanations for this was that visceral obesity was linked to overactivity of the body's stress response mechanisms, which raise blood pressure, blood sugar levels, and cardiac risk.

A newer explanation relies on the concept of *lipotoxicity*. Unlike subcutaneous fat, visceral fat cells release their metabolic products directly into the *portal circulation*, which carries blood straight to the liver. As a result, visceral fat cells that are enlarged and stuffed with excess triglycerides pour free fatty acids into the liver. Free fatty acids also accumulate in the pancreas, heart, and other organs. In all these locations, the free fatty acids accumulate in cells that are not engineered to store fat. The result is organ dysfunction, which produces impaired regulation of insulin, blood sugar, and cholesterol, as well as abnormal heart function.

These explanations are not mutually exclusive; all may help account for the hazards of visceral fat. All in all, clinical observations and basic research results agree that excessive fat inside the abdomen is a major contributor to cardiovascular disease.

Evaluating Abdominal Obesity

The most accurate method is to use computed tomography (CT) or magnetic resonance imaging (MRI) to measure the amount of visceral fat. But they're expensive and require sophisticated equipment.

A far simpler method is to determine the waist-to-hip ratio. With your abdomen relaxed, measure your waist at the navel. Next, measure your hips at their widest point, usually at the bony prominences. Finally, divide your waist size by your hip size: waist (in inches) / hips (in inches) = ratio.

How does your ratio translate into health risk? The chance of suffering a heart attack or stroke increases steadily as a man's ratio rises above 0.95; for women, risk begins to rise above 0.85.

The waist-to-hip ratio is a very useful tool. But many experts are now turning to an even simpler technique: waist circumference.

Because it involves one measurement instead of two, it's more accurate and reproducible than the waist-to-hip ratio.

To measure your waist circumference properly, take your shoes off and stand with your feet together. Be sure your belly is bare. Relax and exhale. Using a cloth measuring tape that can't be stretched, not the stiff metal tape from your toolbox, measure your waist at the navel. Be sure to keep the tape parallel to the ground. Record the measurement to the nearest one-tenth of an inch.

Table 48.1. Interpreting Your Waist Circumference

	Men	**Women**
Low risk	37 inches and below	31.5 inches and below
Intermediate risk	37.1–39.9 inches	31.6–34.9 inches
High risk	40 inches and above	35 inches and above

Girth Control

Measuring your waist to learn if you have abdominal obesity and excess visceral fat is easy—but doing something about it is much harder.

Remember the basics. The only way to reduce visceral fat is to lose weight—and the only way to do that is to burn up more calories with exercise than you take in from food. Sustained weight loss requires both caloric restriction and increased exercise.

BMI versus Waist Circumference

The BMI is more complex, but waist measurement is more prone to errors than measuring height and weight. So for the time being, you should use both standards. Your BMI will give you the best estimate of your total body fatness, while your waist measurement will give you the best estimate of your visceral fat and risk of obesity-related disease.

Chapter 49

Physical Fitness for People with Heart Conditions

Physical Activity: The Heart Connection

Chances are, you already know that physical activity is good for you. "Sure," you may say, "When I get out and move around, I know it helps me to look and feel better." But you may not realize just how important regular physical activity is to your health. Inactive people are nearly twice as likely to develop heart disease as those who are active. Lack of physical activity also leads to more visits to the doctor, more hospitalizations, and more use of medicines for a variety of illnesses. The good news is that physical activity can protect your heart in a number of important ways and keep you healthy overall.

Heart Disease Risk Factors

Risk factors are conditions or habits that make a person more likely to develop a disease. They can also increase the chances that an existing disease will get worse. Certain risk factors for heart disease, such as getting older or having a family history of early heart disease, can't be changed. But physical inactivity is a major risk factor for heart disease that you can control.

Other major risk factors for heart disease that you can control are smoking, high blood pressure, high blood cholesterol, overweight, and

---

This chapter excerpted from "In Brief: Your Guide to Physical Activity and Your Heart," National Heart, Lung, and Blood Institute (www.nhlbi.nih.gov), January 2008.

diabetes. Every risk factor greatly increases the chances of developing heart disease and having a heart attack. A damaged heart can keep you from doing simple, enjoyable things, such as taking a walk or climbing steps. But it's important to know that you have a lot of power to protect your heart health. Getting regular physical activity is especially important because it directly reduces your heart disease risk and your chances of developing other risk factors for heart disease. Physical activity can also protect your heart by helping to prevent and control diabetes. Finally, physical activity can help you to lose excess weight or to stay at a healthy weight, which will also help to lower your risk of heart disease.

You Have Control

Physical inactivity is one of several major risk factors for heart disease that you can do something about. The other major risk factors are the following:

Smoking: People who smoke are up to six times more likely to have a heart attack than nonsmokers. Check with local community groups for free or low-cost programs designed to help people stop smoking.

High blood pressure increases your risk of heart disease, stroke, and other conditions. It can be controlled by getting regular physical activity, losing excess weight, cutting down on alcohol, and changing eating habits, such as using less salt and other forms of sodium. For some people, medication is also needed.

High blood cholesterol can lead to a buildup of plaque in your arteries, which raises your risk for a heart attack. You can lower high blood cholesterol by getting regular physical activity, eating less saturated fat and trans fat, and managing your weight. For some people, medication is also needed.

Overweight: If you're overweight or obese, you're more likely to develop heart disease even if you have no other risk factors. However, there is good news: Losing just 5–10% of your current weight will help to lower your risk for heart disease and many other medical disorders.

Type 2 diabetes greatly increases your risk for heart disease, stroke, and other serious diseases. Ask your health care provider whether you should be tested for diabetes. Many people at high risk for diabetes can prevent or delay the disease by reducing calories as part of a healthy eating plan and by becoming more physically active.

The Benefits Keep Coming

In addition to protecting your heart, staying active has other effects:

- May help to prevent cancers of the breast, uterus, and colon
- Strengthens your lungs and helps them to work more efficiently
- Tones and strengthens your muscles
- Builds your stamina
- Keeps your joints in good condition
- Improves your balance
- May slow bone loss

Regular physical activity can also boost the way you feel in these ways:

- Give you more energy
- Help you to relax, cope better with stress, and beat the blues
- Build your confidence
- Allow you to fall asleep more quickly and sleep more soundly
- Provide you with an enjoyable way to share time with friends or family

Physical Activity: The Calorie Connection

One way that regular physical activity protects against heart disease is by burning extra calories, which can help you to lose excess weight or stay at your healthy weight. To understand how physical activity affects calories, it's helpful to consider the concept of "energy balance." Energy balance is the amount of calories you take in relative to the amount of calories you burn. If you need to lose weight for your health, eating fewer calories and being more active is the best approach. You're more likely to be successful by combining a healthful, lower calorie diet with physical activity. For example, a 200-pound person who consumes 250 fewer calories per day and walks briskly each day for 1 1/2 miles will lose about 40 pounds in one year. Most of the energy you burn each day—about three-quarters of it—goes to activities that your body automatically engages in for survival, such as breathing, sleeping, and digesting food. The part of your energy output that you control is daily physical activity. Any activity you take part in beyond your body's automatic activities will burn extra calories. Even seated activities, such as using the computer or watching TV, will burn calories—but only a very small number. That's why it's important to make time each day for moderate-to vigorous-intensity physical activity.

If you are just starting or significantly increasing your physical activity, take proper precautions and check with your doctor first.

Great Moves

Given the numerous benefits of regular physical activity, you may be ready to get in motion! Three types of activity are important for a complete physical activity program: aerobic activity, resistance training, and flexibility exercises.

Aerobic activity is any physical activity that uses large muscle groups and causes your body to use more oxygen than it would while resting. Aerobic activity is the type of movement that most benefits the heart.

Examples of aerobic activity are brisk walking, jogging, and bicycling. If you're just starting to be active, try brisk walking for short periods such as 5 or 10 minutes, and build up gradually to 30 to 60 minutes at least five days per week. Always start with a 5-minute, slower paced walk to warm up, and end with a 5-minute, slower paced walk to cool down.

Resistance training—also called strength training—can firm, strengthen, and tone your muscles, as well as improve bone strength, balance, and coordination. Examples of resistance training are push-ups, lunges, and bicep curls using dumbbells.

Flexibility exercises stretch and lengthen your muscles. These activities help improve joint flexibility and keep muscles limber, thereby preventing injury. An example of a flexibility exercise is sitting cross-legged on the floor and gently pushing down on the tops of your legs to stretch the inner-thigh muscles.

Family Fitness

When it comes to getting in shape, what's good for you is good for your whole family. Children and teenagers should be physically active for at least 60 minutes per day. A great way to pry kids off the couch—and help you to stay fit as well—is to do enjoyable activities together.

Some ideas include the following:

- Kick up your heels. Take turns picking out your favorite music, and dance up a storm in the living room.

- Explore the outdoors. Hit your local trail on weekends for some biking or hiking. Pack a healthy lunch, and let the kids choose the picnic spot.

- Get classy. Join family members in an active class, such as martial arts, yoga, or aerobics.

- Play pupil. Ask one of your children or grandchildren to teach you an active game or sport. Kids love to be the experts, and you'll get a work out learning a new activity!

- Use online resources. Check out the We Can! website at wecan. nhlbi.nih.gov. You'll find more family-friendly ideas for making smart food choices, increasing physical activity, and reducing "screen time" in front of the TV and other electronic attractions.

Creating Opportunities

It's easier to stay physically active over time if you take advantage of everyday opportunities to move around.

- Use the stairs—both up and down—instead of the elevator. Start with one flight of stairs and gradually build up to more.

- Park a few blocks from the office or store and walk the rest of the way. If you take public transportation, get off a stop or two early and walk a few blocks.

- While working, take frequent activity breaks. Get up and stretch, walk around, and give your muscles and mind a chance to relax.

- Instead of eating that extra snack, take a brisk stroll around the neighborhood or your office building.

- Do housework, gardening, or yard work at a more vigorous pace.

- When you travel, walk around the train station, bus station, or airport rather than sitting and waiting.

Chapter 50

Physical Fitness for People with Bone Disorders

Chapter Contents

Section 50.1

Arthritis and Fitness

This section excerpted from "Exercise and Arthritis," Federal Occupational Health, Department of Health and Human Services (www.foh.dhhs.gov), February 2004, reviewed by David A. Cooke, MD, FACP, May 2010, and "Arthritis Basics: Frequently Asked Questions," Centers for Disease Control and Prevention (www.cdc.gov), October 28, 2009.

Arthritis and Exercise

Arthritis is one of the most pervasive diseases in the United States and is the leading cause of disability. According to the National Institutes of Health, an estimated 43 million people in the United States have arthritis or other rheumatic conditions. In general, people who have arthritis feel pain and stiffness in their joints, and, because of this pain, they often tend to limit activity. However, a diagnosis of arthritis does not have to signal an end to enjoyable physical activities.

It was thought for many years that people with arthritis should limit their exercise because it would increase the risk of damage to their joints. This kind of thinking has changed dramatically because recent research has shown that exercise is actually an essential part of a comprehensive disease management plan. And while people with arthritis should first discuss exercise options with their health care providers, it is now widely believed that arthritis sufferers actually benefit greatly from a variety of sensible exercises designed for them. For example, gentle range-of-motion exercises help maintain normal joint movement, and strength training can strengthen muscles that support affected joints.

Properly executed, exercise may reduce joint pain and stiffness, strengthens muscles, helps bone and cartilage stay strong and healthy, and improves the ability to manage everyday activities. In conjunction with medicine, rest, and a prescribed treatment program, regular exercise can help keep joints in working order and vastly improve the quality of one's life. In order to select from the many types of exercises that will best meet individual needs, the Arthritis Foundation suggests finding a nationally certified fitness professional. Certified fitness professionals are trained to design safe and effective exercise programs with regard to physical limitations and medical conditions.

Questions about Arthritis and Exercise

How can I manage arthritis pain?

Both medical treatment and self-management strategies are very important. The Arthritis Foundation Self Help Program and the Chronic Disease Self-Management Program, both developed by Dr. Kate Lorig of Stanford University, are effective self-management education programs. These programs help people learn the techniques needed to manage their arthritis on a day-to-day basis and gain the confidence to carry it out.

Physical activity can also help reduce pain. Programs like the Arthritis Foundation Exercise Program and Enhance Fitness can help can help you safely increase your physical activity.

What does the CDC recommend for people with arthritis?

The CDC recommends the following:

Early diagnosis and appropriate management of arthritis, including self-management activities, can help people with arthritis decrease pain, improve function, stay productive, and lower health care costs. Key self-management activities include the following:

Learn arthritis management strategies: Learning techniques to reduce pain and limitations can be beneficial to people with arthritis. Self-management education, such as the Arthritis Foundation Self Help Program (AFSHP) or the Chronic Disease Self Management Program (CDSMP), help you learn the strategies and develop the confidence to manage your arthritis on a day-to-day basis. For example, AFSHP has been shown to reduce pain even four years after participating in the program.

Be active: Research has shown that physical activity decreases pain, improves function, and delays disability. Make sure you get at least 30 minutes of moderate physical activity five days a week. You can get activity in 10-minute intervals.

Watch your weight: The prevalence of arthritis increases with increasing weight. Research suggests that maintaining a healthy weight reduces the risk of developing arthritis and may decrease disease progression. A loss of just 11 pounds can decrease the occurrence (incidence) of new knee osteoarthritis.

See your doctor: Although there is no cure for most types of arthritis, early diagnosis and appropriate management are important, especially for inflammatory types of arthritis. For example, early use of disease-modifying drugs can affect the course of rheumatoid arthritis. If you have symptoms of arthritis, see your doctor and begin appropriate management of your condition.

Protect your joints: Joint injury can lead to osteoarthritis. People who experience sports or occupational injuries or have jobs with repetitive motions like repeated knee bending have more osteoarthritis. Avoid joint injury to reduce your risk of developing osteoarthritis.

Is exercise recommended for people who have arthritis?

Recent studies have shown that moderate physical activity five or more days a week can help to relieve arthritis pain and stiffness and give you more energy. Regular physical activity can also lift your mood and make you feel more positive.

An activity that produces a slight increase in heart rate or breathing is considered moderate physical activity. Low-impact activities performed at a moderate pace work best for people with arthritis. These include walking, swimming, and riding a bicycle. Everyday activities such as dancing, gardening, and washing the car can be good if done at a moderate pace that produces slight breathing and heart rate changes.

If you are having an acute flare-up of your inflammatory arthritis, it may be better to restrict your exercise to simple range of motion (carefully moving the joint as far as it can go) during the flare-up.

How does body weight influence arthritis?

Weight control is essential; research suggests that maintaining a healthy weight reduces the risk of developing osteoarthritis and may decrease disease progression. A loss of just 11 pounds can decrease the occurrence (incidence) of new knee osteoarthritis.

Section 50.2

Exercising Safely with Osteoporosis

This section excerpted from "Once Is Enough: A Guide to Preventing Future Fractures," National Institute of Arthritis and Musculoskeletal and Skin Diseases (www.niams.nih.gov), January 2009.

Many people are unaware of the link between a broken bone and osteoporosis. Osteoporosis, or "porous bone," is a disease characterized by low bone mass. It makes bones fragile and more prone to fractures, especially the bones of the hip, spine, and wrist. Osteoporosis is called a "silent disease" because bone loss occurs without symptoms. People typically do not know that they have osteoporosis until their bones become so weak that a sudden strain, twist, or fall results in a fracture. The following concerns address fitness for those who have had a fracture or who are at risk for a fracture.

I've always been active, but I don't want to risk breaking another bone. Maybe I need to spend more time "on the sidelines" from now on.

It is perfectly understandable that you want to avoid another fracture. No one who has broken a bone wants to revisit that pain and loss of independence. However, living your life "on the sidelines" is not an effective way to protect your bones. Remaining physically active reduces your risk of heart disease, colon cancer, and type 2 diabetes. It may also protect you against prostate and breast cancer, high blood pressure, obesity, and mood disorders such as depression and anxiety. If that isn't enough to convince you to stay active, consider this: exercise is one of the best ways to preserve your bone density and prevent falls as you age.

What type of exercise is best to reduce my risk of another fracture?

Exercise can reduce your risk of fracturing in two ways—by helping you build and maintain bone density and by enhancing your balance, flexibility, and strength, all of which reduce your chance of falling.

- **Building and maintaining bone density:** Bone is a living tissue that responds to exercise by becoming stronger. Just as a muscle gets stronger and bigger with use, a bone becomes stronger and denser when it is called upon to bear weight. Two types of exercise are important for building and maintaining bone density: weight bearing and resistance. Weight-bearing exercises are those in which your bones and muscles work against gravity. Examples include walking, climbing stairs, dancing, and playing tennis. Resistance exercises are those that use muscular strength to improve muscle mass and strengthen bone. The best example of a resistance exercise is weight training, with either free weights or weight machines.

- **Reducing the risk of falling:** You can significantly reduce your risk of falling by engaging in activities that enhance your balance, flexibility, and strength.

  - **Balance** is the ability to maintain your body's stability while moving or standing still. You can improve your balance with activities such as tai chi and yoga.

  - **Flexibility** refers to the range of motion of a muscle or group of muscles. You can improve your flexibility through tai chi, swimming, yoga, and gentle stretching exercises.

  - **Strength** refers to your body's ability to develop and maintain strong muscles. Lifting weights will increase your strength.

Smart Moves

- Walking
- Strength training
- Dancing
- Tai chi
- Stair climbing
- Hiking
- Bicycling
- Swimming
- Gardening

How can I exercise safely if I have osteoporosis?

If you have osteoporosis, it is important for you to get plenty of exercise. However, you will need to choose your activities carefully. Be sure to avoid activities with a high risk of falling, such as skiing or skating; those that have too much impact, such as jogging and jumping rope; and those that cause you to twist or bend, such as golf.

Unfortunately, some people become so afraid of breaking another bone that they become more sedentary, which leads to further loss of bone and muscle. Rest assured, however, that by practicing proper posture and learning the correct way to move, you can protect your bones while remaining physically active. Every activity can be adapted to meet your age, ability, lifestyle, and strength. Your doctor or a physical therapist can help you design a safe and effective exercise program. In the meantime, here are some general guidelines for safe movement.

Don't do the following:

- Wear shoes with slippery soles

- Slouch when standing, walking, or sitting at a desk

- Move too quickly

- Engage in sports or activities that require twisting the spine or bending forward from the waist, such as conventional sit-ups, toe touches, or swinging a golf club

Do take the following precautions:

- Pay attention to proper posture. This includes lifting your breastbone, keeping your head erect and eyes forward, keeping your shoulders back, lightly "pinching" your shoulder blades, and tightening your abdominal muscles and buttocks.

- Make sure to use a handrail when climbing stairs.

- Bend from the hips and knees and never from the waist, especially when lifting.

Before embarking on any exercise program, be sure to consult your doctor.

Chapter 51

Physical Fitness for People with Asthma

Chapter Contents

Section 51.1

Exercise for People with Asthma

Fit to Breathe

Be honest. You're among friends—you can admit the truth. That New Year's resolution to be fit and healthy is teetering just a wee bit, right? After all, this has been a tough asthma, cold, and flu season for most of the country, and darned near impossible to keep up with work, kids, and running errands—much less running a mile.

The good news is that it's never too late to regroup and get back on track. The key is knowing that a fit and healthy body means more than fitting into your jeans or getting rid of that muffin top from your kids. The more fit the family, the better everyone breathes.

The Catch-22 for adults and parents of children with asthma is that we're taught to slow down and rest during asthma flares. While this advice may be accurate, it was never intended as a long-term solution to controlling asthma.

It's no secret that asthma rates have doubled in the past two decades. It's the fifth leading chronic disease among children under 18 in the United States, and it's the third most common cause of child hospitalization for children 15 years and younger.

But the lesser appreciated stats concern the correlation between obesity and asthma. Factor in the escalating rate of obesity—which tripled from 6.1 to 17.6% over the past three decades, according to the Centers for Disease Control and Prevention (CDC)—and it's hard to ignore this dual issue.

Obesity doesn't just happen overnight. It sneaks up on you, and in the case of adults and children with asthma and COPD [chronic obstructive pulmonary disease], the consequences are even more serious. So how do you fix things?

Contrary to what many parents might think, exercise is great for children with asthma. A Johns Hopkins study found that 20% of all children with asthma don't exercise enough, primarily due to parents' fear of exercise-induced episodes. And while kids may prefer to watch TV or play video and computer games rather than run the risk of an attack, there are ways for parents to encourage them to explore safe and fun ways to exercise to keep their bodies and minds fit.

It doesn't happen overnight—whether you're starting a healthy new routine for yourself or helping a child with a respiratory issue, including exercise in one's daily routine is a process.

First step is to talk with your doctor and get a written asthma action plan that includes being able to exercise without fear of an asthma flare-up. Next, you need your body to be well-fed and hydrated. Eat a balanced diet and drink enough fluid to support physical activity (especially for people with food allergies!). A healthy diet paired with exercise has been shown to strengthen bones, the heart, and the immune system, which means fewer cases of colds, flu, and other viruses.

The Mind-Body Connection

A healthy diet-and-exercise combo improves moods and stress levels. Being able to participate in school and community sports programs like their peers is also a way for kids with asthma to shake off the stigma of isolation and feeling like the last person anyone wants on their team. Healthy eating and an active lifestyle also boost concentration.

An upbeat attitude toward exercise can make all the difference in sticking with a healthy new lifestyle change. Studies show that people develop habits in childhood, good or bad—and these tend to last a lifetime. Rather than accommodating asthma, families can plan together to overcome it!

Experiment with exercise. During a flare, try yoga. Doesn't burn many calories but simple positions and deep-breathing exercises ease your airways into higher levels of performance.

Experiment with food! When you expand your horizons, opening up to activities and healthy foods—you're giving your body beneficial new nutrients, getting fit, and having fun!

Don't get bummed out over food allergies either! It's possible to eat a healthy balanced diet even though it may not be the one you grew up eating or consider normal. About 90% of all food allergies are typically caused by only eight foods—tree nuts, shellfish, milk, soy, wheat, egg, peanuts, and fish. This leaves hundreds of different foods to choose from when creating healthy meals. Think fresh. Think whole foods versus packaged. Saves money, leaves less waste, and tastes better! Saves time reading food labels as well!

About the Authors

First published: *Allergy & Asthma Today,* Spring 2010 (www.aanma. org/publication/aat-subscription).

Chef Michelle Austin is a chef, founder of On Thyme Consulting and contributor to *SOBeFiT* magazine (www.sobefitmagazine.com). She's also co-owner and creative director of Just to Please You Productions, an event production and consulting company, and has been featured on food and design segments on NBC and CBS. Michelle lives in Miami with her daughter, Gabrielle.

Lisa Dorfman, MS, RD, CSSD, LMHC, is a licensed nutritionist, board-certified specialist in sports dietetics and counseling, and author of five books. Lisa is also an adjunct professor at the University of Miami's Department of Exercise and Sports Science, nutritionist for the Miami Hurricanes and the U.S. Olympic and Paralympic sailing teams, and nutrition editor for *SOBeFiT* magazine. She lives in Miami with her husband and three children.

Medical editors: Robert Bahadori, MD, and Neil MacIntyre Jr., MD.

Smart Starts

Fuel up before and refuel after exercise. We lose fluids through sweat and our muscles use up carbohydrate energy. In order for our bodies to recover completely after exercise, we need to replenish these resources. Post-exercise fuel should be consumed within 30 minutes to two hours after exercising. An easy way to refuel is with a healthy shake.

Chef Michelle's Recovery Shake

You can make this shake with any favorite fruits and vegetables in place of the berries. There's no need to add sugar—fruits have natural sugars of their own.

4 oz vanilla Greek yogurt*

1/4 cup quinoa*

1/2 cup mixed berries (like strawberries and blueberries)

1/2 kiwi*

2 oz beet juice

2 oz filtered water

*Greek yogurt has more protein, less lactose, and fewer carbs than regular yogurt. Substitute tofu-, soy- or any milk-based yogurt if you like.

*Quinoa is a wheat-free grain from Africa. Many ancient civilizations used it, but most Americans are unfamiliar with this tasty treat. It has the consistency of small couscous, a mild flavor that cooks in minutes, and is great for shakes, salads, and side dishes.

*Kiwi—do you have latex allergies? Allergic to bananas? Substitute the kiwi with a fruit you enjoy.

View the nutrition facts online at www.aanma.org/wordpress/wp-content/uploads/Shake_nutritional_facts.pdf.

Step by Step

Studies show that exercising on a routine basis reduces the amount of medication needed to control asthma symptoms, and also reduces the number of asthma attacks. Exercise improves lung capacity—the more fit you are, the less likely you are to experience an asthma attack. Resistance training (working out with weights and doing exercises that work your muscles) most likely won't provoke asthma attacks. Here's a customized routine created by Marta Montenegro, founder, CEO, publisher, and editor-in-chief of SOBeFiT magazine, specifically for people with asthma and other respiratory conditions.

Before you begin any workout regimen, check with your doctor to determine how much you can exercise based on your fitness level and asthma condition. People with well-controlled asthma should be able to sleep, work, and play like everyone else.

- Keep asthma medications (such as a bronchodilator) handy when working out in case you become short of breath.

- Take plenty of time to warm up and cool down—at least 10 minutes for each.

- Walking, baseball, gymnastics, and swimming are great activities for people with asthma!

- For more high-intensity sports and activities (such as running or soccer), start slow. Gradually increase the intensity over time.

- Avoid exercising outside on days when air pollution is high or in cold or dry air. If you have seasonal allergies, you might need to avoid activities on high pollen days, as well. Talk with an allergist about immunotherapy if your allergies keep you from doing your favorite activities.

- If you start to have asthma symptoms during exercise—stop, and follow your asthma action plan, including medication if necessary. When symptoms go away, you can resume your workout. If you still feel short of breath, you should stop exercising, use medication as necessary, and consult your doctor for advice.

Source: Chan Tran, executive staff writer for *SOBeFiT* magazine.

Section 51.2

Exercise-Induced Asthma

Everyone needs to exercise, even people with asthma! A strong healthy body is one of your best defenses against disease. But some people with asthma have "exercise-induced asthma" (EIA). But with proper medical prevention and management you should be able to walk, climb stairs, run, and participate in activities, sports, and exercise without experiencing symptoms. You don't have to let EIA keep you from leading an active life or from achieving your athletic dreams.

What Is Exercise-Induced Asthma?

Exercise is a common cause of asthma symptoms. This is usually called exercise-induced asthma or exercise-induced bronchospasm (EIB). It is estimated that 80 to 90% of all individuals who have allergic asthma will experience symptoms of EIA with vigorous exercise or activity. For teenagers and young adults this is often the most common cause of asthma symptoms. Fortunately with better medications, monitoring, and management you can participate in physical activity and sports and achieve your highest performance level.

What Are the Symptoms of EIA?

Symptoms of exercised-induced asthma include coughing, wheezing, chest tightness, and shortness of breath. Coughing is the most common symptom of EIA and may be the only symptom you have. The symptoms of EIA may begin during exercise and will usually be worse 5 to 10 minutes after stopping exercise. Symptoms most often resolve in another 20 to 30 minutes and can range from mild to severe. Occasionally some individuals will experience "late phase" symptoms 4 to 12 hours after stopping exercise. Late-phase symptoms are frequently less severe and can take up to 24 hours to go away.

What Causes EIA?

When you exercise you breathe faster due to the increased oxygen demands of your body. Usually during exercise you inhale through your mouth, causing the air to be dryer and cooler than when you breathe through your nasal passages. This decrease in warmth and humidity are both causes of bronchospasm. Exercise that exposes you to cold air such as skiing or ice hockey is therefore more likely to cause symptoms than exercise involving warm and humid air such as swimming. Pollution levels, high pollen counts, and exposure to other irritants such as smoke and strong fumes can also make EIA symptoms worse. A recent cold or asthma episode can cause you to have more difficulty exercising.

How Is EIA Diagnosed?

It is important to know the difference between being out of condition and having exercise-induced asthma. A well-conditioned person will usually only experience the symptoms of EIA with vigorous activity or exercise. To make a diagnosis, your doctor will take a thorough history and may perform a series of test. During these tests, which may include running or a treadmill test, your doctor will measure your lung functions using a spirometer before, during, and after exercise. Monitoring your peak flows before, during, and after exercise can also help you and your doctor detect narrowing of your airways. Then, using guidelines established by your doctor you can help prevent asthma symptoms and participate in and enjoy physical activity. Your doctor will also tell you what to do should a full-blown episode occur.

Treatment and Management of EIA

With proper treatment and management people with EIA can participate safely and achieve their full potential. Proper management requires that you take steps to prevent symptoms and carefully monitor your respiratory status before, during, and after exercise. Taking medication prior to exercising is important in preventing EIA. Proper warm-up for 6 to 10 minutes before periods of exercise or vigorous activity will usually help. Individuals who can tolerate continuous exercise with minimal symptoms may find that proper warm-up may prevent the need for repeated medications.

What Types of Medications Treat/Prevent EIA?

There are three types of medications to prevent or treat the symptoms of EIA. Your health care provider can help you determine the best treatment program for you based on your asthma condition and the type of activity or exercise.

The first medication is a short-acting beta2-agonist, also called a bronchodilator. This medication can prevent symptoms and should be taken 10 to 15 minutes before exercise. It will help prevent symptoms for up to four hours. This same medication can also be used to treat and reverse the symptoms of EIA should they occur.

The second medication is a long-acting bronchodilator. It needs to be taken 30 to 60 minutes prior to activity and only once within a 12-hour period. Salmeterol can help prevent EIA symptoms for 10 to 12 hours. This medication should only be used to prevent symptoms and should never be used to relieve symptoms once they occur because it does not offer any quick relief.

The third type of medication is cromolyn or nedocromil. They also need to be taken 15 to 20 minutes prior to exercise. There is also some evidence that taking these medications will also help to prevent the late-phase reaction of EIA that is experienced by some individuals. These medications also should only be used as a preventative measure because they do not relieve symptoms once they begin. Some individuals use one of these medications in combination with a short-acting bronchodilator.

If you have frequent symptoms with usual activity or exercise, talk to your doctor. An increase in your long-term control medications may help. Long-term anti-inflammatory medications, such as inhaled steroids, can reduce the frequency and severity of EIA.

Teachers and coaches should be informed if a child has exercise-induced asthma. They should be told that the child should be able to participate in activities, but that they may require medication prior to activity. Athletes should also disclose their medications and adhere to standards set by the U.S. Olympic Committee. Approved and prohibited medications can be obtained from the committee hotline (800-233-0393).

What Types of Sports Are Best for People with EIA?

Activities that involve only short burst of exercise or intermittent periods of activity are usually better tolerated. Such sports include walking, volleyball, and gymnastics or baseball. Swimming that involves breathing warm and moist air is often well tolerated. Aerobic sports such as distance running, soccer, or basketball are more likely to cause symptoms. In addition cold air sports such as ice hockey or ice-skating may not be tolerated as well.

It is important to consult with your health care provider prior to beginning any exercise program and to pace yourself. With effective management people with EIA can perform and excel in a variety of sports. Many Olympic athletes and professional athletes with exercise-induced asthma have excelled in their sports, many winning Olympic gold medals.

Remember, with proper medical management you should be able to walk, climb stairs, run, and participate in activities, sports, and exercise without experiencing symptoms. Do not let EIA keep you from leading an active life or from achieving your athletic dreams.

Chapter 52

Physical Fitness for People with Diabetes

How can I take care of my diabetes?

Diabetes means your blood glucose, also called blood sugar, is too high. Your body uses glucose for energy. But having too much glucose in your blood can hurt you.

When you take care of your diabetes, you'll feel better. You'll reduce your risk for problems with your kidneys, eyes, nerves, feet and legs, and teeth. You'll also lower your risk for a heart attack or a stroke. You can take care of your diabetes by doing the following:

- Being physically active

- Following a healthy meal plan

- Taking medicines, if prescribed by your doctor

What can a physically active lifestyle do for me?

Research has shown that physical activity can accomplish the following:

- Lower your blood glucose and your blood pressure

- Lower your bad cholesterol and raise your good cholesterol

- Improve your body's ability to use insulin

"What I Need to Know about Physical Activity and Diabetes," National Institute of Diabetes and Digestive and Kidney Diseases (www.niddk.nih.gov), March 2008.

- Lower your risk for heart disease and stroke
- Keep your heart and bones strong
- Keep your joints flexible
- Lower your risk of falling
- Help you lose weight
- Reduce your body fat
- Give you more energy
- Reduce your stress levels

Physical activity also plays an important part in preventing type 2 diabetes. A major government study, the Diabetes Prevention Program (DPP), showed that modest weight loss of 5 to 7%—for example, 10 to 15 pounds for a 200-pound person—can delay and possibly prevent type 2 diabetes. People in the study used diet and exercise to lose weight.

For more information about the study, read the DPP fact sheet online. Go to www.diabetes.niddk.nih.gov/intro and click on Diabetes Prevention Program under "Pre-diabetes." Or call the National Diabetes Information Clearinghouse at 800-860-8747 to request a printed copy.

What kinds of physical activity can help me?

Be extra active every day: Being extra active can increase the number of calories you burn. Try these ways to be extra active, or think of other things you can do.

- Walk around while you talk on the phone.
- Play with the kids.
- Take the dog for a walk.
- Get up to change the TV channel instead of using the remote control.
- Work in the garden or rake leaves.
- Clean the house.
- Wash the car.
- Stretch out your chores. For example, make two trips to take the laundry downstairs instead of one.
- Park at the far end of the shopping center parking lot and walk to the store.

- At the grocery store, walk down every aisle.
- At work, walk over to see a co-worker instead of calling or emailing.
- Take the stairs instead of the elevator.
- Stretch or walk around instead of taking a coffee break and eating.
- During your lunch break, walk to the post office or do other errands.

Do aerobic exercise: Aerobic exercise is activity that requires the use of large muscles and makes your heart beat faster. You will also breathe harder during aerobic exercise. Doing aerobic exercise for 30 minutes a day at least five days a week provides many benefits. You can even split up those 30 minutes into several parts. For example, you can take three brisk 10-minute walks, one after each meal.

If you haven't exercised lately, see your doctor first to make sure it's okay for you to increase your level of physical activity. Talk with your doctor about how to warm up and stretch before you exercise and how to cool down after you exercise. Then start slowly with 5 to 10 minutes a day. Add a little more time each week, aiming for at least 150 minutes per week. Try these activities:

- Walking briskly
- Hiking
- Climbing stairs
- Swimming or taking a water-aerobics class
- Dancing
- Riding a bicycle outdoors or a stationary bicycle indoors
- Taking an aerobics class
- Playing basketball, volleyball, or other sports
- In-line skating, ice skating, or skate boarding
- Playing tennis
- Cross-country skiing

The National Institute on Aging offers a free booklet, "Exercise: A Guide From the National Institute on Aging." To read it online, go to www.nia.nih.gov/HealthInformation/Publications, click on "Healthy Aging," and then choose "Exercise Guide (only)." Or call 800–222–2225 to request a printed copy.

Do strength training: Doing exercises with hand weights, elastic bands, or weight machines three times a week builds muscle. When you have more muscle and less fat, you'll burn more calories because muscle burns more calories than fat, even between exercise sessions. Strength training can help make daily chores easier, improving your balance and coordination, as well as your bones' health. You can do strength training at home, at a fitness center, or in a class. Your health care team can tell you more about strength training and what kind is best for you.

Stretch: Stretching increases your flexibility, lowers stress, and helps prevent muscle soreness after other types of exercise. Your health care team can tell you what kind of stretching is best for you.

Can I exercise any time I want?

Your health care team can help you decide the best time of day for you to exercise. Together, you and your team will consider your daily schedule, your meal plan, and your diabetes medicines.

If you have type 1 diabetes, avoid strenuous exercise when you have ketones in your blood or urine. Ketones are chemicals your body might make when your blood glucose level is too high and your insulin level is too low. Too many ketones can make you sick. If you exercise when you have ketones in your blood or urine, your blood glucose level may go even higher.

If you have type 2 diabetes and your blood glucose is high but you don't have ketones, light or moderate exercise will probably lower your blood glucose. Ask your health care team whether you should exercise when your blood glucose is high.

Are there any types of physical activity I shouldn't do?

If you have diabetes complications, some kinds of exercise can make your problems worse. For example, activities that increase the pressure in the blood vessels of your eyes, such as lifting heavy weights, can make diabetic eye problems worse. If nerve damage from diabetes has made your feet numb, your doctor may suggest that you try swimming instead of walking for aerobic exercise.

When you have numb feet, you might not feel pain in your feet. Sores or blisters might get worse because you don't notice them. Without proper care, minor foot problems can turn into serious conditions, sometimes leading to amputation. Make sure you exercise in cotton socks and comfortable, well-fitting shoes designed for the activity you are doing. After you exercise, check your feet for cuts, sores, bumps, or redness. Call your doctor if any foot problems develop.

Can physical activity cause low blood glucose?

Physical activity can cause low blood glucose, also called hypoglycemia, in people who take insulin or certain types of diabetes medicines. Ask your health care team whether your diabetes medicines can cause low blood glucose.

Low blood glucose can happen while you exercise, right afterward, or even up to a day later. It can make you feel shaky, weak, confused, grumpy, hungry, or tired. You may sweat a lot or get a headache. If your blood glucose drops too low, you could pass out or have a seizure.

However, you should still be physically active. These steps can help you be prepared for low blood glucose:

Before Exercise

- Ask your health care team whether you should check your blood glucose level before exercising.

- If you take diabetes medicines that can cause low blood glucose, ask your health care team whether you should take the following precautions:

  - Change the amount you take before you exercise

  - Have a snack if your blood glucose level is below 100

During Exercise

- Wear your medical identification (ID) bracelet or necklace or carry your ID in your pocket.

- Always carry food or glucose tablets so you'll be ready to treat low blood glucose.

- If you'll be exercising for more than an hour, check your blood glucose at regular intervals. You may need snacks before you finish.

After Exercise

- Check to see how exercise affected your blood glucose level. If your blood glucose is below 70, have one of the following right away:

  - 3 or 4 glucose tablets

  - 1 serving of glucose gel—the amount equal to 15 grams of carbohydrate

  - 1/2 cup (4 ounces) of any fruit juice

- 1/2 cup (4 ounces) of a regular—not diet—soft drink
- 1 cup (8 ounces) of milk
- 5 or 6 pieces of hard candy
- 1 tablespoon of sugar or honey

After 15 minutes, check your blood glucose again. If it's still too low, have another serving. Repeat until your blood glucose is 70 or higher. If it will be an hour or more before your next meal, have a snack as well.

What should I do before I start a physical activity program?

Check with your doctor. Always talk with your doctor before you start a new physical activity program. Ask about your medicines—prescription and over-the-counter—and whether you should change the amount you take before you exercise. If you have heart disease, kidney disease, eye problems, or foot problems, ask which types of physical activity are safe for you.

Decide exactly what you'll do and set some goals. Choose the following:

- The type of physical activity you want to do
- The clothes and items you'll need to get ready
- The days and times you'll add activity
- The length of each session
- Your plan for warming up, stretching, and cooling down for each session
- A backup plan, such as where you'll walk if the weather is bad
- Your measures of progress

Find an exercise buddy. Many people find they are more likely to do something active if a friend joins them. If you and a friend plan to walk together, for example, you may be more likely to do it.

Keep track of your physical activity. Write down when you exercise and for how long in your blood glucose record book. You'll be able to track your progress and see how physical activity affects your blood glucose.

Decide how you'll reward yourself. Do something nice for yourself when you reach your activity goals. For example, treat yourself to a movie or buy a new plant for the garden.

What can I do to make sure I stay active?

One of the keys to staying on track is finding some activities you like to do. If you keep finding excuses not to exercise, think about why. Are your goals realistic? Do you need a change in activity? Would another time be more convenient? Keep trying until you find a routine that works for you. Once you make physical activity a habit, you'll wonder how you lived without it.

Chapter 53

Physical Fitness and Cancer

Chapter Contents

Section 53.1

Physical Fitness and Cancer Prevention

"Physical Activity and Cancer," National Cancer
Institute (www.cancer.gov), July 2009.

What is physical activity?

Physical activity is any bodily movement produced by skeletal muscles; such movement results in an expenditure of energy. Physical activity is a critical component of energy balance, a term used to describe how weight, diet, and physical activity influence health, including cancer risk.

How is physical activity related to health?

Researchers have established that regular physical activity can improve health in the following ways:

• Helping to control weight

• Maintaining healthy bones, muscles, and joints

• Reducing the risk of developing high blood pressure and diabetes

• Promoting psychological well-being

• Reducing the risk of death from heart disease

• Reducing the risk of premature death[1]

In addition to these health benefits, researchers are learning that physical activity can also affect the risk of cancer. There is convincing evidence that physical activity is associated with a reduced risk of cancers of the colon and breast. Several studies also have reported links between physical activity and a reduced risk of cancers of the prostate, lung, and lining of the uterus (endometrial cancer). Despite these health benefits, recent studies have shown that more than 50% of Americans do not engage in enough regular physical activity.[2]

How much physical activity do adults need?

The Centers for Disease Control and Prevention (CDC) recommend that adults "engage in moderate-intensity physical activity for at least 30 minutes on five or more days of the week," or "engage in vigorous-intensity physical activity for at least 20 minutes on three or more days of the week."[1] Examples of moderate-intensity and vigorous-intensity physical activities can be found on the CDC Physical Activity website at www.cdc.gov/nccdphp/dnpa/physical/pdf/PA_Intensity_table_2_1.pdf.

What is the relationship between physical activity and colon cancer risk?

Colorectal cancer has been one of the most extensively studied cancers in relation to physical activity, with more than 50 studies examining this association. Many studies in the United States and around the world have consistently found that adults who increase their physical activity, either in intensity, duration, or frequency, can reduce their risk of developing colon cancer by 30 to 40% relative to those who are sedentary regardless of body mass index (BMI), with the greatest risk reduction seen among those who are most active.[3-7] The magnitude of the protective effect appears greatest with high-intensity activity, although the optimal levels and duration of exercise are still difficult to determine due to differences between studies, making comparisons difficult. It is estimated that 30 to 60 minutes of moderate to vigorous physical activity per day is needed to protect against colon cancer.[6,7] It is not yet clear at this time whether physical activity has a protective effect for rectal cancer, adenomas, or polyp recurrence.[3]

Physical activity most likely influences the development of colon cancer in multiple ways. Physical activity may protect against colon cancer and tumor development through its role in energy balance, hormone metabolism, insulin regulation, and by decreasing the time the colon is exposed to potential carcinogens. Physical activity has also been found to alter a number of inflammatory and immune factors, some of which may influence colon cancer risk.

What is the relationship between physical activity and breast cancer risk?

The relationship between physical activity and breast cancer incidence has been extensively studied, with over 60 studies published in North America, Europe, Asia, and Australia. Most studies indicate that physically active women have a lower risk of developing breast cancer than inactive women; however, the amount of risk reduction achieved through physical activity varies widely (between 20 to 80%).[6,7] Although most evidence suggests that physical activity reduces breast cancer risk in both premenopausal and postmenopausal women,[6] high levels of moderate and vigorous physical activity during adolescence may be especially protective. Although a lifetime of regular, vigorous activity is thought to be of greatest benefit, women who increase their physical activity after menopause may also experience a reduced risk compared with inactive women. A number of studies also suggest that the effect of physical activity may be different across levels of BMI, with the greatest benefit seen in women in the normal weight range (generally a BMI under 25 kg/m-squared) in some studies. Existing evidence shows a decreasing risk of breast cancer as the frequency and duration of physical activity increase. Most studies suggest that 30 to 60 minutes per day of moderate- to high-intensity physical activity is associated with a reduction in breast cancer risk.[4,6]

Researchers have proposed several biological mechanisms to explain the relationship between physical activity and breast cancer development. Physical activity may prevent tumor development by lowering hormone levels, particularly in premenopausal women; lowering levels of insulin and insulin-like growth factor I (IGF-I), improving the immune response; and assisting with weight maintenance to avoid a high body mass and excess body fat.[7]

What is the relationship between physical activity and risk of endometrial cancer?

About 20 studies have examined the role of physical activity on endometrial cancer risk. The results suggest an inverse relationship between physical activity and endometrial cancer incidence. These studies suggest that women who are physically active have a 20 to 40% reduced risk of endometrial cancer,[6] with the greatest reduction in risk among those with the highest levels of physical activity. Risk does not appear to vary by age.[4]

Changes in body mass and changes in the levels and metabolism of sex hormones, such as estrogen, are the major biological mechanisms thought to explain the association between physical activity and endometrial cancer. However, fewer than half of the studies in this area have also adjusted for the potential effect of postmenopausal hormone use, which may increase the risk of endometrial cancer. A few studies have examined whether the effect of physical activity varies according to the weight of the woman, but the results have been inconsistent.

What is the relationship between physical activity and lung cancer risk?

At least 21 studies have examined the impact of physical activity on the risk of lung cancer. Overall, these studies suggest an inverse association between physical activity and lung cancer risk, with the most physically active individuals experiencing about a 20% reduction in risk.[4,6] An analysis of many existing studies found evidence that higher levels of physical activity protect against lung cancer, but was unable to fully control for the effects of smoking or respiratory disease in estimating the magnitude of the potential benefit.[6,8] The relationship between physical activity and lung cancer risk is less clear for women than it is for men.

What is the relationship between physical activity and risk of prostate cancer?

Research findings are less consistent about the effect of physical activity on prostate cancer, with at least 36 studies in North America, Europe, and Asia. Overall, the epidemiologic research does not indicate that there is an inverse relationship between physical activity and prostate cancer.[4,7] Although it is possible that men who are physically active experience a reduction in risk of prostate cancer, the potential biological mechanisms that may explain this association are unknown, but may be related to changes in hormones, energy balance, insulin-like growth factors, immunity, and antioxidant defense mechanisms.[7] One recent study suggested that regular vigorous activity could slow the progression of prostate cancer in men age 65 or older.[9]

How might physical activity affect cancer survivorship?

Research indicates that physical activity after a diagnosis of breast cancer may be beneficial in improving quality of life, reducing fatigue,[7] and assisting with energy balance. Both reduced physical activity and the side effects of treatment have been linked to weight gain after a breast cancer diagnosis. One study found that women who exercised moderately (the equivalent of walking three to five hours per week at an average pace) after a diagnosis of breast cancer had improved survival rates compared with more sedentary women. The benefit was particularly pronounced in women with hormone responsive tumors.[10] Another study found that a home-based physical activity program had a beneficial effect on the fitness and psychological well-being of previously sedentary women who had completed treatment for early-stage through stage II breast cancer.[11] Increasing physical activity may influence insulin and leptin levels and influence breast cancer prognosis. Although there are several promising studies, it is too early to draw any strong conclusions regarding physical activity and breast cancer survival.

Two additional studies have suggested a protective association of physical activity after colon cancer diagnosis and survival. Researchers examined the relationship between levels of physical activity both before and after a diagnosis of colon cancer in two different observational studies. Whereas levels of pre-diagnosis physical activity were not related to survival, participants with higher levels of physical activity post-diagnosis were less likely to have a cancer recurrence and had increased survival.[12] Although these studies suggest protective effects of physical activity, more research is needed to understand what levels of physical activity provide these benefits.

Is the National Cancer Institute (NCI) exploring the role of physical activity in the prognosis and quality of life of cancer patients?

NCI-funded studies are exploring the ways in which physical activity may improve the prognosis and quality of life of cancer patients and survivors. For more information about current research in this area, please visit NCI's Cancer Survivorship Research website at cancercontrol.cancer.gov/ocs.

Is NCI studying the role of physical activity in cancer risk?

A number of NCI-funded studies are answering questions about the relationship between physical activity and the risk of developing cancer. NCI has established the Transdisciplinary Research on Energetics and Cancer (TREC) initiative, which links four research centers investigating how energy balance and physical activity modify the risk of cancer and influence the process of carcinogenesis. The TREC initiative also incorporates a broad range of scientists, ranging from experts in basic biological science to those with expertise in community behavioral interventions to increase physical activity. This combination of scientists and expertise will allow exploration of the role of physical activity across the full spectrum of cancer prevention. More information about TREC can be found at cancercontrol.cancer.gov/trec/.

Do any of these studies focus on special populations who are at increased risk of cancer?

NCI funds a number of research projects and interventions aimed at helping vulnerable populations reduce their risk of cancer by becoming more active, changing their nutritional behavior, and/or maintaining an optimal weight. Populations included in these projects include multiethnic working poor populations, African American women, rural communities, overweight or obese individuals, and cancer survivors. Several NCI-funded studies have started examining the factors related to long-term behavior change and increases in physical activity.

NCI is supporting national and regional surveys, as well as research methodology development, to gain more accurate information about physical activity across all age groups and diverse populations, as defined by race, ethnicity, income, and other factors known to influence levels of physical activity. This information will help identify groups who may benefit from programs to increase physical activity.

Selected References

1. National Center for Chronic Disease Prevention and Health Promotion and Centers for Disease Control and Prevention (1996). *Physical Activity and Health: A Report of the Surgeon General.* Retrieved June 26, 2009, from www.cdc.gov/nccdphp/sgr/sgr.htm.

2. National Center for Chronic Disease Prevention and Health Promotion and Centers for Disease Control and Prevention (2008). *Preventing Obesity and Chronic Diseases through Good Nutrition and Physical Activity.* Retrieved June 26, 2009, from www.cdc.gov/nccdphp/publications/factsheets/Prevention/obesity.htm.

3. Slattery, ML. Physical activity and colorectal cancer. *Sports Medicine* 2004; 34(4): 239–252.

4. IARC Handbooks of Cancer Prevention. *Weight Control and Physical Activity.* Vol. 6. 2002.

5. Ballard-Barbash R, Friedenreich C, Slattery M, Thune L. Obesity and body composition. In: Schottenfeld D, Fraumeni JF, editors. *Cancer Epidemiology and Prevention.* 3rd ed. New York: Oxford University Press, 2006.

6. Lee I, Oguma Y. Physical activity. In: Schottenfeld D, Fraumeni JF, editors. *Cancer Epidemiology and Prevention.* 3rd ed. New York: Oxford University Press, 2006.

7. McTiernan A, editor. *Cancer Prevention and Management through Exercise and Weight Control.* Boca Raton: Taylor & Francis Group, LLC, 2006.

8. Tardon A, Lee WJ, Delgado-Rodriguez M, et al. Leisure-time physical activity and lung cancer: A meta-analysis. *Cancer Causes and Control* 2005; 16(4):389–397.

9. Giovannucci EL, Liu Y, Leitzmann MF, Stampfer MJ, Willett WC. A prospective study of physical activity and incident and fatal prostate cancer. *Archives of Internal Medicine* 2005; 165(9):1005–1010.

10. Holmes MD, Chen WY, Feskanich D, Kroenke CH, Colditz GA. Physical activity and survival after breast cancer diagnosis. *Journal of the American Medical Association* 2005; 293(20):2479–2486.

11. Pinto BM, Frierson GM, Rabin C, Trunzo JJ, Marcus BH. Home-based physical activity intervention for breast cancer patients. *Journal of Clinical Oncology* 2005; 23(15): 3577–3587.

12. Meyerhardt JA, Giovannucci EL, Holmes MD, et al. Physical activity and survival after colorectal cancer diagnosis. *Journal of Clinical Oncology* 2006; 24(22):3527–3534.

Section 53.2

Exercise during Cancer Treatment

"Exercise during Cancer Treatment," by Kerry Courneya, PhD, and Margaret McNeely, PhD. © 2009. Reprinted with permission of the American College of Sports Medicine, ACSM Fit Society® Page, Spring 2009, p 3.

What Is Cancer?

According to the American Cancer Society (ACS), there are more than 100 different diseases that are classified as "cancer." The common thread among these different types of cancers is that they all start as abnormal cells that grow out of control in some part of the body. The ACS estimates that more than 1.4 million Americans were newly diagnosed with cancer and more than a half million were expected to die of the disease in 2008. The three most common cancers occurring in men are prostate, lung, and colorectal cancers; in women, breast, lung, and colorectal cancers are the three most common. Cancer may be treated by a number of methods, either alone or in combination. These treatments include surgery, radiation, chemotherapy, hormonal therapy, and biological therapy.

How Exercise Helps

An increasing number of studies have examined the benefits of exercising during cancer treatment. Although the majority of studies have examined women with early-stage breast cancer, research evidence suggests that exercise can have a positive impact on body weight, overall fitness, muscle strength, flexibility, and quality of life, as well as on symptoms such as pain and fatigue. A recent study by Kerry Courneya, PhD, and colleagues found benefits from exercise for chemotherapy completion. In the study, women with breast cancer participating in a resistance training program during chemotherapy had dose reductions and fewer delays in their chemotherapy treatments.

Physical Activity Recommendations

The optimal form of exercise training for cancer patients undergoing treatment still remains unclear. Research studies have generally examined moderate-intensity aerobic exercise, resistance exercise, and/ or combined programs. Further research is needed to determine the best type, timing, and intensity of exercise for the different types and stages of cancer. Despite these limitations, for the most part, exercise prescriptions have closely followed the published guidelines of the American College of Sports Medicine.

Special Considerations

Individuals are potentially different in their responses to cancer treatment. Exercise programs may need to be modified to allow for "down" days in the treatment cycle. In the case of chemotherapy or biological therapy, this may mean avoiding or scaling back exercise on days when side effects from treatment are more pronounced. In the case of radiation therapy, exercise may need to be reduced, or in some cases avoided, toward the end of treatment and/or in the early weeks following treatment.

If an individual is not regularly active and wishes to start an exercise program during cancer treatment, they may need to start with low-intensity exercise, consisting of slow walks, and gradually progress exercise over time. If they will be receiving chemotherapy, it may be wise to wait one chemotherapy cycle to see the response to treatment prior to starting an exercise program.

Individuals undergoing cancer treatment should:

- obtain approval from their oncologist (cancer doctor) before starting an exercise program;

- have vital signs (temperature, pulse/ heart rate, blood pressure, respiration rate) monitored regularly (if participating in moderate-to-vigorous exercise, have their blood pressure and heart rate monitored before, during, and after exercise to ensure that participation in exercise is appropriate and safe);

- exercise with a partner, caregiver, or exercise professional for safety reasons;

- avoid public fitness facilities and activities (e.g., swimming), where there may be an increased risk of exposure to viral and/or bacterial infection;

- avoid swimming if undergoing radiation therapy treatments or if they have an indwelling catheter (a tube that goes in the body), such as a central venous catheter or peripherally inserted central catheter;

- stop exercise and contact their doctor if they have any of the following symptoms during exercise or after an exercise session:

  - Disorientation, dizziness, blurred vision, or fainting

  - Sudden onset of nausea, vomiting

  - Unusual or sudden shortness of breath

  - Irregular heart beat, palpitations, chest pain

  - Leg/calf pain, bone pain, unusual joint pain, or pain not caused by injury

  - Muscle cramps or sudden onset of muscular weakness or fatigue

Exercise Precautions

Although exercise may be an effective intervention for cancer patients undergoing treatment, it is important to recognize there may be factors that make it unwise to exercise. In these cases, exercise may be still beneficial; however, the risks may be higher, and close medical supervision may be required.

According to the ACS, the following are specific precautions to be aware of during cancer treatment:

- Anemia (low red blood cell count): If the red blood cell count is low, the body's ability to carry oxygen to the tissues is reduced. Exercise may need to be scaled back and possibly avoided.

- Neutropenia (low white blood cell count): If the white blood cell count is low, the body's ability to fight infection is reduced. Exercise should be avoided if there is a fever above 100.4° F (>38° C).

- Thrombocytopenia (low platelet count): If platelet count is low, there is an increased risk of bruising and bleeding. Avoid contact sports or activities with high risk of injury or falling. Report any unusual bruising or symptoms, such as nose bleeds, to a doctor.

- Side effects such as vomiting and diarrhea, and symptoms such as swollen ankles, unexplained weight loss/gain, or shortness of breath with low levels of exertion may make exercise unsafe. Check with a doctor before exercising.

Conclusion

Research evidence suggests that individuals with cancer who follow recommended guidelines and observe specific precautions can safely exercise during cancer treatment.

Did You Know...

The American College of Sports Medicine and the American Cancer Society recently launched a specialty certification for fitness professionals, enabling to work with patients suffering or recovering from cancer. Visit www.acsm.org/certification for more details.

Part Seven

Additional Help
and Information

Chapter 54

Glossary of Fitness Terms

accumulate: The concept of meeting a specific physical activity dose or goal by performing activity in short bouts, then adding together the time spent during each of these bouts. For example, a goal of 30 minutes a day could be met by performing three bouts of 10 minutes each throughout the day.

adaptation: The body's response to exercise or activity. Some of the body's structures and functions favorably adjust to the increase in demands placed on them whenever physical activity of a greater amount or higher intensity is performed than what is usual for the individual. These adaptations are the basis for much of the improved health and fitness associated with increases in physical activity.

aerobic exercise: Any continuous activity of large muscle groups that forces your heart and lungs to work harder. Aerobic means your heart and lungs are using oxygen. Examples include walking, swimming, stair climbing, and jumping rope.[2]

anaerobic exercise: Exercise that requires your body to perform at a great effort for a relatively short duration. This type of exercise

---

This glossary contains terms excerpted from glossaries produced by the following government agencies: Centers for Disease Control and Prevention (www.cdc.gov); National Women's Health Information Center (www.womenshealth.gov), marked with a superscript 1; U.S. Department of Agriculture Center for Nutrition Policy and Promotion (www.mypyramidtracker.gov), marked with a superscript 2; and the Weight-Control Information Network, National Institute of Diabetes and Digestive and Kidney Diseases (www.win.niddk.gov), marked with a superscript 3.

583

requires your body to use stored energy that does not need oxygen to be released. Examples include weight training or sprinting.[2]

balance training: Static and dynamic exercises that are designed to improve individuals' ability to withstand challenges from postural sway or destabilizing stimuli caused by self-motion, the environment, or other objects.

baseline activity: The light-intensity activities of daily life, such as standing, walking slowly, and lifting lightweight objects. People who do only baseline activity are considered to be inactive.

body composition: A health-related component of physical fitness that applies to body weight and the relative amounts of muscle, fat, bone, and other vital tissues of the body. Most often, the components are limited to fat and lean body mass (or fat-free mass).

body mass index (BMI): A measure of body weight relative to height. BMI is a tool that is often used to determine if a person is at a healthy weight, overweight, or obese, and whether a person's health is at risk due to his or her weight. To figure out BMI, use the following formula: (weight in pounds times 703) divided by (height in inches squared). A BMI of 18.5 to 24.9 is considered healthy. A person with a BMI of 25 to 29.9 is considered overweight, and a person with a BMI of 30 or more is considered obese.[3]

bone-strengthening activity: Physical activity primarily designed to increase the strength of specific sites in bones that make up the skeletal system. Bone-strengthening activities produce an impact or tension force on the bones that promotes bone growth and strength. Running, jumping rope, and lifting weights are examples of bone-strengthening activities.

calisthenics: Physical exercises done without equipment to build muscular strength, endurance, and flexibility.[2]

calorie: A unit of energy in food. Foods have carbohydrates, proteins, and/or fats. Some beverages have alcohol. Carbohydrates and proteins have four calories per gram. Fat has nine calories per gram. Alcohol has seven calories per gram.[3]

calorie balance: The difference between how many calories (energy intake) you eat from food and how many you burn (calorie expenditure). When the calories you eat from food equal the calories you burn, you maintain your weight. Eating more calories than you burn results in weight gain. Burning more calories than you eat results in weight loss. During periods of growth and development, you need to eat more calories than you burn to meet the energy needs of increased body tissue.[2]

calorie expenditure: The amount of energy your body uses to do anything. For example, you burn or expend calories when you walk, swim, sleep, read, and breathe.[2]

carbohydrate: A major source of energy in the diet. There are two kinds of carbohydrates—simple carbohydrates and complex carbohydrates: simple carbohydrates are sugars and complex carbohydrates include both starches and fiber. Carbohydrates have four calories per gram. They are found naturally in foods such as breads, pasta, cereals, fruits, vegetables, and milk and dairy products. Foods such as sugary cereals, soft drinks, fruit drinks, fruit punch, lemonade, cakes, cookies, pies, ice cream, and candy are very high in sugars.[3]

cardiorespiratory endurance: The ability of the circulatory and respiratory systems to adjust to and recover from the effects of whole body exercise or work. The circulatory and respiratory systems deliver oxygen and nutrients to tissues and remove waste products. Long runs and swims are example of endurance activities.[2]

cholesterol: A fatty substance present in all parts of the body. It is a component of cell membranes and is used to make vitamin D and some hormones. Some cholesterol in the body is produced by the liver and some is derived from food, particularly animal products. A high level of cholesterol in the blood can help cause atherosclerosis and coronary artery disease. In the blood, cholesterol is bound to chemicals called lipoproteins. Cholesterol attached to low-density lipoprotein (LDL) harms health and is often called "bad cholesterol." Cholesterol attached to high-density lipoprotein (HDL) is good for health and is often called "good cholesterol."[1]

cool down: A gradual reduction of the intensity of physical activity to allow physiological processes to return to normal.[2]

dehydration: Excessive loss of body water that the body needs to carry on normal functions at an optimal level. Signs include increasing thirst, dry mouth, weakness or lightheadedness (particularly if worse on standing), and a darkening of the urine or a decrease in urination.[1]

diabetes: A disease in which blood glucose (blood sugar) levels are above normal. There are two main types of diabetes. Type 1 diabetes is caused by a problem with the body's defense system, called the immune system. This form of diabetes usually starts in childhood or adolescence. Type 2 diabetes is the most common form of diabetes. It starts most often in adulthood.[1]

duration: The length of time in which an activity or exercise is performed. Duration is generally expressed in minutes.

exercise: A subcategory of physical activity that is planned, structured, repetitive, and purposive in the sense that the improvement or maintenance of one or more components of physical fitness is the objective. "Exercise" and "exercise training" frequently are used interchangeably and generally refer to physical activity performed during leisure time with the primary purpose of improving or maintaining physical fitness, physical performance, or health.

fat: A major source of energy in the diet. All food fats have nine calories per gram. Fat helps the body absorb fat-soluble vitamins, such as vitamins A, D, E, and K, and carotenoids. Some kinds of fats, especially saturated fats and trans fats, may raise blood cholesterol and increase the risk for heart disease. Other fats, such as unsaturated fats, do not raise blood cholesterol. Fats that are in foods are combinations of monounsaturated, polyunsaturated, and saturated fatty acids.[3]

flexibility: A health- and performance-related component of physical fitness that is the range of motion possible at a joint. Flexibility is specific to each joint and depends on a number of specific variables, including but not limited to the tightness of specific ligaments and tendons. Flexibility exercises enhance the ability of a joint to move through its full range of motion.

healthy weight: Compared to overweight or obese, a body weight that is less likely to be linked with any weight-related health problems, such as type 2 diabetes, heart disease, high blood pressure, and high blood cholesterol. A body mass index (BMI) of 18.5 to 24.9 is considered a healthy weight, though not all individuals with a BMI in this range may be at a healthy level of body fat; they may have more body fat tissue and less muscle. A person with a BMI of 25 to 29.9 is considered overweight, and a person with a BMI of 30 or more is considered obese.[3]

heart disease: A number of abnormal conditions affecting the heart and the blood vessels in the heart. The most common type of heart disease is coronary artery disease, which is the gradual buildup of plaques in the coronary arteries, the blood vessels that bring blood to the heart. This disease develops slowly and silently, over decades. It can go virtually unnoticed until it produces a heart attack.[1]

heart rate: Reserve is the difference between the resting heart rate and the maximal heart rate.[2]

hydration: The amount of fluid in your body. It is important to replace any fluid your body loses during physical activity.[2]

hypertension: Also called high blood pressure, it is having blood pressure greater than 140 over 90 mmHg (millimeters of mercury). Long-term high blood pressure can damage blood vessels and organs, including the heart, kidneys, eyes, and brain.[1]

intensity: Intensity refers to how much work is being performed or the magnitude of the effort required to perform an activity or exercise. Intensity can be expressed either in absolute or relative terms.

- **absolute intensity:** The absolute intensity of an activity is determined by the rate of work being performed and does not take into account the physiologic capacity of the individual. For aerobic activity, absolute intensity typically is expressed as the rate of energy expenditure (for example, milliliters per kilogram per minute of oxygen being consumed, kilocalories per minute, or METs) or, for some activities, simply as the speed of the activity (for example, walking at three miles an hour, jogging at six miles an hour), or physiologic response to the intensity (for example, heart rate). For resistance activity or exercise, intensity frequently is expressed as the amount of weight lifted or moved.

- **relative intensity:** Relative intensity takes into account or adjusts for a person's exercise capacity. For aerobic exercise, relative intensity is expressed as a percent of a person's aerobic capacity (VO2max) or VO2 reserve, or as a percent of a person's measured or estimated maximum heart rate (heart rate reserve). It also can be expressed as an index of how hard the person feels he or she is exercising (for example, a 0 to 10 scale).

interval training: An exercise session in which the intensity and duration of exercise are consciously alternated between harder and easier work. Often used to improve aerobic capacity and/or anaerobic endurance in people who exercise regularly or who are physically well trained.[2]

leisure-time physical activity: A recreational activity generally associated with pleasure and/or health and fitness. Such activities are varied as to type and intensity. Some leisure-time activities are of light intensity such as sitting in a boat fishing; others are of moderate activity, such as low impact aerobics. Those that are classified as vigorous intensity are more strenuous, such as high impact aerobics or running.[2]

lifestyle activities: This term is frequently used to encompass activities that a person carries out in the course of daily life and that can contribute to sizeable energy expenditure. Examples include taking the stairs instead of using the elevator, walking to do errands instead of driving, getting off a bus one stop early, or parking farther away than usual to walk to a destination.

maximal oxygen uptake (VO2 max): The body's capacity to transport and use oxygen during a maximal exertion involving dynamic contraction of large muscle groups, such as during running or cycling. Also known as maximal aerobic power and cardiorespiratory endurance capacity.

metabolic equivalents (METs): A ratio of work metabolic rate to standard resting metabolic rate. Resting energy expenditure is considered 1 MET. Therefore, a 3 MET activity (equivalent to walking the dog or bowling) would require energy expenditure at a level equal to three times resting.[2]

metabolism: All of the processes in the body that make and use energy, such as digesting food and nutrients and removing waste through urine and feces.[1]

muscle-strengthening activity: Physical activity, including exercise that increases skeletal muscle strength, power, endurance, and mass.

muscular endurance: The ability of the muscle to perform repetitive contractions over a prolonged period of time. Push-ups are often used to test endurance of arm and shoulder muscles.[2]

obesity: Excess body fat. Because body fat is usually not measured, a ratio of body weight to height is often used instead. It is defined as BMI. An adult who has a BMI of 30 or higher is considered obese.[3]

osteoarthritis: A joint disease that mostly affects cartilage, the slippery tissue that covers the ends of bones in a joint. The top layer of cartilage breaks down and wears away. This allows bones under the cartilage to rub together, which causes pain, swelling, and loss of motion of the joint.[1]

osteoporosis: A bone disease that is characterized by progressive loss of bone density and thinning of bone tissue, causing bones to break easily.[1]

overload: The amount of new activity added to a person's usual level of activity. The risk of injury to bones, muscles, and joints is directly related to the size of the gap between these two levels. This gap is called the amount of overload.

overweight: A body mass index (BMI) of 25 to 29.9. Body weight comes from fat, muscle, bone, and body water. It is important to remember that although BMI correlates with the amount of body fat, BMI does not directly measure body fat. As a result, some people, such as athletes, may have a BMI that identifies them as overweight even though they do not have excess body fat.[3]

pedometer: A step counter that is worn at the waist or on a person's waistband. It tallies the number of steps a person takes each day. Walking 2,000 steps is equal to about one mile and roughly 100 calories are burned over and above calories for resting metabolism.[2]

physical fitness: The ability to carry out daily tasks with vigor and alertness, without undue fatigue, and with ample energy to enjoy leisure-time pursuits and respond to emergencies. Physical fitness includes a number of components consisting of cardiorespiratory endurance (aerobic power), skeletal muscle endurance, skeletal muscle strength, skeletal muscle power, flexibility, balance, speed of movement, reaction time, and body composition.

progression: The process of increasing the intensity, duration, frequency, or amount of activity or exercise as the body adapts to a given activity pattern.

repetitions: The number of times a person lifts a weight in muscle-strengthening activities. Repetitions are analogous to duration in aerobic activity.

resting heart rate: The rate that your heart beats at rest.[2]

stretching: Stretching includes movements that lengthen muscles to their maximum extension and move joints to the limits of their extension.[2]

target heart rate: A safe heart rate recommended for fitness workouts; it depends on age and gender. It is the rate you want the heart to work (beats per minute) during a certain activity. You can use it to help determine the intensity of an activity.[2]

transportation-related activity: Physical activity undertaken for the purpose of getting from place to place, which may include walking, jogging, biking, or any other physically active method of getting from one place to another.

warm-up: A gradual increase in the intensity of exercise to allow physiological processes to prepare for greater energy outputs. Changes include a rise in body temperature, cardiorespiratory changes (i.e., increased heart and ventilation rate), and increase in muscle elasticity and contractility.[2]

Chapter 55

Directory of Fitness Resources

Government Agencies That Provide Information about Fitness and Exercise

Americans with Disabilities Act Hotline
United States Access Board
1331 F Street, NW
Suite 1000
Washington, DC 20004-1111
Toll-Free: 800-USA-ABLE
(872-2253)
Toll-Free TTY: 800-993-2822
Phone: 202-272-0080
TTY: 202-272-0082
Fax: 202-272-0081
Website: http://www.access-board
.gov
E-mail: info@access-board.gov

Centers for Disease Control and Prevention (CDC)
Division of Nutrition, Physical Activity, and Obesity (DNPAO)
1600 Clifton Road
Atlanta, GA 30333
Toll-Free: 800-CDC-INFO
(232-4636)
Toll-Free TTY: 888-232-6348
Website: http://www.cdc.gov/
nccdphp/dnpao/index.html
E-mail: cdcinfo@cdc.gov

The resources listed in this chapter were compiled from many sources deemed accurate. Inclusion does not constitute endorsement and there is no implication associated with omission. All contact information was verified in April 2010.

National Cancer Institute (NCI)
NCI Public Inquiries Office
6116 Executive Boulevard
Suite 300
Bethesda, MD 20892-8322
Toll-Free: 800-4-CANCER
(422-6237), Monday through
Friday 9:00 a.m. to 4:30 p.m., EST
Live chat: http://cissecure.nci
.nih.gov/livehelp/welcome.asp
Website: http://www.cancer.gov

National Center for Complementary and Alternative Medicine (NCCAM)
NCCAM Clearinghouse
P.O. Box 7923
Gaithersburg, MD 20898
Toll-Free: 888-644-6226
TTY: 866-464-3615
Fax: 866-464-3616
Website: http://nccam.nih.gov

National Diabetes Information Clearinghouse
1 Information Way
Bethesda, MD 20892-3560
Toll-Free: 800-860-8747
Toll-Free TTY: 866-569-1162
Fax: 703-738-4929
Website: http://diabetes.niddk
.nih.gov
E-mail: ndic@info.niddk.nih.gov

National Heart, Lung, and Blood Institute (NHLBI)
NHLBI Health Information
Center
Attention: Web site
P.O. Box 30105
Bethesda, MD 20824-0105
Phone: 301-592-8573
TTY: 240-629-3255
Fax: 240-629-3246
Website: http://www.nhlbi.nih
.gov
E-mail: nhlbiinfo@rover.nhlbi
.nih.gov

National Institute of Arthritis and Musculoskeletal and Skin Diseases (NIAMS)
Information Clearinghouse
National Institutes of Health
1 AMS Circle
Bethesda, MD 20892-3675
Toll Free: 877-22-NIAMS
(226-4267)
Phone: 301-495-4484
TTY: 301-565-2966
Fax: 301-718-6366
Website: http://www.niams.nih
.gov
E-mail: NIAMSinfo@mail.nih
.gov

National Institute of Diabetes and Digestive and Kidney Diseases (NIDDK)
Office of Communications & Public Liaison
Building 31, Room 9A06
31 Center Drive, MSC 2560
Bethesda, MD 20892-2560
Phone: 301-496-3583
Website: http://www.niddk.nih.gov

National Institute of Mental Health (NIMH)
6001 Executive Boulevard
Room 8184, MSC 9663
Bethesda, MD 20892-9663
Toll-Free: 866-615-NIMH (615-6464)
Toll-Free TTY: 866-415-8051
Phone: 301-443-4513
TTY: 301-443-8431
Fax: 301-443-4279
Website: http://www.nimh.nih.gov
E-mail: nimhinfo@nih.gov

National Institute on Aging (NIA)
Building 31, Room 5C27
31 Center Drive, MSC 2292
Bethesda, MD 20892
Toll-Free: 800-222-2225 (Publications Only)
Toll-Free TTY: 800-222-4225
Phone: 301-496-1752
Fax: 301-496-1072
Website: http://www.nia.nih.gov

National Institutes of Health (NIH)
9000 Rockville Pike
Bethesda, MD 20892
Phone: 301-496-4000
TTY: 301-402-9612
Website: http://www.nih.gov
E-mail: NIHinfo@od.nih.gov

National Library of Medicine
Reference and Web Services
8600 Rockville Pike
Bethesda, MD 20894
Toll-Free: 888-FIND-NLM (346-3656)
Toll-Free TDD: 800-735-2258 (via Maryland Relay Service)
Phone: 301-594-5983
Fax: 301-402-1384
Interlibrary loan fax: 301-496-2809
Website: http://www.nlm.nih.gov
E-mail: custserv@nlm.nih.gov

National Women's Health Information Center
U.S. Department of Health and Human Services
8270 Willow Oaks Corporate Drive
Fairfax, VA 22031
Toll-Free: 800-994-9662
Toll-Free TTD: 888-220-5446
Website: http://www.womenshealth.gov

President's Council on Physical Fitness and Sports (PCPFS)

Department W
Tower Building, Suite 560
1101 Wootton Parkway
Rockville, MD 20852
Phone: 240-276-9567
Fax: 240-276-9860
Website: http://www.fitness.gov
E-mail: fitness@hhs.gov

Smallstep

U.S. Department of Health and Human Services
200 Independence Avenue, SW
Washington, D.C. 20201
Toll-Free: 877-696-6775 (Hotline)
Website: http://www.smallstep
.gov

U.S. Consumer Product Safety Commission

4330 East West Highway
Bethesda, MD 20814
Toll-Free: 800-638-2772 (Hotline; 8:00 a.m.–5:30 p.m. EST)
Toll-Free TTY: 800-638-8270 (Hotline; 8:00 a.m.–5:30 p.m. EST)
Phone: 301-504-7923 (General Information; Monday–Friday 8:00 a.m.–4:30 p.m. EST)
Fax: 301-504-0124 and 301-504-0025
Website: http://www.cpsc.gov

U.S. Department of Health and Human Services (HHS)

200 Independence Avenue, SW
Washington, DC 20201
Toll-Free: 877-696-6775 (Hotline)
Website: http://www.hhs.gov

Weight-Control Information Network (WIN)

National Institute of Diabetes and Digestive and Kidney Diseases
1 WIN Way
Bethesda, MD 20892-3665
Toll-Free: 877-946-4627
Fax: 202-828-1028
Website: http://win.niddk.nih.gov
E-mail: win@info.niddk.nih.gov

Private Organizations That Provide Information about Fitness and Exercise

Action for Healthy Kids

4711 West Golf Road
Suite 625
Skokie, IL 60076
Toll-Free: 800-416-5136
Fax: 847-329-1849
Website: http://www
.actionforhealthykids.org

Aerobics and Fitness Association of America

15250 Ventura Boulevard
Suite 200
Sherman Oaks, CA 91403
Toll-Free: 877-YOUR-BODY (968-7263), Mon.–Fri 6:30 a.m.–6:30 p.m., Sat 9 a.m.–1 p.m. PST
Website: http://www.afaa.com

*American Academy of
Orthopaedic Surgeons
(AAOS)*
6300 North River Road
Rosemont, IL 60018-4262
Phone: 847-823-7186
Fax: 847-823-8125
Website: http://www.aaos.org
E-mail: custserv@aaos.org

*American Alliance for
Health, Physical Education,
Recreation, & Dance*
1900 Association Drive
Reston, VA 20191-1598
Toll-Free: 800-213-7193
Phone: 703-476-3400
Website: http://www.aahperd.org

*American College of Sports
Medicine (ACSM)*
P.O. Box 1440
Indianapolis, IN 46206-1440
Phone: 317-637-9200
Fax: 317-634-7817
Website: http://www.acsm.org

*American Council on
Exercise (ACE)*
4851 Paramount Drive
San Diego, CA 92123
Toll-Free: 888-825-3636
Phone: 858-279-8227
Fax: 858-576-6564
Website: http://www.acefitness
.org
E-mail: support@acefitness.org

*American Diabetes
Association*
1701 North Beauregard Street
Alexandria, VA 22311
Phone: 800-DIABETES
(342-2383)
Website: http://www.diabetes
.com

American Heart Association
7272 Greenville Avenue
Dallas, TX 75231-4596
Toll-Free: 800-AHA-USA1
(242-8721)
Website: www.americanheart
.org

*American Stroke
Association*
7272 Greenville Avenue
Dallas TX 75231
Toll-Free: 888-4-STROKE
(478-7653)
Website: http://www
.americanheart.org

American Lung Association
National Headquarters
1301 Pennsylvania Avenue, NW
Suite 800
Washington, DC 20004
Toll-Free: 800-LUNGUSA
(800-586-4872)
Toll-Free: 800-548-8252 (Helpline)
Phone: 202-785-3355
Fax: 202-452-1805
Website: http://www.lungusa.org
E-mail: info@lungusa.org

American Orthopaedic Society for Sports Medicine (AOSSM)
6300 North River Road
Suite 500
Rosemont, IL 60018
Phone: 847-292-4900
Website: http://www.sportsmed
.org
E-mail: aossm@aossm.org

American Physical Therapy Association (APTA)
1111 North Fairfax Street
Alexandria, VA 22314-1488
Toll-Free: 800-999-2782
Phone: 703-684-APTA (684-2782)
TDD: 703-683-6748
Fax: 703-684-7343
Website: http://www.apta.org
E-mail: Research-dept@apta.org

American Physiological Society
9650 Rockville Pike
Bethesda, MD 20814-3991
Phone: 301-634-7164
Fax: 301-634-7241
Website: http://www.the-aps.org

American Running Association (ARA)
4405 East-West Highway
Suite 405
Bethesda, MD 20814
Phone: 800-776-2732 ext. 13 or
ext. 12
Fax: 301-913-9520
Website: http://www
.americanrunning.org

Arthritis Foundation (AF)
P.O. Box 7669
Atlanta, GA 30357-0669
Toll-Free: 800-283-7800
Website: http://www.arthritis.org

Asthma and Allergy Foundation of America (AAFA)
8201 Corporate Drive, Suite 1000
Landover, MD 20785
Toll-Free: 800-7-ASTHMA
(727-8462)
Website: http://www.aafa.org
E-mail: info@aafa.org

Aquatic Exercise Association (AEA)
P.O. Box 1609
Nokomis, FL 34274-1609
Website: http://www.aeawave
.com

Cleveland Clinic
9500 Euclid Avenue
Cleveland, OH 44195
Toll-Free: 800-223-2273
Phone: 216-444-2200
TTY: 216-444-0261
Website: http://www
.clevelandclinic.org

Disabled Sports USA (DS/USA)
451 Hungerford Drive
Suite 100
Rockville, MD 20850
Phone: 301-217-0960
Fax: 301-217-0968
Website: http://www.dsusa.org
E-mail: information@dsusa.org

HealthyWomen
157 Broad Street
Suite 106
Red Bank, NJ 07701
Toll-Free: 877-986-9472
Fax: 732-530-3347
Website: http://www
.healthywomen.org

IDEA Health & Fitness Association
10455 Pacific Center Court
San Diego, CA 92121
Toll-Free: 800-999-4332, ext. 7
Phone: 858-535-8979, ext. 7
Fax: 858-535-8234
Website: http://www.ideafit.com
E-mail: contact@ideafit.com

International Fitness Association (IFA)
12472 Lake Underhill Road
#341
Orlando, FL 32828
Toll-Free: 800-227-1976
Phone: 407-579-8610
Website: http://www.ifafitness
.com

Kidshealth.org
Nemours Foundation
Website: http://www.kidshealth
.org

National Alliance for Youth Sports (NAYS)
National Headquarters
2050 Vista Parkway
West Palm Beach, FL 33411
Toll-Free: 800-688-KIDS
(729-2057)
Phone: 561-684-1141
Fax: 561-684-2546
Website: http://www.nays.org
E-mail: nays@nays.org

National Association for Health and Fitness (NAHF)
c/o Be Active New York State
65 Niagara Square
Room 607
Buffalo, NY 14202
Phone: 716-583-0521
Fax: 716-851-4309
Website: http://www
.physicalfitness.org
E-mail: wellness@city-buffalo
.org

National Center on Physical Activity and Disability (NCPAD)
University of Illinois at Chicago
Department of Disability and
Human Development
Toll-Free: 800-900-8086
Website: http://www.ncpad.org
E-mail: ncpad@uic.edu

National Coalition for Promoting Physical Activity
1100 H Street, NW
Suite 510
Washington, DC 20005
Phone: 202-454-7521
Fax: 202-454-7598
Website: http://www.ncppa.org
E-mail: info@ncppa.org

National Osteoporosis Foundation (NOF)
1150 17th Street, NW
Suite 850
Washington, DC 20036
Toll-Free: 800-231-4222
Phone: 202-223-2226
Website: http://www.nof.org

National Recreation and Park Association (NRPA)
22377 Belmont Ridge Road
Ashburn, VA 20148-4501
Toll-Free: 800-626-NRPA
(626-6772)
Website: http://www.nrpa.org

National Strength and Conditioning Association (NSCA)
1885 Bob Johnson Drive
Colorado Springs, CO 80906
Toll-Free: 800-815-6826
Phone: 719-632-6722
Fax: 719-632-6367
Website: http://www.nsca-lift.org
E-mail: nsca@nsca-lift.org

PE Central
P.O. Box 10262
1995 South Main Street
Suite 902
Blacksburg, VA 24062
Phone: 540-953-1043
Fax: 540-301-0112
Website: http://www.pecentral
.org
E-mail: pec@pecentral.org

Shape Up America
P.O. Box 149
506 Brackett Creek Road
Clyde Park, MT 59018-0149
Phone: 406-686-4844
Website: http://www.shapeup.org

Women's Sports Foundation
National Office
Eisenhower Park
1899 Hempstead Turnpike
Suite 400
East Meadow, NY 11554
Toll-Free: 800-227-3988
Phone: 516-542-4700
Fax: 516-542-4716
Website: http://www
.womenssportsfoundation.org
E-mail: Info@
WomensSportsFoundation.org

World Health Organization
Avenue Appia 20
1211 Geneva 27
Switzerland
Phone: +41 22 791 21 11
Fax: +41 22 791 31 11
Website: http://www.who.int
E-mail: info@who.int

Index

Index

Health Reference Series
Complete Catalog
List price $93 per volume. School and library price $84 per volume.

Adolescent Health Sourcebook, 3rd Edition

Basic Consumer Health Information about Adolescent Growth and Development, Puberty, Sexuality, Reproductive Health, and Physical, Emotional, Social, and Mental Health Concerns of Teens and Their Parents, Including Facts about Nutrition, Physical Activity, Weight Management, Acne, Allergies, Cancer, Diabetes, Growth Disorders, Juvenile Arthritis, Infections, Substance Abuse, and More

Along with Information about Adolescent Safety Concerns, Youth Violence, a Glossary of Related Terms, and a Directory of Resources

Edited by Amy L. Sutton. 600 pages. 2010. 978-0-7808-1140-9.

Adult Health Concerns Sourcebook

Basic Consumer Health Information about Medical and Mental Concerns of Adults, Including Facts about Choosing Healthcare Providers, Navigating Insurance Options, Maintaining Wellness, Preventing Cancer, Heart Disease, Stroke, Diabetes, and Osteoporosis, and Understanding Aging-Related Health Concerns, Including Menopause, Cognitive Changes, and Changes in the Coronary and Vascular Systems

Along with Tips on Caring for Aging Parents and Dealing with Health-Related Work and Travel Issues, a Glossary, and a Directory of Resources for Additional Help and Information

Edited by Sandra J. Judd. 648 pages. 2008. 978-0-7808-0999-4.

"Provides a thorough list of topics that are important to adult health and for caregivers."
—CHOICE, Nov '08

"Written in easy-to-understand language... the content is well-organized and is intended to aid adults in making health care-related decisions."
—AORN Journal, Dec '08

AIDS Sourcebook, 4th Edition

Basic Consumer Health Information about Human Immunodeficiency Virus (HIV) and Acquired Immunodeficiency Syndrome (AIDS), Featuring Updated Statistics and Facts about Risks, Prevention, Screening, Diagnosis, Treatments, Side Effects, and Complications, and Including a Section about the Impact of HIV/AIDS on the Health of Women, Children, and Adolescents

Along with Tips on Managing Life with AIDS, Reports on Current Research Initiatives and Clinical Trials, a Glossary of Related Terms, and Resource Directories for Further Help and Information

Edited by Ivy L. Alexander. 680 pages. 2008. 978-0-7808-0997-0.

SEE ALSO *Contagious Diseases Sourcebook, 2nd Edition*

Alcoholism Sourcebook, 3rd Edition

Basic Consumer Health Information about Alcohol Use, Abuse, and Dependence, Featuring Facts about the Physical, Mental, and Social Health Effects of Alcohol Addiction, Including Alcoholic Liver Disease, Pancreatic Disease, Cardiovascular Disease, Neurological Disorders, and the Effects of Drinking during Pregnancy

Along with Information about Alcohol Treatment, Medications, and Recovery Programs, in Addition to Tips for Reducing the Prevalence of Underage Drinking, Statistics about Alcohol Use, a Glossary of Related Terms, and Directories of Resources for More Help and Information

Edited by Joyce Brennfleck Shannon. 600 pages. 2010. 978-0-7808-1141-6.

SEE ALSO *Drug Abuse Sourcebook, 3rd Edition*

Allergies Sourcebook, 3rd Edition

Basic Consumer Health Information about Allergic Disorders, Such as Anaphylaxis, Hives,

Eczema, Rhinitis, Sinusitis, and Conjunctivitis, and Their Triggers, Including Pollen, Mold, Dust Mites, Animal Dander, Insects, Chemicals, Food, Food Additives, and Medications

Along with Advice about the Diagnosis and Treatment of Allergy Symptoms, a Glossary of Related Terms, a Directory of Resources for Help and Information, and Suggestions for Additional Reading

Edited by Amy L. Sutton. 588 pages. 2007. 978-0-7808-0950-5.

SEE ALSO Asthma Sourcebook, 2nd Edition

Alzheimer Disease Sourcebook, 4th Edition

Basic Consumer Health Information about Alzheimer Disease, Other Dementias, and Related Disorders, Including Multi-Infarct Dementia, Dementia with Lewy Bodies, Frontotemporal Dementia (Pick Disease), Wernicke-Korsakoff Syndrome (Alcohol-Related Dementia), AIDS Dementia Complex, Huntington Disease, Creutzfeldt-Jacob Disease, and Delirium

Along with Information about Coping with Memory Loss and Forgetfulness, Maintaining Skills, and Long-Term Planning for People with Dementia, and Suggestions Addressing Common Caregiver Concerns, Updated Information about Current Research Efforts, a Glossary of Related Terms, and Directories of Sources for Additional Help and Information

Edited by Karen Bellenir. 603 pages. 2008. 978-0-7808-1001-3.

"An invaluable resource for persons who have received a diagnosis, for caregivers, and for family members dealing with this insidious disease. It is recommended for public, community college, and ready-reference sections in academic libraries."
—American Reference Books Annual, 2009

SEE ALSO Brain Disorders Sourcebook, 3rd Edition

Arthritis Sourcebook, 3rd Edition

Basic Consumer Health Information about the Risk Factors, Symptoms, Diagnosis, and

Treatment of Osteoarthritis, Rheumatoid Arthritis, Juvenile Arthritis, Gout, Infectious Arthritis, and Autoimmune Disorders Associated with Arthritis

Along with Facts about Medications, Surgeries, and Self-Care Techniques to Manage Pain and Disability, Tips on Living with Arthritis, a Glossary of Related Terms, and Resources for Additional Help and Information

Edited by Amy L. Sutton. 600 pages. 2010. 978-0-7808-1077-8.

Asthma Sourcebook, 2nd Edition

Basic Consumer Health Information about the Causes, Symptoms, Diagnosis, and Treatment of Asthma in Infants, Children, Teenagers, and Adults, Including Facts about Different Types of Asthma, Common Co-Occurring Conditions, Asthma Management Plans, Triggers, Medications, and Medication Delivery Devices

Along with Asthma Statistics, Research Updates, a Glossary, a Directory of Asthma-Related Resources, and More

Edited by Karen Bellenir. 581 pages. 2006. 978-0-7808-0866-9.

SEE ALSO Lung Disorders Sourcebook; Respiratory Disorders Sourcebook, 2nd Edition

Attention Deficit Disorder Sourcebook

Basic Consumer Health Information about Attention Deficit/Hyperactivity Disorder in Children and Adults, Including Facts about Causes, Symptoms, Diagnostic Criteria, and Treatment Options Such as Medications, Behavior Therapy, Coaching, and Homeopathy

Along with Reports on Current Research Initiatives, Legal Issues, and Government Regulations, and Featuring a Glossary of Related Terms, Internet Resources, and a List of Additional Reading Material

Edited by Dawn D. Matthews. 447 pages. 2002. 978-0-7808-0624-5.

"Recommended reference source."
—Booklist, Jan '03

SEE ALSO Learning Disabilities Sourcebook, 3rd Edition

Autism and Pervasive Developmental Disorders Sourcebook

Basic Consumer Health Information about Autism Spectrum and Pervasive Developmental Disorders, Such as Classical Autism, Asperger Syndrome, Rett Syndrome, and Childhood Disintegrative Disorder, Including Information about Related Genetic Disorders and Medical Problems and Facts about Causes, Screening Methods, Diagnostic Criteria, Treatments and Interventions, and Family and Education Issues

Along with a Glossary of Related Terms, Tips for Evaluating the Validity of Health Claims, and a Directory of Resources for Additional Help and Information

Edited by Sandra J. Judd. 603 pages. 2007. 978-0-7808-0953-6.

"This book provides a current overview of disorders on the autism spectrum and information about various therapies, educational resources, and help for families with practical issues such as workplace adjustments, living arrangements, and estate planning. It is a useful resource for public and consumer health libraries."
— American Reference Books Annual, 2009

SEE ALSO Learning Disabilities Sourcebook, 3rd Edition

Back and Neck Disorders Sourcebook, 2nd Edition

Basic Consumer Health Information about Spinal Pain, Spinal Cord Injuries, and Related Disorders, Such as Degenerative Disk Disease, Osteoarthritis, Scoliosis, Sciatica, Spina Bifida, and Spinal Stenosis, and Featuring Facts about Maintaining Spinal Health, Self-Care, Pain Management, Rehabilitative Care, Chiropractic Care, Spinal Surgeries, and Complementary Therapies

Along with Suggestions for Preventing Back and Neck Pain, a Glossary of Related Terms, and a Directory of Resources

Edited by Amy L. Sutton. 607 pages. 2004. 978-0-7808-0738-9.

"Recommended... An easy to use, comprehensive medical reference book."
— E-Streams, Sep '05

"For anyone who has back or neck problems, this book is ideal. Its easy-to-understand language and variety of topics makes this sourcebook a worthwhile read. The price... is reasonable for the amount of information contained in the book"
— Occupational Therapy in Health Care, 2007

Blood & Circulatory Disorders Sourcebook, 3rd Edition

Basic Consumer Health Information about Blood and Circulatory System Disorders, Such as Anemia, Leukemia, Lymphoma, Rh Disease, Hemophilia, Thrombophilia, Other Bleeding and Clotting Deficiencies, and Artery, Vascular, and Venous Diseases, Including Facts about Blood Types, Blood Donation, Bone Marrow and Stem Cell Transplants, Tests and Medications, and Tips for Maintaining Circulatory Health

Along with a Glossary of Related Terms and a List of Resources for Additional Help and Information

Edited by Sandra J. Judd. 600 pages. 2010. 978-0-7808-1081-5.

SEE ALSO Leukemia Sourcebook

Brain Disorders Sourcebook, 3rd Edition

Basic Consumer Health Information about Acquired and Traumatic Brain Injuries, Brain Tumors, Cerebral Palsy and Other Genetic and Congenital Brain Disorders, Infections of the Brain, Epilepsy, and Degenerative Neurological Disorders Such as Dementia, Huntington Disease, and Amyotrophic Lateral Sclerosis (ALS)

Along with Information on Brain Structure and Function, Treatment and Rehabilitation Options, a Glossary of Terms Related to Brain Disorders, and a Directory of Resources for More Information

Edited by Joyce Brennfleck Shannon. 600 pages. 2010. 978-0-7808-1083-9.

SEE ALSO Alzheimer Disease Sourcebook, 4th Edition

Breast Cancer Sourcebook, 3rd Edition

Basic Consumer Health Information about Breast Health and Breast Cancer, Including Facts about Environmental, Genetic, and Other Risk Factors, Prevention Efforts, Screening and Diagnostic Methods, Surgical Treatment Options and Other Care Choices, Complementary and Alternative Therapies, and Post-Treatment Concerns

Along with Statistical Data, News about Research Advances, a Glossary of Related Terms, and Directories of Resources for Additional Information and Support

Edited by Karen Bellenir. 606 pages. 2009. 978-0-7808-1030-3.

"A very useful reference for people wanting to learn more about breast cancer and how to negotiate their care or the care of a loved one. The third edition is necessary as information/treatment options continue to evolve."
—*Doody's Review Service, 2009*

SEE ALSO Cancer Sourcebook for Women, 3rd Edition, Women's Health Concerns Sourcebook, 3rd Edition

Breastfeeding Sourcebook

Basic Consumer Health Information about the Benefits of Breastmilk, Preparing to Breastfeed, Breastfeeding as a Baby Grows, Nutrition, and More, Including Information on Special Situations and Concerns Such as Mastitis, Illness, Medications, Allergies, Multiple Births, Prematurity, Special Needs, and Adoption

Along with a Glossary and Resources for Additional Help and Information

Edited by Jenni Lynn Colson. 367 pages. 2002. 978-0-7808-0332-9.

SEE ALSO Pregnancy and Birth Sourcebook, 3rd Edition

Burns Sourcebook

Basic Consumer Health Information about Various Types of Burns and Scalds, Including Flame, Heat, Cold, Electrical, Chemical, and Sun Burns

Along with Information on Short-Term and Long-Term Treatments, Tissue Reconstruction, Plastic Surgery, Prevention Suggestions, and First Aid

Edited by Allan R. Cook. 604 pages. 1999. 978-0-7808-0204-9.

"This is an exceptional addition to the series and is highly recommended for all consumer health collections, hospital libraries, and academic medical centers."
—*E-Streams, Mar '00*

"This key reference guide is an invaluable addition to all health care and public libraries in confronting this ongoing health issue."
—*American Reference Books Annual, 2000*

SEE ALSO Dermatological Disorders Sourcebook, 2nd Edition

Cancer Sourcebook, 5th Edition

Basic Consumer Health Information about Major Forms and Stages of Cancer, Featuring Facts about Head and Neck Cancers, Lung Cancers, Gastrointestinal Cancers, Genitourinary Cancers, Lymphomas, Blood Cell Cancers, Endocrine Cancers, Skin Cancers, Bone Cancers, Metastatic Cancers, and More

Along with Facts about Cancer Treatments, Cancer Risks and Prevention, a Glossary of Related Terms, Statistical Data, and a Directory of Resources for Additional Information

Edited by Karen Bellenir. 1105 pages. 2007. 978-0-7808-0947-5.

"The 5th, updated edition of Cancer Sourcebook should be in every public and health lending library collection... An unparalleled discussion essential for any health collections considering an all-in-one basic general reference."
—*California Bookwatch, Aug '07*

SEE ALSO Breast Cancer Sourcebook, 3rd Edition, Cancer Survivorship Sourcebook, Leukemia Sourcebook

Cancer Sourcebook for Women, 4th Edition

Basic Consumer Health Information about Gynecologic Cancers and Other Cancers of Special Concern to Women, Including Cancers of the Breast, Cervix, Colon, Lung, Ovaries, Thyroid, and Uterus

Along with Facts about Benign Conditions of the Female Reproductive System, Cancer Risk

Factors, Diagnostic and Treatment Procedures, Side Effects of Cancer and Cancer Treatments, Women's Issues in Cancer Survivorship, a Glossary of Related Terms, and a Directory of Resources for Additional Help and Information

Edited by Karen Bellenir. 600 pages. 2010. 978-0-7808-1139-3.

SEE ALSO Breast Cancer Sourcebook, 3rd Edition, Women's Health Concerns Sourcebook, 3rd Edition

Cancer Survivorship Sourcebook

Basic Consumer Health Information about the Physical, Educational, Emotional, Social, and Financial Needs of Cancer Patients from Diagnosis, through Cancer Treatment, and Beyond, Including Facts about Researching Specific Types of Cancer and Learning about Clinical Trials and Treatment Options, and Featuring Tips for Coping with the Side Effects of Cancer Treatments and Adjusting to Life after Cancer Treatment Concludes

Along with Suggestions for Caregivers, Friends, and Family Members of Cancer Patients, a Glossary of Cancer Care Terms, and Directories of Related Resources

Edited by Karen Bellenir. 633 pages. 2007. 978-0-7808-0985-7.

"Well organized and comprehensive in coverage, the book speaks to issues encountered both during and after cancer treatment. Recommended for consumer health and public libraries."
—Library Journal, Aug 1 '07

"Cancer Survivorship Sourcebook will be useful to anyone who has a friend or loved one with a cancer diagnosis."
—American Reference Books Annual, 2008

SEE ALSO Cancer Sourcebook, 5th Edition, Disease Management Sourcebook

Cardiovascular Disorders Sourcebook, 4th Edition

Basic Consumer Health Information about Heart and Blood Vessel Diseases and Disorders, Such as Angina, Heart Attack, Heart Failure, Cardiomyopathy, Arrhythmias, Valve Disease, Atherosclerosis, Aneurysms, and

Congenital Heart Defects, Including Information about Cardiovascular Disease in Women, Men, Children, Adolescents, and Minorities

Along with Facts about Diagnosing, Managing, and Preventing Cardiovascular Disease, a Glossary of Related Medical Terms, and a Directory of Resources for Additional Information

Edited by Amy L. Sutton. 600 pages. 2010. 978-0-7808-1080-8.

Caregiving Sourcebook

Basic Consumer Health Information for Caregivers, Including a Profile of Caregivers, Caregiving Responsibilities and Concerns, Tips for Specific Conditions, Care Environments, and the Effects of Caregiving

Along with Facts about Legal Issues, Financial Information, and Future Planning, a Glossary, and a Listing of Additional Resources

Edited by Joyce Brennfleck Shannon. 583 pages. 2001. 978-0-7808-0331-2.

"Essential for most collections."
—Library Journal, Apr 1 '02

"An ideal addition to the reference collection of any public library. Health sciences information professionals may also want to acquire the Caregiving Sourcebook for their hospital or academic library for use as a ready reference tool by health care workers interested in aging and caregiving."
—E-Streams, Jan '02

Child Abuse Sourcebook, 2nd Edition

Basic Consumer Health Information about the Physical, Sexual, and Emotional Abuse of Children, Neglect, Münchhausen Syndrome by Proxy (MSBP), and Shaken Baby Syndrome, and Featuring Facts about Withholding Medical Care, Corporal Punishment, Child Maltreatment in Youth Sports, and Parental Substance Abuse

Along with Information about Child Protective Services, Foster Care, Adoption, Parenting Challenges, Abuse Prevention Programs, and Intervention, Treatment, and Recovery Guidelines, a Glossary of Related Terms, and Resources for Additional Help and Information

Edited by Joyce Brennfleck Shannon. 600 pages. 2009. 978-0-7808-1037-2.

SEE ALSO Domestic Violence Sourcebook, 3rd Edition

Childhood Diseases and Disorders Sourcebook, 2nd Edition

Basic Consumer Health Information about the Physical, Mental, and Developmental Health of Pre-Adolescent Children, Including Facts about Infectious Diseases, Asthma, Allergies, Diabetes, and Other Acute and Chronic Conditions Affecting the Gastrointestinal Tract, Ears, Nose, Throat, Liver, Kidneys, Heart, Blood, Brain, Muscles, Bones, and Skin

Along with Reports on Recommended Childhood Vaccinations, Wellness Guidelines, a Glossary of Related Medical Terms, and a List of Resources for Parents

Edited by Sandra J. Judd. 694 pages. 2009. 978-0-7808-1031-0.

"The strength of this source is the wide range of information given about childhood health issues... It is most appropriate for public libraries and academic libraries that field medical questions."
—American Reference Books Annual, 2009

SEE ALSO Healthy Children Sourcebook

Colds, Flu and Other Common Ailments Sourcebook

Basic Consumer Health Information about Common Ailments and Injuries, Including Colds, Coughs, the Flu, Sinus Problems, Headaches, Fever, Nausea and Vomiting, Menstrual Cramps, Diarrhea, Constipation, Hemorrhoids, Back Pain, Dandruff, Dry and Itchy Skin, Cuts, Scrapes, Sprains, Bruises, and More

Along with Information about Prevention, Self-Care, Choosing a Doctor, Over-the-Counter Medications, Folk Remedies, and Alternative Therapies, and Including a Glossary of Important Terms and a Directory of Resources for Further Help and Information

Edited by Chad T. Kimball. 622 pages. 2001. 978-0-7808-0435-7.

"A good starting point for research on common illnesses. It will be a useful addition to public and consumer health library collections."
—American Reference Books Annual, 2002

"Will prove valuable to any library seeking to maintain a current, comprehensive reference collection of health resources... Excellent reference."
—The Bookwatch, Aug '01

SEE ALSO Contagious Diseases Sourcebook, 2nd Edition

Communication Disorders Sourcebook

Basic Information about Deafness and Hearing Loss, Speech and Language Disorders, Voice Disorders, Balance and Vestibular Disorders, and Disorders of Smell, Taste, and Touch

Edited by Linda M. Ross. 533 pages. 1996. 978-0-7808-0077-9.

"This is skillfully edited and is a welcome resource for the layperson. It should be found in every public and medical library."
—Booklist Health Sciences Supplement, Oct '97

Complementary & Alternative Medicine Sourcebook, 4th Edition

Basic Consumer Health Information about Ayurveda, Acupuncture, Aromatherapy, Chiropractic Care, Diet-Based Therapies, Guided Imagery, Herbal and Vitamin Supplements, Homeopathy, Hypnosis, Massage, Meditation, Naturopathy, Pilates, Reflexology, Reiki, Shiatsu, Tai Chi, Traditional Chinese Medicine, Yoga, and Other Complementary and Alternative Medical Therapies

Along with Statistics, Tips for Selecting a Practitioner, Treatments for Specific Health Conditions, a Glossary of Related Terms, and a Directory of Resources for Additional Help and Information

Edited by Amy L. Sutton. 600 pages. 2010. 978-0-7808-1082-2.

Congenital Disorders Sourcebook, 2nd Edition

Basic Consumer Health Information about Nonhereditary Birth Defects and Disorders

Related to Prematurity, Gestational Injuries, Congenital Infections, and Birth Complications, Including Heart Defects, Hydrocephalus, Spina Bifida, Cleft Lip and Palate, Cerebral Palsy, and More

Along with Facts about the Prevention of Birth Defects, Fetal Surgery and Other Treatment Options, Research Initiatives, a Glossary of Related Terms, and Resources for Additional Information and Support

Edited by Sandra J. Judd. 619 pages. 2007. 978-0-7808-0945-1.

"Congenital Disorders Sourcebook provides an excellent, non-technical overview of many aspects of pregnancy with the focus on congenital disorders."
—American Reference Books Annual, 2008

"An excellent readable reference aimed at the lay public for difficult to understand medical problems. An excellent starting point for the interested parent or family member who may then be motivated to seek more information."
—Doody's Review Service, 2007

SEE ALSO Pregnancy and Birth Sourcebook, 3rd Edition

Contagious Diseases Sourcebook, 2nd Edition

Basic Consumer Health Information about Diseases Spread from Person to Person through Direct Physical Contact, Airborne Transmissions, Sexual Contact, or Contact with Blood or Other Body Fluids, Including Pneumococcal, Staphylococcal, and Streptococcal Diseases, Colds, Influenza, Lice, Measles, Mumps, Tuberculosis, and Others

Along with Facts about Self-Care and Over-the-Counter Medications, Antibiotics and Drug Resistance, Disease Prevention, Vaccines, and Bioterrorism, a Glossary, and a Directory of Resources for More Information

Edited by Joyce Brennfleck Shannon. 600 pages. 2010. 978-0-7808-1075-4.

SEE ALSO AIDS Sourcebook, 4th Edition, Hepatitis Sourcebook

Cosmetic and Reconstructive Surgery Sourcebook, 2nd Edition

Basic Consumer Information about Plastic Surgery and Non-Surgical Appearance-Enhancing Procedures, Including Facts about Botulinum Toxin, Collagen Replacement, Dermabrasion, Chemical Peels, Eyelid Surgery, Nose Reshaping, Lip Augmentation, Liposuction, Breast Enlargement and Reduction, Tummy Tucking, and Other Skin, Hair, Facial, and Body Shaping Procedures

Along with Information about Reconstructive Procedures for Congenital Disorders, Disfiguring Diseases, Burns, and Traumatic Injuries, a Glossary of Related Terms, and a Directory of Additional Resources

Edited by Karen Bellenir. 483 pages. 2007. 978-0-7808-0951-2.

"A comprehensive source for people considering cosmetic surgery... also recommended for medical students who will perform these procedures later in their careers; and public librarians and academic medical librarians who may assist patrons interested in this information."
—Medical Reference Services Quarterly, Fall '08

"A practical guide for health care consumers and health care workers... This easy-to-read reference guide would be useful for novice and veteran health care consumers, surgical technology students, nursing students, and perioperative nurses new to plastic and reconstructive surgery. It also may be helpful for medical-surgical nurses as a guide for patient teaching in their practices."
—AORN Journal, Aug '08

SEE ALSO Surgery Sourcebook, 2nd Edition

Death and Dying Sourcebook, 2nd Edition

Basic Consumer Health Information about End-of-Life Care and Related Perspectives and Ethical Issues, Including End-of-Life Symptoms and Treatments, Pain Management, Quality-of-Life Concerns, the Use of Life Support, Patients' Rights and Privacy Issues, Advance Directives, Physician-Assisted Suicide, Caregiving, Organ and Tissue Donation, Autopsies, Funeral Arrangements, and Grief

Along with Statistical Data, Information about the Leading Causes of Death, a Glossary, and Directories of Support Groups and Other Resources

Edited by Joyce Brennfleck Shannon. 626 pages. 2006. 978-0-7808-0871-3.

Dental Care and Oral Health Sourcebook, 3rd Edition

Basic Consumer Health Information about Dental Care and Oral Health Throughout the Lifespan, Including Facts about Cavities, Bad Breath, Cold and Canker Sores, Dry Mouth, Toothaches, Gum Disease, Malocclusion, Temporomandibular Joint and Muscle Disorders, Oral Cancers, and Dental Emergencies

Along with Information about Mouth Hygiene, Crowns, Bridges, Implants, and Fillings, Surgical, Orthodontic, and Cosmetic Dental Procedures, Pain Management, Health Conditions that Impact Oral Care, a Glossary of Related Terms, and a Directory of Additional Resources

Edited by Amy L. Sutton. 619 pages. 2008. 978-0-7808-1032-7.

"Could serve as turning point in the battle to educate consumers in issues concerning oral health. Tightly written in terms the average person can understand, yet comprehensive in scope and authoritative in tone, it is another excellent sourcebook in the Health Reference Series... Should be in the reference department of all public libraries, and in academic libraries that have a public constituency."
—*American Reference Books Annual, 2009*

Depression Sourcebook, 2nd Edition

Basic Consumer Health Information about Unipolar Depression, Bipolar Disorder, Dysthymia, Seasonal Affective Disorder, Postpartum Depression, and Other Depressive Disorders, Including Facts about Populations at Special Risk, Coexisting Medical Conditions, Symptoms, Treatment Options, and Suicide Prevention

Along with Statistical Data, a Glossary of Related Terms, and a Directory of Resources for Additional Help and Information

Edited by Sandra J. Judd. 646 pages. 2008. 978-0-7808-1003-7.

"Recommended for public libraries."
—*American Reference Books Annual, 2009*

SEE ALSO Mental Health Disorders Sourcebook, 4th Edition

Dermatological Disorders Sourcebook, 2nd Edition

Basic Consumer Health Information about Conditions and Disorders Affecting the Skin, Hair, and Nails, Such as Acne, Rosacea, Rashes, Dermatitis, Pigmentation Disorders, Birthmarks, Skin Cancer, Skin Injuries, Psoriasis, Scleroderma, and Hair Loss, Including Facts about Medications and Treatments for Dermatological Disorders and Tips for Maintaining Healthy Skin, Hair, and Nails

Along with Information about How Aging Affects the Skin, a Glossary of Related Terms, and a Directory of Resources for Additional Help and Information

Edited by Amy L. Sutton. 617 pages. 2006. 978-0-7808-0795-2.

"Well organized... presents a plethora of information in a manner that is appropriate in style and readability for the intended audience."
—*Physical Therapy, Nov '06*

"Helpfully brings together... sources in one convenient place, saving the user hours of research time."
—*American Reference Books Annual, 2006*

SEE ALSO Burns Sourcebook

Diabetes Sourcebook, 4th Edition

Basic Consumer Health Information about Type 1 and Type 2 Diabetes Mellitus, Gestational Diabetes, Monogenic Forms of Diabetes, and Insulin Resistance, with Guidelines for Lifestyle Modifications and the Medical Management of Diabetes, Including Facts about Insulin, Insulin Delivery Devices, Oral Diabetes Medications, Self-Monitoring of Blood Glucose, Meal Planning, Physical Activity Recommendations, Foot Care, and Treatment Options for People with Kidney Failure

Along with a Section about Diabetes Complications and Co-Occurring Conditions, a Glossary of Related Terms, and Directories of Resources for Additional Help and Information

Edited by Karen Bellenir. 627 pages. 2008. 978-0-7808-1005-1.

"Completely and comprehensively covering almost everything a student or physician would need to know... well worth the investment."
— *Internet Bookwatch*, Dec '08

SEE ALSO Endocrine and Metabolic Disorders Sourcebook, 2nd Edition

Diet and Nutrition Sourcebook, 3rd Edition

Basic Consumer Health Information about Dietary Guidelines and the Food Guidance System, Recommended Daily Nutrient Intakes, Serving Proportions, Weight Control, Vitamins and Supplements, Nutrition Issues for Different Life Stages and Lifestyles, and the Needs of People with Specific Medical Concerns, Including Cancer, Celiac Disease, Diabetes, Eating Disorders, Food Allergies, and Cardiovascular Disease

Along with Facts about Federal Nutrition Support Programs, a Glossary of Nutrition and Dietary Terms, and Directories of Additional Resources for More Information about Nutrition

Edited by Joyce Brennfleck Shannon. 605 pages. 2006. 978-0-7808-0800-3.

"A valuable resource tool for any individual."
— *Journal of Dental Hygiene*, Apr '07

"From different recommended eating habits to reduce disease and common ailments to nutrition advice for those with specific conditions, Diet and Nutrition Sourcebook is especially important because so much is changing in this area, and so rapidly."
— *California Bookwatch*, Jun '06

SEE ALSO Eating Disorders Sourcebook, 2nd Edition, Vegetarian Sourcebook

Digestive Diseases and Disorders Sourcebook

Basic Consumer Health Information about Diseases and Disorders that Impact the Upper and Lower Digestive System, Including Celiac

Disease, Constipation, Crohn's Disease, Cyclic Vomiting Syndrome, Diarrhea, Diverticulosis and Diverticulitis, Gallstones, Heartburn, Hemorrhoids, Hernias, Indigestion (Dyspepsia), Irritable Bowel Syndrome, Lactose Intolerance, Ulcers, and More

Along with Information about Medications and Other Treatments, Tips for Maintaining a Healthy Digestive Tract, a Glossary, and Directory of Digestive Diseases Organizations

Edited by Karen Bellenir. 323 pages. 2000. 978-0-7808-0327-5.

"An excellent addition to all public or patient-research libraries."
— *American Reference Books Annual*, 2001

"Recommended reference source."
— *Booklist*, May '00

SEE ALSO Gastrointestinal Diseases and Disorders Sourcebook, 2nd Edition

Disabilities Sourcebook

Basic Consumer Health Information about Physical and Psychiatric Disabilities, Including Descriptions of Major Causes of Disability, Assistive and Adaptive Aids, Workplace Issues, and Accessibility Concerns

Along with Information about the Americans with Disabilities Act, a Glossary, and Resources for Additional Help and Information

Edited by Dawn D. Matthews. 602 pages. 2000. 978-0-7808-0389-3.

"A must for libraries with a consumer health section."
— *American Reference Books Annual*, 2002

"A much needed addition to the Omnigraphics Health Reference Series. A current reference work to provide people with disabilities, their families, caregivers or those who work with them, a broad range of information in one volume, has not been available until now... It is recommended for all public and academic library reference collections."
— *E-Streams*, May '01

"An excellent source book in easy-to-read format covering many current topics; highly recommended for all libraries."
— *CHOICE*, Jan '01

Disease Management Sourcebook

Basic Consumer Health Information about Coping with Chronic and Serious Illnesses, Navigating the Health Care System, Communicating with Health Care Providers, Assessing Health Care Quality, and Making Informed Health Care Decisions, Including Facts about Second Opinions, Hospitalization, Surgery, and Medications

Along with a Section about Children with Chronic Conditions, Information about Legal, Financial, and Insurance Issues, a Glossary of Related Terms, and Directories of Additional Resources

Edited by Joyce Brennfleck Shannon. 621 pages. 2008. 978-0-7808-1002-0.

"Consumers need to know how to manage their health care the same way they manage anything else in their lives. The text is very readable and is written for the layperson and consumer. The cost is not prohibitive. This book should be in all collections of health care libraries and public libraries."
— *American Reference Books Annual, 2009*

"The information is very current, and the selection of font and layout make the book easy to read. A hardback that will stand up to much usage, this is an excellent resource for consumers... Recommended. General readers."
—*CHOICE, Nov '08*

"Intended for lay readers, this resource clarifies the many confusing and overwhelming details associated with chronic disease care. Meticulous and clearly explained, the book even includes diagrams intended to ease comprehension of over-the-counter medication labels. An essential guide to navigating the health-care rapids."
—*Library Journal, Aug '08*

Domestic Violence Sourcebook, 3rd Edition

Basic Consumer Health Information about Warning Signs, Risk Factors, and Health Consequences of Intimate Partner Violence, Sexual Violence and Rape, Stalking, Human Trafficking, Child Maltreatment, Teen Dating Violence, and Elder Abuse

Along with Facts about Victims and Perpetrators, Strategies for Violence Prevention, and Emergency Interventions, Safety Plans, and Financial and Legal Tips for Victims, a Glossary of Related Terms, and Directories of Resources for Additional Information and Support

Edited by Joyce Brennfleck Shannon. 634 pages. 2009. 978-0-7808-1038-9.

"A recommended pick for any library interested in consumer health and social issues... A 'must' for any serious health collection."
—*California Bookwatch, Jul '09*

SEE ALSO Child Abuse Sourcebook, 2nd Edition

Drug Abuse Sourcebook, 3rd Edition

Basic Consumer Health Information about the Abuse of Cocaine, Club Drugs, Hallucinogens, Heroin, Inhalants, Marijuana, and Other Illicit Substances, Prescription Medications, and Over-the-Counter Medicines

Along with Facts about Addiction and Related Health Effects, Drug Abuse Treatment and Recovery, Drug Testing, Prevention Programs, Glossaries of Drug-Related Terms, and Directories of Resources for More Information

Edited by Joyce Brennfleck Shannon. 600 pages. 2010. 978-0-7808-1079-2.

SEE ALSO Alcoholism Sourcebook, 3rd Edition

Ear, Nose, and Throat Disorders Sourcebook, 2nd Edition

Basic Consumer Health Information about Disorders of the Ears, Hearing Loss, Vestibular Disorders, Nasal and Sinus Problems, Throat and Vocal Cord Disorders, and Otolaryngologic Cancers, Including Facts about Ear Infections and Injuries, Genetic and Congenital Deafness, Sensorineural Hearing Disorders, Tinnitus, Vertigo, Ménière Disease, Rhinitis, Sinusitis, Snoring, Sore Throats, Hoarseness, and More

Along with Reports on Current Research Initiatives, a Glossary of Related Medical Terms, and a Directory of Sources for Further Help and Information

Edited by Sandra J. Judd. 631 pages. 2007. 978-0-7808-0872-0.

"A resource book for the general public that provides comprehensive coverage of basic up-to-date medical information about the causes, symptoms, diagnosis, and treatment of diseases and disorders that affect the ears, nose, sinuses, throat, and voice... The majority of information is presented in question and answer format, much like questions a patient might ask of a health care provider. An extensive index facilitates the reader's ability to easily access information on any specific topic."
—*Journal of Dental Hygiene, Oct '07*

"A handy compilation of information on common and some not so common ailments of the ears, nose, and throat."
—*Doody's Review Service, 2007*

■

Eating Disorders Sourcebook, 2nd Edition

Basic Consumer Health Information about Anorexia Nervosa, Bulimia, Binge Eating, Compulsive Exercise, Female Athlete Triad, and Other Eating Disorders, Including Facts about Body Image and Other Cultural and Age-Related Risk Factors, Prevention Efforts, Adverse Health Effects, Treatment Options, and the Recovery Process

Along with Guidelines for Healthy Weight Control, a Glossary, and Directories of Additional Resources

Edited by Joyce Brennfleck Shannon. 557 pages. 2007. 978-0-7808-0948-2.

"Recommended for the reference collection of large public libraries."
—*American Reference Books Annual, 2008*

"A basic health reference any health or general library needs."
—*Internet Bookwatch, Jun '07*

SEE ALSO *Diet and Nutrition Sourcebook, 3rd Edition, Mental Health Disorders Sourcebook, 4th Edition*

■

Emergency Medical Services Sourcebook

Basic Consumer Health Information about Preventing, Preparing for, and Managing Emergency Situations, When and Who to Call for Help, What to Expect in the Emergency Room, the Emergency Medical Team,

Patient Issues, and Current Topics in Emergency Medicine

Along with Statistical Data, a Glossary, and Sources of Additional Help and Information

Edited by Jenni Lynn Colson. 472 pages. 2002. 978-0-7808-0420-3.

"Handy and convenient for home, public, school, and college libraries. Recommended."
—*CHOICE, Apr '03*

"This reference can provide the consumer with answers to most questions about emergency care in the United States, or it will direct them to a resource where the answer can be found."
—*American Reference Books Annual, 2003*

SEE ALSO *Injury and Trauma Sourcebook*

■

Endocrine and Metabolic Disorders Sourcebook, 2nd Edition

Basic Consumer Health Information about Hormonal and Metabolic Disorders that Affect the Body's Growth, Development, and Functioning, Including Disorders of the Pancreas, Ovaries and Testes, and Pituitary, Thyroid, Parathyroid, and Adrenal Glands, with Facts about Growth Disorders, Addison Disease, Cushing Syndrome, Conn Syndrome, Diabetic Disorders, Multiple Endocrine Neoplasia, Inborn Errors of Metabolism, and More

Along with Information about Endocrine Functioning, Diagnostic and Screening Tests, a Glossary of Related Terms, and Directories of Additional Resources

Edited by Joyce Brennfleck Shannon. 597 pages. 2007. 978-0-7808-0952-9.

SEE ALSO *Diabetes Sourcebook, 4th Edition*

■

Environmental Health Sourcebook, 3rd Edition

Basic Consumer Health Information about the Environment and Its Effects on Human Health, Including Facts about Air, Water, and Soil Contamination, Hazardous Chemicals, Foodborne Hazards and Illnesses, Household Hazards Such as Radon, Mold, and Carbon Monoxide, Consumer Hazards from Toxic Products and Imported Goods, and Disorders

Linked to Environmental Causes, Including Chemical Sensitivity, Cancer, Allergies, and Asthma

Along with Information about the Impact of Environmental Hazards on Specific Populations, a Glossary of Related Terms, and Resources for Additional Help and Information.

Edited by Laura Larsen. 600 pages. 2010. 978-0-7808-1078-5

Ethnic Diseases Sourcebook

Basic Consumer Health Information for Ethnic and Racial Minority Groups in the United States, Including General Health Indicators and Behaviors, Ethnic Diseases, Genetic Testing, the Impact of Chronic Diseases, Women's Health, Mental Health Issues, and Preventive Health Care Services

Along with a Glossary and a Listing of Additional Resources

Edited by Joyce Brennfleck Shannon. 648 pages. 2001. 978-0-7808-0336-7.

"Not many books have been written on this topic to date, and the Ethnic Diseases Sourcebook is a strong addition to the list. It will be an important introductory resource for health consumers, students, health care personnel, and social scientists. It is recommended for public, academic, and large hospital libraries."
— American Reference Books Annual, 2002

"Will prove valuable to any library seeking to maintain a current, comprehensive reference collection of health resources... An excellent source of health information about genetic disorders which affect particular ethnic and racial minorities in the U.S."
—The Bookwatch, Aug '01

Eye Care Sourcebook, 3rd Edition

Basic Consumer Health Information about Eye Care and Eye Disorders, Including Facts about the Diagnosis, Prevention, and Treatment of Refractive Disorders, Cataracts, Glaucoma, Macular Degeneration, and Problems Affecting the Cornea, Retina, and Lacrimal Glands

Along with Advice about Preventing Eye Injuries and Tips for Living with Low Vision or Blindness, a Glossary of Related Terms, and Directories of Resources for More Help and Information

Edited by Amy L. Sutton. 646 pages. 2008. 978-0-7808-1000-6.

"A solid reference tool for eye care and a valuable addition to a collection."
—American Reference Books Annual, 2009

Family Planning Sourcebook

Basic Consumer Health Information about Planning for Pregnancy and Contraception, Including Traditional Methods, Barrier Methods, Hormonal Methods, Permanent Methods, Future Methods, Emergency Contraception, and Birth Control Choices for Women at Each Stage of Life

Along with Statistics, a Glossary, and Sources of Additional Information

Edited by Amy Marcaccio Keyzer. 503 pages. 2001. 978-0-7808-0379-4.

"Recommended for public, health, and undergraduate libraries as part of the circulating collection."
—E-Streams, Mar '02

"Will prove valuable to any library seeking to maintain a current, comprehensive reference collection of health resources... Excellent reference."
—The Bookwatch, Aug '01

SEE ALSO Pregnancy and Birth Sourcebook, 3rd Edition

Fitness and Exercise Sourcebook, 3rd Edition

Basic Consumer Health Information about the Physical and Mental Benefits of Fitness, Including Cardiorespiratory Endurance, Muscular Strength, Muscular Endurance, and Flexibility, with Facts about Sports Nutrition and Exercise-Related Injuries and Tips about Physical Activity and Exercises for People of All Ages and for People with Health Concerns

Along with Advice on Selecting and Using Exercise Equipment, Maintaining Exercise Motivation, a Glossary of Related Terms, and a Directory of Resources for More Help and Information

Edited by Amy L. Sutton. 635 pages. 2007. 978-0-7808-0946-8.

"Updates the consumer information on the physical and mental benefits of physical activity throughout the lifespan offered in earlier editions... Recommended. All readers; all levels."
—CHOICE, Oct '07

"An exceptionally well-rounded coverage perfect for any concerned about developing and understanding a fitness program."
—California Bookwatch, Jun '07

SEE ALSO Sports Injuries Sourcebook, 3rd Edition

Food Safety Sourcebook

Basic Consumer Health Information about the Safe Handling of Meat, Poultry, Seafood, Eggs, Fruit Juices, and Other Food Items, and Facts about Pesticides, Drinking Water, Food Safety Overseas, and the Onset, Duration, and Symptoms of Foodborne Illnesses, Including Types of Pathogenic Bacteria, Parasitic Protozoa, Worms, Viruses, and Natural Toxins

Along with the Role of the Consumer, the Food Handler, and the Government in Food Safety, a Glossary, and Resources for Additional Help and Information

Edited by Dawn D. Matthews. 327 pages. 1999. 978-0-7808-0326-8.

"Recommended reference source."
—Booklist, May '00

"This book takes the complex issues of food safety and foodborne pathogens and presents them in an easily understood manner. [It does] an excellent job of covering a large and often confusing topic."
— American Reference Books Annual, 2000

Forensic Medicine Sourcebook

Basic Consumer Information for the Layperson about Forensic Medicine, Including Crime Scene Investigation, Evidence Collection and Analysis, Expert Testimony, Computer-Aided Criminal Identification, Digital Imaging in the Courtroom, DNA Profiling, Accident Reconstruction, Autopsies, Ballistics, Drugs and Explosives Detection, Latent Fingerprints, Product Tampering, and Questioned Document Examination

Along with Statistical Data, a Glossary of Forensics Terminology, and Listings of Sources for Further Help and Information

Edited by Annemarie S. Muth. 574 pages. 1999. 978-0-7808-0232-2.

"Given the expected widespread interest in its content and its easy to read style, this book is recommended for most public and all college and university libraries."
—E-Streams, Feb '01

"A wealth of information, useful statistics, references are up-to-date and extremely complete. This wonderful collection of data will help students who are interested in a career in any type of forensic field. It is a great resource for attorneys who need information about types of expert witnesses needed in a particular case. It also offers useful information for fiction and nonfiction writers whose work involves a crime. A fascinating compilation. All levels."
—CHOICE, Jan '00

"There are several items that make this book attractive to consumers who are seeking certain forensic data... This is a useful current source for those seeking general forensic medical answers."
—American Reference Books Annual, 2000

Gastrointestinal Diseases and Disorders Sourcebook, 2nd Edition

Basic Consumer Health Information about the Upper and Lower Gastrointestinal (GI) Tract, Including the Esophagus, Stomach, Intestines, Rectum, Liver, and Pancreas, with Facts about Gastroesophageal Reflux Disease, Gastritis, Hernias, Ulcers, Celiac Disease, Diverticulitis, Irritable Bowel Syndrome, Hemorrhoids, Gastrointestinal Cancers, and Other Diseases and Disorders Related to the Digestive Process

Along with Information about Commonly Used Diagnostic and Surgical Procedures, Statistics, Reports on Current Research Initiatives and Clinical Trials, a Glossary, and Resources for Additional Help and Information

Edited by Sandra J. Judd. 654 pages. 2006. 978-0-7808-0798-3.

"The text is designed for the general reader seeking information on prevention, disease warning signs, diagnostic and therapeutic questions... It is an excellent resource for the general reader to conveniently locate credible, coordinated and indexed information... The sourcebook will prove very helpful for patients, caregivers and should be available in every physician waiting room."
—*Doody's Review Service, 2006*

SEE ALSO Diet and Nutrition Sourcebook, 3rd Edition, Digestive Diseases and Disorders Sourcebook

Genetic Disorders Sourcebook, 4th Edition

Basic Consumer Health Information about Hereditary Diseases and Disorders, Including Facts about the Human Genome, Genetic Inheritance Patterns, Disorders Associated with Specific Genes, Such as Sickle Cell Disease, Hemophilia, and Cystic Fibrosis, Chromosome Disorders, Such as Down Syndrome, Fragile X Syndrome, and Turner Syndrome, and Complex Diseases and Disorders Resulting from the Interaction of Environmental and Genetic Factors, Such as Allergies, Cancer, and Obesity

Along with Facts about Genetic Testing, Suggestions for Parents of Children with Special Needs, Reports on Current Research Initiatives, a Glossary of Genetic Terminology, and Resources for Additional Help and Information

Edited by Sandra J. Judd. 600 pages. 2010. 978-0-7808-1076-1.

Head Trauma Sourcebook

Basic Information for the Layperson about Open-Head and Closed-Head Injuries, Treatment Advances, Recovery, and Rehabilitation

Along with Reports on Current Research Initiatives

Edited by Karen Bellenir. 414 pages. 1997. 978-0-7808-0208-7.

Headache Sourcebook

Basic Consumer Health Information about Migraine, Tension, Cluster, Rebound and Other Types of Headaches, with Facts about the Cause and Prevention of Headaches, the Effects of Stress and the Environment, Headaches during Pregnancy and Menopause, and Childhood Headaches

Along with a Glossary and Other Resources for Additional Help and Information

Edited by Dawn D. Matthews. 342 pages. 2002. 978-0-7808-0337-4.

"Highly recommended for academic and medical reference collections."
—*Library Bookwatch, Sep '02*

SEE ALSO Pain Sourcebook, 3rd Edition

Healthy Aging Sourcebook

Basic Consumer Health Information about Maintaining Health through the Aging Process, Including Advice on Nutrition, Exercise, and Sleep, Help in Making Decisions about Midlife Issues and Retirement, and Guidance Concerning Practical and Informed Choices in Health Consumerism

Along with Data Concerning the Theories of Aging, Different Experiences in Aging by Minority Groups, and Facts about Aging Now and Aging in the Future; and Featuring a Glossary, a Guide to Consumer Help, Additional Suggested Reading, and Practical Resource Directory

Edited by Jenifer Swanson. 537 pages. 1999. 978-0-7808-0390-9.

"Recommended reference source."
—*Booklist, Feb '00*

SEE ALSO Adult Health Sourcebook, Physical and Mental Issues in Aging Sourcebook

Healthy Children Sourcebook

Basic Consumer Health Information about the Physical and Mental Development of Children between the Ages of 3 and 12, Including Routine Health Care, Preventative Health Services, Safety and First Aid, Healthy Sleep, Dental Care, Nutrition, and Fitness, and Featuring Parenting Tips on Such Topics as Bedwetting, Choosing Day Care, Monitoring TV and Other Media, and Establishing a Foundation for Substance Abuse Prevention

Along with a Glossary of Commonly Used Pediatric Terms and Resources for Additional Help and Information.

Edited by Chad T. Kimball. 624 pages. 2003. 978-0-7808-0247-6.

"Should be required reading for parents and teachers."
—*E-Streams, Jun '04*

"It is hard to imagine that any other single resource exists that would provide such a comprehensive guide of timely information on health promotion and disease prevention for children aged 3 to 12."
—*American Reference Books Annual, 2004*

"This easy-to-read volume is a tremendous resource."
—*AORN Journal, May '05*

SEE ALSO Childhood Diseases and Disorders Sourcebook, 2nd Edition

Healthy Heart Sourcebook for Women

Basic Consumer Health Information about Cardiac Issues Specific to Women, Including Facts about Major Risk Factors and Prevention, Treatment and Control Strategies, and Important Dietary Issues

Along with a Special Section Regarding the Pros and Cons of Hormone Replacement Therapy and Its Impact on Heart Health, and Additional Help, Including Recipes, a Glossary, and a Directory of Resources

Edited by Dawn D. Matthews. 321 pages. 2000. 978-0-7808-0329-9.

"A good reference source and recommended for all public, academic, medical, and hospital libraries."
—*Medical Reference Services Quarterly, Summer '01*

"Contains very important information about coronary artery disease that all women should know. The information is current and presented in an easy-to-read format. The book will make a good addition to any library."
—*American Medical Writers Association Journal, Summer '00*

SEE ALSO Cardiovascular Diseases and Disorders Sourcebook, 4th Edition, Women's Health Concerns Sourcebook, 3rd Edition

Hepatitis Sourcebook

Basic Consumer Health Information about Hepatitis A, Hepatitis B, Hepatitis C, and Other Forms of Hepatitis, Including Autoimmune Hepatitis, Alcoholic Hepatitis, Nonalcoholic Steatohepatitis, and Toxic Hepatitis, with Facts about Risk Factors, Screening Methods, Diagnostic Tests, and Treatment Options

Along with Information on Liver Health, Tips for People Living with Chronic Hepatitis, Reports on Current Research Initiatives, a Glossary of Terms Related to Hepatitis, and a Directory of Sources for Further Help and Information

Edited by Sandra J. Judd. 570 pages. 2006. 978-0-7808-0749-5.

"The breadth of information found in this one book would not be readily found in another source. Highly recommended."
—*American Reference Books Annual, 2006*

SEE ALSO Contagious Diseases Sourcebook, 2nd Edition

Household Safety Sourcebook

Basic Consumer Health Information about Household Safety, Including Information about Poisons, Chemicals, Fire, and Water Hazards in the Home

Along with Advice about the Safe Use of Home Maintenance Equipment, Choosing Toys and Nursery Furniture, Holiday and Recreation Safety, a Glossary, and Resources for Further Help and Information

Edited by Dawn D. Matthews. 587 pages. 2002. 978-0-7808-0338-1.

"As a sourcebook on household safety this book meets its mark. It is encyclopedic in scope and covers a wide range of safety issues that are commonly seen in the home."
—*E-Streams, Jul '02*

Hypertension Sourcebook

Basic Consumer Health Information about the Causes, Diagnosis, and Treatment of High Blood Pressure, with Facts about Consequences, Complications, and Co-Occurring Disorders, Such as Coronary Heart Disease, Diabetes, Stroke, Kidney Disease, and Hypertensive Retinopathy, and Issues in Blood Pressure

Control, Including Dietary Choices, Stress Management, and Medications

Along with Reports on Current Research Initiatives and Clinical Trials, a Glossary, and Resources for Additional Help and Information

Edited by Dawn D. Matthews and Karen Bellenir. 588 pages. 2004. 978-0-7808-0674-0.

"Academic, public, and medical libraries will want to add the Hypertension Sourcebook to their collections."
— E-Streams, Aug '05

"The strength of this source is the wide range of information given about hypertension."
— American Reference Books Annual, 2005

SEE ALSO Stroke Sourcebook, 2nd Edition

Immune System Disorders Sourcebook, 2nd Edition

Basic Consumer Health Information about Disorders of the Immune System, Including Immune System Function and Response, Diagnosis of Immune Disorders, Information about Inherited Immune Disease, Acquired Immune Disease, and Autoimmune Diseases, Including Primary Immune Deficiency, Acquired Immunodeficiency Syndrome (AIDS), Lupus, Multiple Sclerosis, Type 1 Diabetes, Rheumatoid Arthritis, and Graves' Disease

Along with Treatments, Tips for Coping with Immune Disorders, a Glossary, and a Directory of Additional Resources

Edited by Joyce Brennfleck Shannon. 643 pages. 2005. 978-0-7808-0748-8.

"Highly recommended for academic and public libraries."
— American Reference Books Annual, 2006

"The updated second edition is a 'must' for any consumer health library seeking a solid resource covering the treatments, symptoms, and options for immune disorder sufferers... An excellent guide."
— MBR Bookwatch, Jan '06

SEE ALSO AIDS Sourcebook, 4th Edition, Arthritis Sourcebook, 3rd Edition

Infant and Toddler Health Sourcebook

Basic Consumer Health Information about the Physical and Mental Development of Newborns, Infants, and Toddlers, Including Neonatal Concerns, Nutrition Recommendations, Immunization Schedules, Common Pediatric Disorders, Assessments and Milestones, Safety Tips, and Advice for Parents and Other Caregivers

Along with a Glossary of Terms and Resource Listings for Additional Help

Edited by Jenifer Swanson. 570 pages. 2000. 978-0-7808-0246-9.

"As a reference for the general public, this would be useful in any library."
— E-Streams, May '01

"Recommended reference source."
— Booklist, Feb '01

Infectious Diseases Sourcebook

Basic Consumer Health Information about Non-Contagious Bacterial, Viral, Prion, Fungal, and Parasitic Diseases Spread by Food and Water, Insects and Animals, or Environmental Contact, Including Botulism, E. Coli, Encephalitis, Legionnaires' Disease, Lyme Disease, Malaria, Plague, Rabies, Salmonella, Tetanus, and Others, and Facts about Newly Emerging Diseases, Such as Hantavirus, Mad Cow Disease, Monkeypox, and West Nile Virus

Along with Information about Preventing Disease Transmission, the Threat of Bioterrorism, and Current Research Initiatives, with a Glossary and Directory of Resources for More Information

Edited by Karen Bellenir. 610 pages. 2004. 978-0-7808-0675-7.

"This reference continues the excellent tradition of the Health Reference Series in consolidating a wealth of information on a selected topic into a format that is easy to use and accessible to the general public."
— American Reference Books Annual, 2005

"Recommended for public and academic libraries."
— E-Streams, Jan '05

SEE ALSO Environmental Health Sourcebook, 3rd Edition

Injury and Trauma Sourcebook

Basic Consumer Health Information about the Impact of Injury, the Diagnosis and Treatment of Common and Traumatic Injuries, Emergency Care, and Specific Injuries Related to Home, Community, Workplace, Transportation, and Recreation

Along with Guidelines for Injury Prevention, a Glossary, and a Directory of Additional Resources

Edited by Joyce Brennfleck Shannon. 675 pages. 2002. 978-0-7808-0421-0.

"Practitioners should be aware of guides such as this in order to facilitate their use by patients and their families."
—*Doody's Health Sciences Book Review Journal, Sep-Oct '02*

"Recommended reference source."
—*Booklist, Sep '02*

"Highly recommended for academic and medical reference collections."
—*Library Bookwatch, Sep '02*

SEE ALSO Emergency Medical Services Sourcebook, Sports Injuries Sourcebook, 3rd Edition

Learning Disabilities Sourcebook, 3rd Edition

Basic Consumer Health Information about Dyslexia, Auditory and Visual Processing Disorders, Communication Disorders, Dyscalculia, Dysgraphia, and Other Conditions That Impede Learning, Including Attention Deficit/ Hyperactivity Disorder, Autism Spectrum Disorders, Hearing and Visual Impairments, Chromosome-Based Disorders, and Brain Injury

Along with Facts about Brain Function, Assessment, Therapy and Remediation, Accommodations, Assistive Technology, Legal Protections, and Tips about Family Life, School Transitions, and Employment Strategies, a Glossary of Related Terms, and Directories of Additional Resources

Edited by Joyce Brennfleck Shannon. 613 pages. 2009. 978-0-7808-1039-6.

"Intended to be a starting point for people who need to know about learning disabilities. Each chapter on a specific disability includes readable,

well-organized descriptions... The book is well indexed and a glossary is included. Chapters on organizations and helpful websites will aid the reader who needs more information."
—*American Reference Books Annual, 2009*

"This book provides the necessary information to better understand learning disabilities and work with children who have them... It would be difficult to find another book that so comprehensively explains learning disabilities without becoming incomprehensible to the average parent who needs this information."
—*Doody's Review Service, 2009*

SEE ALSO Attention Deficit Disorder Sourcebook, Autism and Pervasive Developmental Disorders Sourcebook

Leukemia Sourcebook

Basic Consumer Health Information about Adult and Childhood Leukemias, Including Acute Lymphocytic Leukemia (ALL), Chronic Lymphocytic Leukemia (CLL), Acute Myelogenous Leukemia (AML), Chronic Myelogenous Leukemia (CML), and Hairy Cell Leukemia, and Treatments Such as Chemotherapy, Radiation Therapy, Peripheral Blood Stem Cell and Marrow Transplantation, and Immunotherapy

Along with Tips for Life During and After Treatment, a Glossary, and Directories of Additional Resources

Edited by Joyce Brennfleck Shannon. 564 pages. 2003. 978-0-7808-0627-6.

"Unlike other medical books for the layperson... the language does not talk down to the reader... This volume is highly recommended for all libraries."
—*American Reference Books Annual, 2004*

"A fine title which ranges from diagnosis to alternative treatments, staging, and tips for life during and after diagnosis."
—*The Bookwatch, Dec '03*

SEE ALSO Blood & Circulatory Disorders Sourcebook, 3rd Edition, Cancer Sourcebook, 5th Edition

Liver Disorders Sourcebook

Basic Consumer Health Information about the Liver and How It Works; Liver Diseases, Including Cancer, Cirrhosis, Hepatitis, and

Toxic and Drug Related Diseases; Tips for Maintaining a Healthy Liver; Laboratory Tests, Radiology Tests, and Facts about Liver Transplantation

Along with a Section on Support Groups, a Glossary, and Resource Listings

Edited by Joyce Brennfleck Shannon. 580 pages. 2000. 978-0-7808-0383-1.

"This title is recommended for health sciences and public libraries with consumer health collections."
—E-Streams, Oct '00

"Recommended reference source."
—Booklist, Jun '00

SEE ALSO Gastrointestinal Diseases and Disorders Sourcebook, 2nd Edition, Hepatitis Sourcebook

■

Lung Disorders Sourcebook

Basic Consumer Health Information about Emphysema, Pneumonia, Tuberculosis, Asthma, Cystic Fibrosis, and Other Lung Disorders, Including Facts about Diagnostic Procedures, Treatment Strategies, Disease Prevention Efforts, and Such Risk Factors as Smoking, Air Pollution, and Exposure to Asbestos, Radon, and Other Agents

Along with a Glossary and Resources for Additional Help and Information

Edited by Dawn D. Matthews. 657 pages. 2002. 978-0-7808-0339-8.

"Highly recommended for academic and medical reference collections."
—Library Bookwatch, Sep '02

SEE ALSO Asthma Sourcebook, 2nd Edition, Respiratory Disorders Sourcebook, 2nd Edition

■

Medical Tests Sourcebook, 3rd Edition

Basic Consumer Health Information about X-Rays, Blood Tests, Stool and Urine Tests, Biopsies, Mammography, Endoscopic Procedures, Ultrasound Exams, Computed Tomography, Magnetic Resonance Imaging (MRI), Nuclear Medicine, Genetic Testing, Home-Use Tests, and More

Along with Facts about Preventive Care and Screening Test Guidelines, Screening and

Assessment Tests Associated with Such Specific Concerns as Cancer, Heart Disease, Allergies, Diabetes, Thyroid Disfunction, and Infertility, a Glossary of Related Terms, and a Directory of Resources for Additional Help and Information

Edited by Karen Bellenir. 627 pages. 2008. 978-0-7808-1040-2

"This volume has a wide scope that makes it useful... Can be a valuable reference guide."
—American Reference Books Annual, 2009

"Would be a valuable contribution to any consumer health or public library."
—Doody's Book Review Service, 2009

■

Men's Health Concerns Sourcebook, 3rd Edition

Basic Consumer Health Information about Wellness in Men and Gender-Related Differences in Health, With Facts about Heart Disease, Cancer, Traumatic Injury, and Other Leading Causes of Death in Men, Reproductive Concerns, Sexual Dysfunction, Disorders of the Prostate, Penis, and Testes, Sex-Linked Genetic Disorders, and Other Medical and Mental Concerns of Men

Along with Statistical Data, a Glossary of Related Terms, and a Directory of Resources for Additional Information

Edited by Sandra J. Judd. 632 pages. 2009. 978-0-7808-1033-4.

"A good addition to any reference shelf in academic, consumer health, or hospital libraries."
—ARBAOnline, Oct '09

SEE ALSO Prostate and Urological Disorders Sourcebook

■

Mental Health Disorders Sourcebook, 4th Edition

Basic Consumer Health Information about the Causes and Symptoms of Mental Health Problems, Including Depression, Bipolar Disorder, Anxiety Disorders, Posttraumatic Stress Disorder, Obsessive-Compulsive Disorder, Eating Disorders, Addictions, and Personality and Psychotic Disorders

Along with Information about Medications and Treatments, Mental Health Concerns in

Children, Adolescents, and Adults, Tips on Living with Mental Health Disorders, a Glossary of Related Terms, and a Directory of Resources for Additional Help and Information

Edited by Amy L. Sutton. 680 pages. 2009. 978-0-7808-1041-9.

"Mental health concerns are presented in everyday language and intended for patients and their families as well as the general public... This resource is comprehensive and up to date... The easy-to-understand writing style helps to facilitate assimilation of needed facts and specifics on often challenging topics."
—*ARBAOnline, Oct '09*

"No health collection should be without this resource, which will reach into many a general lending library as well."
—*Internet Bookwatch, Oct '09*

SEE ALSO *Depression Sourcebook, 2nd Edition, Stress-Related Disorders Sourcebook, 2nd Edition*

Mental Retardation Sourcebook

Basic Consumer Health Information about Mental Retardation and Its Causes, Including Down Syndrome, Fetal Alcohol Syndrome, Fragile X Syndrome, Genetic Conditions, Injury, and Environmental Sources

Along with Preventive Strategies, Parenting Issues, Educational Implications, Health Care Needs, Employment and Economic Matters, Legal Issues, a Glossary, and a Resource Listing for Additional Help and Information

Edited by Joyce Brennfleck Shannon. 627 pages. 2000. 978-0-7808-0377-0.

"Public libraries will find the book useful for reference and as a beginning research point for students, parents, and caregivers."
—*American Reference Books Annual, 2001*

"The strength of this work is that it compiles many basic fact sheets and addresses for further information in one volume. It is intended and suitable for the general public."
—*E-Streams, Nov '00*

"An invaluable overview."
—*Reviewer's Bookwatch, Jul '00*

Movement Disorders Sourcebook, 2nd Edition

Basic Consumer Health Information about the Symptoms and Causes of Movement Disorders, Including Parkinson Disease, Amyotrophic Lateral Sclerosis, Cerebral Palsy, Muscular Dystrophy, Multiple Sclerosis, Myasthenia, Myoclonus, Spina Bifida, Dystonia, Essential Tremor, Choreatic Disorders, Huntington Disease, Tourette Syndrome, and Other Disorders That Cause Slowed, Absent, or Excessive Movements

Along with Information about Surgical and Nonsurgical Interventions, Physical Therapies, Strategies for Independent Living, a Glossary of Related Terms, and a Directory of Resources for Additional Help and Information

Edited by Amy L. Sutton. 618 pages. 2009. 978-0-7808-1034-1.

"The second updated edition of Movement Disorders Sourcebook is a winner, providing the latest research and health findings on all kinds of movement disorders in children and adults... a top pick for any health or general lending library's health reference collection."
—*California Bookwatch, Aug '09*

SEE ALSO *Muscular Dystrophy Sourcebook*

Multiple Sclerosis Sourcebook

Basic Consumer Health Information about Multiple Sclerosis (MS) and Its Effects on Mobility, Vision, Bladder Function, Speech, Swallowing, and Cognition, Including Facts about Risk Factors, Causes, Diagnostic Procedures, Pain Management, Drug Treatments, and Physical and Occupational Therapies

Along with Guidelines for Nutrition and Exercise, Tips on Choosing Assistive Equipment, Information about Disability, Work, Financial, and Legal Issues, a Glossary of Related Terms, and a Directory of Additional Resources

Edited by Joyce Brennfleck Shannon. 553 pages. 2007. 978-0-7808-0998-7.

Muscular Dystrophy Sourcebook

Basic Consumer Health Information about Congenital, Childhood-Onset, and Adult-Onset

Forms of Muscular Dystrophy, Such as Duchenne, Becker, Emery-Dreifuss, Distal, Limb-Girdle, Facioscapulohumeral (FSHD), Myotonic, and Ophthalmoplegic Muscular Dystrophies, Including Facts about Diagnostic Tests, Medical and Physical Therapies, Management of Co-Occurring Conditions, and Parenting Guidelines

Along with Practical Tips for Home Care, a Glossary, and Directories of Additional Resources

Edited by Joyce Brennfleck Shannon. 552 pages. 2004. 978-0-7808-0676-4.

"This book is highly recommended for public and academic libraries as well as health care offices that support the information needs of patients and their families."
—E-Streams, Apr '05

"Excellent reference."
—The Bookwatch, Jan '05

SEE ALSO Movement Disorders Sourcebook, 2nd Edition

Obesity Sourcebook

Basic Consumer Health Information about Diseases and Other Problems Associated with Obesity, and Including Facts about Risk Factors, Prevention Issues, and Management Approaches

Along with Statistical and Demographic Data, Information about Special Populations, Research Updates, a Glossary, and Source Listings for Further Help and Information

Edited by Wilma Caldwell and Chad T. Kimball. 360 pages. 2001. 978-0-7808-0333-6.

"The book synthesizes the reliable medical literature on obesity into one easy-to-read and useful resource for the general public."
—American Reference Books Annual, 2002

"Well suited for the health reference collection of a public library or an academic health science library that serves the general population."
—E-Streams, Sep '01

Osteoporosis Sourcebook

Basic Consumer Health Information about Primary and Secondary Osteoporosis and Juvenile Osteoporosis and Related Conditions, Including Fibrous Dysplasia, Gaucher Disease, Hyperthyroidism, Hypophosphatasia,

Myeloma, Osteopetrosis, Osteogenesis Imperfecta, and Paget's Disease

Along with Information about Risk Factors, Treatments, Traditional and Non-Traditional Pain Management, a Glossary of Related Terms, and a Directory of Resources

Edited by Allan R. Cook. 568 pages. 2001. 978-0-7808-0239-1.

"This resource is recommended as a great reference source for public, health, and academic libraries, and is another triumph for the editors of Omnigraphics."
—American Reference Books Annual, 2002

"Will prove valuable to any library seeking to maintain a current, comprehensive reference collection of health resources... From prevention to treatment and associated conditions, this provides an excellent survey."
—The Bookwatch, Aug '01

SEE ALSO Healthy Aging Sourcebook, Women's Health Concerns Sourcebook, 3rd Edition

Pain Sourcebook, 3rd Edition

Basic Consumer Health Information about Acute and Chronic Pain, Including Nerve Pain, Bone Pain, Muscle Pain, Cancer Pain, and Disorders Characterized by Pain, Such as Arthritis, Temporomandibular Muscle and Joint (TMJ) Disorder, Carpal Tunnel Syndrome, Headaches, Heartburn, Sciatica, and Shingles, and Facts about Diagnostic Tests and Treatment Options for Pain, Including Over-the-Counter and Prescription Drugs, Physical Rehabilitation, Injection and Infusion Therapies, Implantable Technologies, and Complementary Medicine

Along with Tips for Living with Pain, a Glossary of Related Terms, and a Directory of Additional Resources

Edited by Joyce Brennfleck Shannon. 644 pages. 2008. 978-0-7808-1006-8.

"Excellent for ready-reference users and can be used for beginning students in health fields... appropriate for the consumer health collection in both public and academic libraries."
—American Reference Books Annual, 2009

SEE ALSO Arthritis Sourcebook, 3rd Edition; Back and Neck Sourcebook, 2nd Edition;

Headache Sourcebook; Sports Injuries Sourcebook, 3rd Edition

SEE ALSO *Healthy Aging Sourcebook*

Pediatric Cancer Sourcebook

Basic Consumer Health Information about Leukemias, Brain Tumors, Sarcomas, Lymphomas, and Other Cancers in Infants, Children, and Adolescents, Including Descriptions of Cancers, Treatments, and Coping Strategies

Along with Suggestions for Parents, Caregivers, and Concerned Relatives, a Glossary of Cancer Terms, and Resource Listings

Edited by Edward J. Prucha. 575 pages. 1999. 978-0-7808-0245-2.

"An excellent source of information. Recommended for public, hospital, and health science libraries with consumer health collections."
—*E-Streams, Jun '00*

"A valuable addition to all libraries specializing in health services and many public libraries."
—*American Reference Books Annual, 2000*

SEE ALSO *Childhood Diseases and Disorders Sourcebook, 2nd Edition, Healthy Children Sourcebook*

Physical and Mental Issues in Aging Sourcebook

Basic Consumer Health Information on Physical and Mental Disorders Associated with the Aging Process, Including Concerns about Cardiovascular Disease, Pulmonary Disease, Oral Health, Digestive Disorders, Musculoskeletal and Skin Disorders, Metabolic Changes, Sexual and Reproductive Issues, and Changes in Vision, Hearing, and Other Senses

Along with Data about Longevity and Causes of Death, Information on Acute and Chronic Pain, Descriptions of Mental Concerns, a Glossary of Terms, and Resource Listings for Additional Help

Edited by Jenifer Swanson. 660 pages. 1999. 978-0-7808-0233-9.

"This is a treasure of health information for the layperson."
—*CHOICE Health Sciences Supplement, May '00*

"Recommended for public libraries."
—*American Reference Books Annual, 2000*

Podiatry Sourcebook, 2nd Edition

Basic Consumer Health Information about Disorders, Diseases, and Deformities that Affect the Foot and Ankle, Including Sprains, Corns, Calluses, Bunions, Plantar Warts, Plantar Fasciitis, Neuromas, Clubfoot, Flat Feet, Achilles Tendonitis, and Much More

Along with Information about Selecting a Foot Care Specialist, Foot Fitness, Shoes and Socks, Diagnostic Tests and Corrective Procedures, Financial Assistance for Corrective Devices, a Glossary of Related Terms, and a Directory of Resources for Additional Help and Information

Edited by Ivy L. Alexander. 516 pages. 2007. 978-0-7808-0944-4.

"An excellent resource... Although there have been various types of 'foot books' published in the past, none are as comprehensive as this one. 5 Stars (out of 5)!"
—*Doody's Review Service, 2007*

"Perfect for both health libraries and general-interest lending collections."
—*Internet Bookwatch, Jul '07*

Pregnancy and Birth Sourcebook, 3rd Edition

Basic Consumer Health Information about Pregnancy and Fetal Development, Including Facts about Fertility and Conception, Physical and Emotional Changes during Pregnancy, Prenatal Care and Diagnostic Tests, High-Risk Pregnancies and Complications, Labor, Delivery, and the Postpartum Period

Along with Tips on Maintaining Health and Wellness during Pregnancy and Caring for Newborn Infants, a Glossary of Related Terms, and Directories of Resources for Additional Help and Information

Edited by Amy L. Sutton. 645 pages. 2009. 978-0-7808-1074-7.

SEE ALSO *Breastfeeding Sourcebook, Congenital Disorders Sourcebook, 2nd Edition, Family Planning Sourcebook, Women's Health Concerns Sourcebook, 3rd Edition*

Prostate and Urological Disorders Sourcebook

Basic Consumer Health Information about Urogenital and Sexual Disorders in Men, Including Prostate and Other Andrological Cancers, Prostatitis, Benign Prostatic Hyperplasia, Testicular and Penile Trauma, Cryptorchidism, Peyronie Disease, Erectile Dysfunction, and Male Factor Infertility, and Facts about Commonly Used Tests and Procedures, Such as Prostatectomy, Vasectomy, Vasectomy Reversal, Penile Implants, and Semen Analysis

Along with a Glossary of Andrological Terms and a Directory of Resources for Additional Information

Edited by Karen Bellenir. 604 pages. 2006. 978-0-7808-0797-6.

"Certain to be a popular pick among library reference holdings... No prior knowledge is assumed for any of the conditions or terms herein, making it a most accessible general-interest reference."
—California Bookwatch, Apr '06

SEE ALSO *Men's Health Concerns Sourcebook, 3rd Edition, Urinary Tract and Kidney Diseases and Disorders Sourcebook, 2nd Edition*

Prostate Cancer Sourcebook

Basic Consumer Health Information about Prostate Cancer, Including Information about the Associated Risk Factors, Detection, Diagnosis, and Treatment of Prostate Cancer

Along with Information on Non-Malignant Prostate Conditions, and Featuring a Section Listing Support and Treatment Centers and a Glossary of Related Terms

Edited by Dawn D. Matthews. 340 pages. 2001. 978-0-7808-0324-4.

"Recommended reference source."
—Booklist, Jan '02

"A valuable resource for health care consumers seeking information on the subject... All text is written in a clear, easy-to-understand language that avoids technical jargon. Any library that collects consumer health resources would strengthen their collection with the addition of the Prostate Cancer Sourcebook."
—American Reference Books Annual, 2002

SEE ALSO *Cancer Sourcebook, 5th Edition, Men's Health Concerns Sourcebook, 3rd Edition*

Rehabilitation Sourcebook

Basic Consumer Health Information about Rehabilitation for People Recovering from Heart Surgery, Spinal Cord Injury, Stroke, Orthopedic Impairments, Amputation, Pulmonary Impairments, Traumatic Injury, and More, Including Physical Therapy, Occupational Therapy, Speech/Language Therapy, Massage Therapy, Dance Therapy, Art Therapy, and Recreational Therapy

Along with Information on Assistive and Adaptive Devices, a Glossary, and Resources for Additional Help and Information

Edited by Dawn D. Matthews. 519 pages. 2000. 978-0-7808-0236-0.

"This is an excellent resource for public library reference and health collections."
—American Reference Books Annual, 2001

"Recommended reference source."
—Booklist, May '00

Respiratory Disorders Sourcebook, 2nd Edition

Basic Consumer Health Information about Infectious, Inflammatory, and Chronic Conditions Affecting the Lungs and Respiratory System, Including Pneumonia, Bronchitis, Influenza, Tuberculosis, Sarcoidosis, Asthma, Cystic Fibrosis, Chronic Obstructive Pulmonary Disease, Lung Abscesses, Pulmonary Embolism, Occupational Lung Diseases, and Other Bacterial, Viral, and Fungal Infections

Along with Facts about the Structure and Function of the Lungs and Airways, Methods of Diagnosing Respiratory Disorders, and Treatment and Rehabilitation Options, a Glossary of Related Terms, and a Directory of Resources for Additional Help and Information

Edited by Sandra L. Judd. 638 pages. 2008. 978-0-7808-1007-5.

"An excellent book for patients, their families, or for those who are just curious about respiratory disease. Public libraries and physician offices would find this a valuable resource as well. 4 Stars! (out of 5)"
—Doody's Review Service, 2009

"A great addition for public and school libraries because it provides concise health information... readers can start with this reference source and get satisfactory answers before proceeding to other medical reference tools for

more in depth information... A good guide for health education on lung disorders."
—*American Reference Books Annual, 2009*

SEE ALSO *Asthma Sourcebook, 2nd Edition, Lung Disorders Sourcebook*

Sexually Transmitted Diseases Sourcebook, 4th Edition

Basic Consumer Health Information about Chlamydial Infections, Gonorrhea, Hepatitis, Herpes, HIV/AIDS, Human Papillomavirus, Pubic Lice, Scabies, Syphilis, Trichomoniasis, Vaginal Infections, and Other Sexually Transmitted Diseases, Including Facts about Risk Factors, Symptoms, Diagnosis, Treatment, and the Prevention of Sexually Transmitted Infections

Along with Updates on Current Research Initiatives, a Glossary of Related Terms, and Resources for Additional Help and Information

Edited by Laura Larsen. 623 pages. 2009. 978-0-7808-1073-0.

"Extremely beneficial... The question-and-answer format along with the index and table of contents make this well-organized resource extremely easy to reference, read, and comprehend... an invaluable medical reference source for lay readers, and a highly appropriate addition for public library collections, health clinics, and any library with a consumer health collection"
—*ARBAOnline, Oct '09*

SEE ALSO *AIDS Sourcebook, 4th Edition, Contagious Diseases Sourcebook, 2nd Edition, Men's Health Concerns Sourcebook, 3rd Edition, Women's Health Concerns Sourcebook, 3rd Edition*

Sleep Disorders Sourcebook, 3rd Edition

Basic Consumer Health Information about Sleep Disorders, Including Insomnia, Sleep Apnea and Snoring, Jet Lag and Other Circadian Rhythm Disorders, Narcolepsy, and Parasomnias, Such as Sleep Walking and Sleep Talking, and Featuring Facts about Other Health Problems that Affect Sleep, Why Sleep Is Necessary, How Much Sleep Is Needed, the Physical and Mental Effects of Sleep Deprivation, and Pediatric Sleep Issues

Along with Tips for Diagnosing and Treating Sleep Disorders, a Glossary of Related Terms, and a List of Resources for Additional Help and Information

Edited by Sandra J. Judd. 600 pages. 2010. 978-0-7808-1084-6.

Smoking Concerns Sourcebook

Basic Consumer Health Information about Nicotine Addiction and Smoking Cessation, Featuring Facts about the Health Effects of Tobacco Use, Including Lung and Other Cancers, Heart Disease, Stroke, and Respiratory Disorders, Such as Emphysema and Chronic Bronchitis

Along with Information about Smoking Prevention Programs, Suggestions for Achieving and Maintaining a Smoke-Free Lifestyle, Statistics about Tobacco Use, Reports on Current Research Initiatives, a Glossary of Related Terms, and Directories of Resources for Additional Help and Information

Edited by Karen Bellenir. 595 pages. 2004. 978-0-7808-0323-7.

"Provides everything needed for the student or general reader seeking practical details on the effects of tobacco use."
—*The Bookwatch, Mar '05*

"Public libraries and consumer health care libraries will find this work useful."
—*American Reference Books Annual, 2005*

SEE ALSO *Respiratory Disorders Sourcebook, 2nd Edition*

Sports Injuries Sourcebook, 3rd Edition

Basic Consumer Health Information about Sprains and Strains, Fractures, Growth Plate Injuries, Overtraining Injuries, and Injuries to the Head, Face, Shoulders, Elbows, Hands, Spinal Column, Knees, Ankles, and Feet, and with Facts about Heat-Related Illness, Steroids and Sport Supplements, Protective Equipment, Diagnostic Procedures, Treatment Options, and Rehabilitation

Along with a Glossary of Related Terms and a Directory of Resources for Additional Help and Information

Edited by Sandra J. Judd. 623 pages. 2007. 978-0-7808-0949-9.

SEE ALSO Fitness and Exercise Sourcebook, 3rd Edition, Podiatry Sourcebook, 2nd Edition

Stress-Related Disorders Sourcebook, 2nd Edition

Basic Consumer Health Information about Stress and Stress-Related Disorders, Including Types of Stress, Sources of Acute and Chronic Stress, the Impact of Stress on the Body's Systems, and Mental and Emotional Health Problems Associated with Stress, Such as Depression, Anxiety Disorders, Substance Abuse, Posttraumatic Stress Disorder, and Suicide

Along with Advice about Getting Help for Stress-Related Disorders, Information about Stress Management Techniques, a Glossary of Stress-Related Terms, and a Directory of Resources for Additional Help and Information

Edited by Amy L. Sutton. 608 pages. 2007. 978-0-7808-0996-3.

"Accessible to the lay reader. Highly recommended for medical and psychiatric collections."
—*Library Journal, Mar '08*

"Well-written for a general readership, the 2nd Edition of Stress-Related Disorders Sourcebook is a useful addition to the health reference literature."
—*American Reference Books Annual, 2008*

SEE ALSO Mental Health Disorders Sourcebook, 4th Edition

Stroke Sourcebook, 2nd Edition

Basic Consumer Health Information about Stroke, Including Ischemic, Hemorrhagic, and Mini Strokes, as Well as Risk Factors, Prevention Guidelines, Diagnostic Tests, Medications and Surgical Treatments, and Complications of Stroke

Along with Rehabilitation Techniques and Innovations, Tips on Staying Healthy and Maintaining Independence after Stroke, a Glossary of Related Terms, and a Directory of Resources for Stroke Survivors and Their Families

Edited by Amy L. Sutton. 626 pages. 2008. 978-0-7808-1035-8.

"An encyclopedic handbook on stroke that is written in a language the layperson can understand... This is one of the most helpful, readable books on stroke. This volume is highly recommended and should be in every medical, hospital and public library; in addition, every family practitioner should have a copy in his or her office."
—*American Reference Books Annual, 2009*

SEE ALSO Brain Disorders Sourcebook, 3rd Edition, Hypertension Sourcebook

Surgery Sourcebook, 2nd Edition

Basic Consumer Health Information about Common Inpatient and Outpatient Surgeries, Including Critical Care and Trauma, Gastrointestinal, Gynecologic and Obstetric, Cardiac and Vascular, Neurologic, Ophthalmologic, Orthopedic, Reconstructive and Cosmetic, and Other Major and Minor Surgeries

Along with Information about Anesthesia and Pain Relief Options, Risks and Complications, Postoperative Recovery Concerns, and Innovative Surgical Techniques and Tools, a Glossary of Related Terms, and a Directory of Additional Resources

Edited by Amy L. Sutton. 645 pages. 2008. 978-0-7808-1004-4.

"Large public libraries and medical libraries would benefit from this material in their reference collections."
—*American Reference Books Annual, 2009*

SEE ALSO Cosmetic and Reconstructive Surgery Sourcebook, 2nd Edition

Thyroid Disorders Sourcebook

Basic Consumer Health Information about Disorders of the Thyroid and Parathyroid Glands, Including Hypothyroidism, Hyperthyroidism, Graves Disease, Hashimoto Thyroiditis, Thyroid Cancer, and Parathyroid Disorders, Featuring Facts about Symptoms, Risk Factors, Tests, and Treatments

Along with Information about the Effects of Thyroid Imbalance on Other Body Systems, Environmental Factors That Affect the Thyroid Gland, a Glossary, and a Directory of Additional Resources

Edited by Joyce Brennfleck Shannon. 573 pages. 2005. 978-0-7808-0745-7.

"Recommended for consumer health collections."
—*American Reference Books Annual, 2006*

"Highly recommended pick for Basic Consumer health reference holdings at all levels."
—*The Bookwatch, Aug '05*

SEE ALSO Endocrine and Metabolic Disorders Sourcebook, 2nd Edition

Transplantation Sourcebook

Basic Consumer Health Information about Organ and Tissue Transplantation, Including Physical and Financial Preparations, Procedures and Issues Relating to Specific Solid Organ and Tissue Transplants, Rehabilitation, Pediatric Transplant Information, the Future of Transplantation, and Organ and Tissue Donation

Along with a Glossary and Listings of Additional Resources

Edited by Joyce Brennfleck Shannon. 610 pages. 2002. 978-0-7808-0322-0.

"Recommended for libraries with an interest in offering consumer health information."
—*E-Streams, Jul '02*

"This is a unique and valuable resource for patients facing transplantation and their families."
—*Doody's Review Service, Jun '02*

Traveler's Health Sourcebook

Basic Consumer Health Information for Travelers, Including Physical and Medical Preparations, Transportation Health and Safety, Essential Information about Food and Water, Sun Exposure, Insect and Snake Bites, Camping and Wilderness Medicine, and Travel with Physical or Medical Disabilities

Along with International Travel Tips, Vaccination Recommendations, Geographical Health Issues, Disease Risks, a Glossary, and a Listing of Additional Resources

Edited by Joyce Brennfleck Shannon. 619 pages. 2000. 978-0-7808-0384-8.

"Recommended reference source."
—*Booklist, Feb '01*

"This book is recommended for any public library, any travel collection, and especially any collection for the physically disabled."
—*American Reference Books Annual, 2001*

SEE ALSO Worldwide Health Sourcebook

Urinary Tract and Kidney Diseases and Disorders Sourcebook, 2nd Edition

Basic Consumer Health Information about the Urinary System, Including the Bladder, Urethra, Ureters, and Kidneys, with Facts about Urinary Tract Infections, Incontinence, Congenital Disorders, Kidney Stones, Cancers of the Urinary Tract and Kidneys, Kidney Failure, Dialysis, and Kidney Transplantation

Along with Statistical and Demographic Information, Reports on Current Research in Kidney and Urologic Health, a Summary of Commonly Used Diagnostic Tests, a Glossary of Related Terms, and a Directory of Resources for Additional Help and Information

Edited by Ivy L. Alexander. 621 pages. 2005. 978-0-7808-0750-1.

"A good choice for a consumer health information library or for a medical library needing information to refer to their patients."
—*American Reference Books Annual, 2006*

SEE ALSO Prostate and Urological Disorders Sourcebook

Vegetarian Sourcebook

Basic Consumer Health Information about Vegetarian Diets, Lifestyle, and Philosophy, Including Definitions of Vegetarianism and Veganism, Tips about Adopting Vegetarianism, Creating a Vegetarian Pantry, and Meeting Nutritional Needs of Vegetarians, with Facts Regarding Vegetarianism's Effect on Pregnant and Lactating Women, Children, Athletes, and Senior Citizens

Along with a Glossary of Commonly Used Vegetarian Terms and Resources for Additional Help and Information

Edited by Chad T. Kimball. 337 pages. 2002. 978-0-7808-0439-5.

"Organizes into one concise volume the answers to the most common questions concerning vegetarian diets and lifestyles. This title is recommended for public and secondary school libraries."

—*E-Streams, Apr '03*

"**Invaluable reference for public and school library collections alike.**"
—*Library Bookwatch, Apr '03*

"**The articles in this volume are easy to read and come from authoritative sources. The book does not necessarily support the vegetarian diet but instead provides the pros and cons of this important decision... Recommended for public libraries and consumer health libraries.**"
—*American Reference Books Annual, 2003*

SEE ALSO *Diet and Nutrition Sourcebook, 3rd Edition*

Women's Health Concerns Sourcebook, 3rd Edition

Basic Consumer Health Information about Issues and Trends in Women's Health and Health Conditions of Special Concern to Women, Including Endometriosis, Uterine Fibroids, Menstrual Irregularities, Menopause, Sexual Dysfunction, Infertility, Cancer in Women, and Other Such Chronic Disorders as Lupus, Fibromyalgia, and Thyroid Disease

Along with Statistical Data, Tips for Maintaining Wellness, a Glossary, and a Directory of Resources for Further Help and Information

Edited by Sandra J. Judd. 679 pages. 2009. 978-0-7808-1036-5.

"**This useful resource provides information about a wide range of topics that will help women understand their bodies, prevent or treat disease, and maintain health... A detailed index helps readers locate information. This is a useful addition to public and consumer health library collections**"
—*ARBAOnline, Jun '09*

SEE ALSO *Breast Cancer Sourcebook, 3rd Edition, Cancer Sourcebook for Women, 4th Edition, Healthy Heart Sourcebook for Women*

Workplace Health and Safety Sourcebook

Basic Consumer Health Information about Workplace Health and Safety, Including the Effect of Workplace Hazards on the Lungs,

Skin, Heart, Ears, Eyes, Brain, Reproductive Organs, Musculoskeletal System, and Other Organs and Body Parts

Along with Information about Occupational Cancer, Personal Protective Equipment, Toxic and Hazardous Chemicals, Child Labor, Stress, and Workplace Violence

Edited by Chad T. Kimball. 610 pages. 2000. 978-0-7808-0231-5.

"**As a reference for the general public, this would be useful in any library.**"
—*E-Streams, Jun '01*

"**Provides helpful information for primary care physicians and other caregivers interested in occupational medicine... General readers; professionals.**"
—*CHOICE, May '01*

Worldwide Health Sourcebook

Basic Information about Global Health Issues, Including Malnutrition, Reproductive Health, Disease Dispersion and Prevention, Emerging Diseases, Risky Health Behaviors, and the Leading Causes of Death

Along with Global Health Concerns for Children, Women, and the Elderly, Mental Health Issues, Research and Technology Advancements, and Economic, Environmental, and Political Health Implications, a Glossary, and a Resource Listing for Additional Help and Information

Edited by Joyce Brennfleck Shannon. 597 pages. 2001. 978-0-7808-0330-5.

"**Named an Outstanding Academic Title.**"
—*CHOICE, Jan '02*

"**Yet another handy but also unique compilation in the extensive Health Reference Series, this is a useful work because many of the international publications reprinted or excerpted are not readily available. Highly recommended.**"
—*CHOICE, Nov '01*

SEE ALSO *Traveler's Health Sourcebook*

Teen Health Series
Complete Catalog
List price $69 per volume. School and library price $62 per volume.

Abuse and Violence Information for Teens
Health Tips about the Causes and Consequences of Abusive and Violent Behavior
Including Facts about the Types of Abuse and Violence, the Warning Signs of Abusive and Violent Behavior, Health Concerns of Victims, and Getting Help and Staying Safe

Edited by Sandra Augustyn Lawton. 411 pages. 2008. 978-0-7808-1008-2.

"A useful resource for schools and organizations providing services to teens and may also be a starting point in research projects."
—*Reference and Research Book News, Aug '08*

"Violence is a serious problem for teens... This resource gives teens the information they need to face potential threats and get help—either for themselves or for their friends."
—*American Reference Books Annual, 2009*

Accident and Safety Information for Teens
Health Tips about Medical Emergencies, Traumatic Injuries, and Disaster Preparedness
Including Facts about Motor Vehicle Accidents, Burns, Poisoning, Firearms, Natural Disasters, National Security Threats, and More

Edited by Karen Bellenir. 420 pages. 2008. 978-0-7808-1046-4.

"Aimed at teenage audiences, this guide provides practical information for handling a comprehensive list of emergencies, from sport injuries and auto accidents to alcohol poisoning and natural disasters."
—*Library Journal, Apr 1, '09*

"Useful in the young adult collections of public libraries as well as high school libraries."
—*American Reference Books Annual, 2009*

SEE ALSO Sports Injuries Information for Teens, 2nd Edition

Alcohol Information for Teens, 2nd Edition
Health Tips about Alcohol and Alcoholism
Including Facts about Alcohol's Effects on the Body, Brain, and Behavior, the Consequences of Underage Drinking, Alcohol Abuse Prevention and Treatment, and Coping with Alcoholic Parents

Edited by Lisa Bakewell. 410 pages. 2009. 978-0-7808-1043-3.

"This handbook, written for a teenage audience, provides information on the causes, effects, and preventive measures related to alcohol abuse among teens... The chapters are quick to make a connection to their teenage reading audience. The prose is straightforward and the book lends itself to spot reading. It should be useful both for practical information and for research, and it is suitable for public and school libraries."
—*ARBAOnline, Jun '09*

SEE ALSO Drug Information for Teens, 2nd Edition

Allergy Information for Teens
Health Tips about Allergic Reactions Such as Anaphylaxis, Respiratory Problems, and Rashes
Including Facts about Identifying and Managing Allergies to Food, Pollen, Mold, Animals, Chemicals, Drugs, and Other Substances

Edited by Karen Bellenir. 410 pages. 2006. 978-0-7808-0799-0.

"This is a comprehensive, readable text on the subject of allergic diseases in teenagers. 5 Stars (out of 5)!"
—*Doody's Review Service, Jun '06*

"This authoritative and useful self-help title is a solid addition to YA collections, whether for personal interest or reports."
—*School Library Journal, Jul '06*

Asthma Information for Teens, 2nd Ed.
Health Tips about Managing Asthma and Related Concerns

Including Facts about Asthma Causes, Triggers and Symptoms, Diagnosis, and Treatment

Edited by Kim Wohlenhaus. 400 pages. 2010. 978-0-7808-1086-0.

Body Information for Teens
Health Tips about Maintaining Well-Being for a Lifetime
Including Facts about the Development and Functioning of the Body's Systems, Organs, and Structures and the Health Impact of Lifestyle Choices

Edited by Sandra Augustyn Lawton. 458 pages. 2007. 978-0-7808-0443-2.

Cancer Information for Teens, 2nd Edition
Health Tips about Cancer Awareness, Symptoms, Prevention, Diagnosis, and Treatment
Including Facts about Common Cancers Affecting Teens, Causes, Detection, Coping Strategies, Clinical Trials, Nutrition and Exercise, Cancer in Friends or Family, and More

Edited by Karen Bellenir and Lisa Bakewell. 445 pages. 2010. 978-0-7808-1085-3.

Complementary and Alternative Medicine Information for Teens
Health Tips about Non-Traditional and Non-Western Medical Practices
Including Information about Acupuncture, Chiropractic Medicine, Dietary and Herbal Supplements, Hypnosis, Massage Therapy, Prayer and Spirituality, Reflexology, Yoga, and More

Edited by Sandra Augustyn Lawton. 407 pages. 2007. 978-0-7808-0966-6.

"This volume covers CAM specifically for teenagers but of general use also. It should be a welcome addition to both public and academic libraries."
—*American Reference Books Annual, 2008*

"This volume provides a solid foundation for further investigation of the subject, making it useful for both public and high school libraries."
—*VOYA: Voice of Youth Advocates, Jun '07*

Diabetes Information for Teens
Health Tips about Managing Diabetes and Preventing Related Complications
Including Information about Insulin, Glucose Control, Healthy Eating, Physical Activity, and Learning to Live with Diabetes

Edited by Sandra Augustyn Lawton. 410 pages. 2006. 978-0-7808-0811-9.

"A comprehensive instructional guide for teens... some of the material may also be directed towards parents or teachers. 5 stars (out of 5)!"
—*Doody's Review Service, 2006*

"Students dealing with their own diabetes or that of a friend or family member or those writing reports on the topic will find this a valuable resource."
—*School Library Journal, Aug '06*

"This text is directed to the teen population and would be an excellent library resource for a health class or for the teacher as a reference for class preparation. It can, however, serve a much wider audience. The clinical educator on diabetes may find it valuable to educate the newly diagnosed client regardless of age. It also would be an excellent reference and education tool for a preventive medicine seminar on diabetes."
—*Physical Therapy, Mar '07*

Diet Information for Teens, 2nd Edition
Health Tips about Diet and Nutrition
Including Facts about Dietary Guidelines, Food Groups, Nutrients, Healthy Meals, Snacks, Weight Control, Medical Concerns Related to Diet, and More

Edited by Karen Bellenir. 432 pages. 2006. 978-0-7808-0820-1.

"A very quick and pleasant read in spite of the fact that it is very detailed in the information it gives... A book for anyone concerned about diet and nutrition."
—*American Reference Books Annual, 2007*

SEE ALSO Eating Disorders Information for Teens, 2nd Edition

Drug Information for Teens, 2nd Edition
Health Tips about the Physical and Mental Effects of Substance Abuse
Including Information about Marijuana, Inhalants, Club Drugs, Stimulants, Hallucinogens, Opiates, Prescription and Over-the-Counter Drugs, Herbal Products, Tobacco, Alcohol, and More

Edited by Sandra Augustyn Lawton. 468 pages. 2006. 978-0-7808-0862-1.

"As with earlier installments in Omnigraphics' Teen Health Series, Drug Information for Teens is designed specifically to meet the needs and interests of middle and high school students... Strongly recommended for both academic and public libraries."
—*American Reference Books Annual, 2007*

"Solid thoughtful advice is given about how to handle peer pressure, drug-related health concerns, and treatment strategies."
—*School Library Journal, Dec '06*

SEE ALSO *Alcohol Information for Teens, 2nd Edition, Tobacco Information for Teens, 2nd Edition*

Eating Disorders Information for Teens, 2nd Edition
Health Tips about Anorexia, Bulimia, Binge Eating, And Other Eating Disorders
Including Information about Risk Factors, Diagnosis and Treatment, Prevention, Related Health Concerns, and Other Issues

Edited by Sandra Augustyn Lawton. 377 pages. 2009. 978-0-7808-1044-0.

"This handy reference offers basic information and addresses specific disorders, consequences, prevention, diagnosis and treatment, healthy eating, and more. It is written in a conversational style that is easy to understand... Will provide plenty of facts for reports as well as browsing potential for students with an interest in the topic."
—*School Library Journal, Jun '09*

"Written in a straightforward style that will appeal to its teenage audience. The author does not play down the danger of living with an eating disorder and urges those struggling with this problem to seek professional help.

This work, as well as others in this series, will be a welcome addition to high school and undergraduate libraries."
—*American Reference Books Annual, 2009*

SEE ALSO *Diet Information for Teens, 2nd Edition*

Fitness Information for Teens, 2nd Edition
Health Tips about Exercise, Physical Well-Being, and Health Maintenance
Including Facts about Conditioning, Stretching, Strength Training, Body Shape and Body Image, Sports Nutrition, and Specific Activities for Athletes and Non-Athletes

Edited by Lisa Bakewell. 432 pages. 2009. 978-0-7808-1045-7.

"This no-nonsense guide packs a great deal into its pages... This is a helpful reference for basic diet and exercise information for health reports or personal use."
—*School Library Journal, April 2009*

"An excellent source for general information on why teens should be active, making time to exercise, the equipment people might need, various types of activities to try, how to maintain health and wellness, and how to avoid barriers to becoming healthier... This would still be an excellent addition to a public library ready-reference collection or a high school health library collection."
—*American Reference Books Annual, 2009*

"This easy to read, well-written, up-to-date overview of fitness for teenagers provides excellent wellness and exercise tips, information, and directions... It is a useful tool for them to obtain a base knowledge in fitness topics and different sports."
—*Doody's Review Service, 2009*

SEE ALSO *Diet Information for Teens, 2nd Edition, Sports Injuries Information for Teens, 2nd Edition*

Learning Disabilities Information for Teens
Health Tips about Academic Skills Disorders and Other Disabilities That Affect Learning

Including Information about Common Signs of Learning Disabilities, School Issues, Learning to Live with a Learning Disability, and Other Related Issues

Edited by Sandra Augustyn Lawton. 400 pages. 2006. 978-0-7808-0796-9.

"This book provides a wealth of information for any reader interested in the signs, causes, and consequences of learning disabilities, as well as related legal rights and educational interventions... Public and academic libraries should want this title for both students and general readers."

—American Reference Books Annual, 2006

Edited by Sandra Augustyn Lawton. 430 pages. 2008. 978-0-7808-1010-5.

"This offering represents the most up-to-date information available on an array of topics including abstinence-only sexual education and pregnancy-prevention methods... The range of coverage—from puberty and anatomy to sexually transmitted diseases—is thorough and extensive. Each chapter includes a bibliographic citation, and the three back sections containing additional resources, further reading, and the index are all first-rate... This volume will be well used by students in need of the facts, whether for educational or personal reasons."

—School Library Journal, Nov '08

Mental Health Information for Teens, 3rd Edition
Health Tips about Mental Wellness and Mental Illness
Including Facts about Mental and Emotional Health, Depression and Other Mood Disorders, Anxiety Disorders, Behavior Disorders, Self-Injury, Psychosis, Schizophrenia, and More

Edited by Karen Bellenir. 400 pages. 2010. 978-0-7808-1087-7.

SEE ALSO *Stress Information for Teens, Suicide Information for Teens, 2nd Edition*

"Presents information related to the emotional, physical, and biological development of both males and females that occurs during puberty. It also strives to address some of the issues and questions that may arise... The text is easy to read and understand for young readers, with satisfactory definitions within the text to explain new terms."

—American Reference Books Annual, 2009

Skin Health Information for Teens, 2nd Edition
Health Tips about Dermatological Concerns and Skin Cancer Risks
Including Facts about Acne, Warts, Hives, and Other Conditions and Lifestyle Choices, Such as Tanning, Tattooing, and Piercing, That Affect the Skin, Nails, Scalp, and Hair

Edited by Edited by Kim Wohlenhaus. 418 pages. 2009. 978-0-7808-1042-6.

"The material in this work will be easily understood by teenagers and young adults. The publisher has liberally used bulleted lists and sidebars to keep the reader's attention... A useful addition to school and public library collections."

—ARBAOnline, Oct '09

Pregnancy Information for Teens
Health Tips about Teen Pregnancy and Teen Parenting
Including Facts about Prenatal Care, Pregnancy Complications, Labor and Delivery, Postpartum Care, Pregnancy-Related Lifestyle Concerns, and More

Edited by Sandra Augustyn Lawton. 434 pages. 2007. 978-0-7808-0984-0.

Sexual Health Information for Teens, 2nd Edition
Health Tips about Sexual Development, Reproduction, Contraception, and Sexually Transmitted Infections
Including Facts about Puberty, Sexuality, Birth Control, Chlamydia, Gonorrhea, Herpes, Human Papillomavirus, Syphilis, and More

Sleep Information for Teens
Health Tips about Adolescent Sleep Requirements, Sleep Disorders, and the Effects of Sleep Deprivation
Including Facts about Why People Need Sleep, Sleep Patterns, Circadian Rhythms, Dreaming, Insomnia, Sleep Apnea, Narcolepsy, and More

Edited by Karen Bellenir. 355 pages. 2008. 978-0-7808-1009-9.

"Clear, concise, and very readable and would be a good source of sleep information for anyone—not just teenagers. This work is highly recommended for medical libraries, public school libraries, and public libraries."
—*American Reference Books Annual, 2009*

SEE ALSO Body Information for Teens

Sports Injuries Information for Teens, 2nd Edition
Health Tips about Acute, Traumatic, and Chronic Injuries in Adolescent Athletes
Including Facts about Sprains, Fractures, and Overuse Injuries, Treatment, Rehabilitation, Sport-Specific Safety Guidelines, Fitness Suggestions, and More

Edited by Karen Bellenir. 429 pages. 2008. 978-0-7808-1011-2.

"An engaging selection of informative articles about the prevention and treatment of sports injuries... The value of this book is that the articles have been vetted and are often augmented with inserts of useful facts, definitions of technical terms, and quick tips. Sensitive topics like injuries to genitalia are discussed openly and responsibly. This revised edition contains updated articles and defines sport more broadly than the first edition."
—*School Library Journal, Nov '08*

"This work will be useful in the young adult collections of public libraries as well as high school libraries... A useful resource for student research."
—*American Reference Books Annual, 2009*

SEE ALSO Accident and Safety Information for Teens

Stress Information for Teens
Health Tips about the Mental and Physical Consequences of Stress
Including Information about the Different Kinds of Stress, Symptoms of Stress, Frequent Causes of Stress, Stress Management Techniques, and More

Edited by Sandra Augustyn Lawton. 392 pages. 2008. 978-0-7808-1012-9.

"Understanding what stress is, what causes it, how the body and the mind are impacted by it, and what teens can do are the general categories addressed here... The chapters are brief but informative, and the list of community-help organizations is exhaustive. Report writers will find information quickly and easily, as will those who have personal concerns. The print is clear and the format is readable, making this an accessible resource for struggling readers and researchers."
—*School Library Journal, Dec '08*

"The articles selected will specifically appeal to young adults and are designed to answer their most common questions."
— *American Reference Books Annual, 2009*

SEE ALSO Mental Health Information for Teens, 3rd Edition

Suicide Information for Teens, 2nd Edition
Health Tips about Suicide Causes and Prevention
Including Facts about Depression, Risk Factors, Getting Help, Survivor Support, and More

Edited by Kim Wohlenhaus. 400 pages. 2010. 978-0-7808-1088-4.

SEE ALSO Mental Health Information for Teens, 3rd Edition

Tobacco Information for Teens, 2nd Edition
Health Tips about the Hazards of Using Cigarettes, Smokeless Tobacco, and Other Nicotine Products
Including Facts about Nicotine Addiction, Nicotine Delivery Systems, Secondhand Smoke, Health Consequences of Tobacco Use, Related Cancers, Smoking Cessation, and Tobacco Use Statistics

Edited by Karen Bellenir. 400 pages. 2010. 978-0-7808-1153-9.

SEE ALSO Drug Information for Teens, 2nd Edition

Health Reference Series

Adolescent Health Sourcebook, 3rd Edition

Adult Health Concerns Sourcebook

AIDS Sourcebook, 4th Edition

Alcoholism Sourcebook, 3rd Edition

Allergies Sourcebook, 3rd Edition

Alzheimer Disease Sourcebook, 4th Edition

Arthritis Sourcebook, 3rd Edition

Asthma Sourcebook, 2nd Edition

Attention Deficit Disorder Sourcebook

Autism & Pervasive Developmental Disorders Sourcebook

Back & Neck Sourcebook, 2nd Edition

Blood & Circulatory Disorders Sourcebook, 3rd Edition

Brain Disorders Sourcebook, 3rd Edition

Breast Cancer Sourcebook, 3rd Edition

Breastfeeding Sourcebook

Burns Sourcebook

Cancer Sourcebook for Women, 4th Edition

Cancer Sourcebook, 5th Edition

Cancer Survivorship Sourcebook

Cardiovascular Disorders Sourcebook, 4th Edition

Caregiving Sourcebook

Child Abuse Sourcebook

Childhood Diseases & Disorders Sourcebook, 2nd Edition

Colds, Flu & Other Common Ailments Sourcebook

Communication Disorders Sourcebook

Complementary & Alternative Medicine Sourcebook, 4th Edition

Congenital Disorders Sourcebook, 2nd Edition

Contagious Diseases Sourcebook

Cosmetic & Reconstructive Surgery Sourcebook, 2nd Edition

Death & Dying Sourcebook, 2nd Edition

Dental Care & Oral Health Sourcebook, 3rd Edition

Depression Sourcebook, 2nd Edition

Dermatological Disorders Sourcebook, 2nd Edition

Diabetes Sourcebook, 4th Edition

Diet & Nutrition Sourcebook, 3rd Edition

Digestive Diseases & Disorder Sourcebook

Disabilities Sourcebook

Disease Management Sourcebook

Domestic Violence Sourcebook, 3rd Edition

Drug Abuse Sourcebook, 3rd Edition

Ear, Nose & Throat Disorders Sourcebook, 2nd Edition

Eating Disorders Sourcebook, 3rd Edition

Emergency Medical Services Sourcebook

Endocrine & Metabolic Disorders Sourcebook, 2nd Edition

Environmental Health Sourcebook, 3rd Edition

Ethnic Diseases Sourcebook

Eye Care Sourcebook, 3rd Edition

Family Planning Sourcebook

Fitness & Exercise Sourcebook, 4th Edition

Food Safety Sourcebook

Forensic Medicine Sourcebook

Gastrointestinal Diseases & Disorders Sourcebook, 2nd Edition

Genetic Disorders Sourcebook, 3rd Edition

Head Trauma Sourcebook

Headache Sourcebook

Health Insurance Sourcebook

Healthy Aging Sourcebook

Healthy Children Sourcebook

Healthy Heart Sourcebook for Women

Hepatitis Sourcebook

Household Safety Sourcebook

Hypertension Sourcebook

Immune System Disorders Sourcebook, 2nd Edition

Infant & Toddler Health Sourcebook

Infectious Diseases Sourcebook

Injury & Trauma Sourcebook